A MEDICATION GUIDE

to Internal Medicine
Tests *and* Procedures

A MEDICATION GUIDE

to Internal Medicine
Tests *and* Procedures

GREGORY J. HUGHES, PharmD, BCPS, BCGP

Associate Clinical Professor
Department of Clinical Health Professions
St. John's University College of Pharmacy
and Health Sciences
Queens, New York, USA

ELSEVIER

Elsevier

1600 John F. Kennedy Blvd.
Ste 1800
Philadelphia, PA 19103-2899

A MEDICATION GUIDE TO INTERNAL MEDICINE TESTS
AND PROCEDURES   ISBN: 978-0-323-79007-9

Library of Congress Control Number: 2021940082

Content Strategist: Charlotta Kryhl
Content Development Specialist: Deborah Poulson
Publishing Services Manager: Deepthi Unni
Project Manager: Haritha Dharmarajan
Design: Bridget Hoette

  Working together
to grow libraries in
developing countries

www.elsevier.com • www.bookaid.org

Printed in India

Last digit is the print number: 9   8   7   6   5   4   3   2   1

To the health care workers who rise to the challenge when duty calls.

Ebtesam Ahmed, PharmD, MS
Clinical Professor
St. John's University College of Pharmacy and
    Health Sciences
Queens, New York, USA
Director, Pharmacy Internship
MJHS Institute for Innovation in Palliative
    Care
New York, USA

Basil E. Akpunonu, MD, MSC, FACP
Professor, Vice Chairman
Department of Medicine
University of Toledo College of Medicine and
    Life Sciences
Toledo, Ohio, USA

Amit Alam, MD
Center for Advanced Heart Failure and
    Transplant Cardiology
Baylor Annette C. and Harold C. Simmons
    Transplant Institute
Baylor University Medical Center
Division of Cardiology
Department of Advanced Heart Failure
Mechanical Support, and Transplant
Baylor Heart and Vascular Hospital
Dallas, Texas, USA
Adjunct Associate Professor
Texas A&M University College of Medicine
Bryan, Texas, USA

Kara E. Bajn, MA, CCC-SLP
Speech Language Pathologist
Rehabilitation Services
North Shore University Hospital
Manhasset, New York, USA
Adjunct Instructor, Department of
    Communication Sciences and Disorders
College of Education and Health Sciences,
    Adelphi University
Garden City, New York, USA

Judith L. Beizer, PharmD, BCGP, FASCP, AGSF
Clinical Professor
Clinical Health Professions
College of Pharmacy and Health Sciences
St. John's University, Queens
New York, USA

David Bernstein, MD, FAASLD, FACG, FACP, AGAF
Head, Liver Sub-Specialty Service Line
Vice Chair of Medicine for Clinical Trials
Chief, Division of Hepatology and Sandra
    Atlas Bass Center for Liver Diseases,
    Northwell Health
Professor of Medicine and Educational Sciences
Zucker School of Medicine at Hofstra/
    Northwell
Manhasset, New York, USA

Frank Cacace, MD, FACP
Associate Chief
Division of General Internal Medicine
Northwell Health
Great Neck, New York, USA
Associate Professor of Medicine
Zucker School of Medicine
Hofstra/Northwell, Hempstead
New York, USA

Wadih Chacra, MD
Assistant Professor of Clinical Medicine
Division of Gastroenterology and
    Hepatology
University of Illinois
Chicago College of Medicine, Chicago
Illinois, USA

Kwan Cheng, MD
Fellow, Department of Endocrinology
Long Island Jewish Medical Center Zucker
    School of Medicine at Hofstra/Northwell
New York, USA

Andrew J. Crannage, PharmD, FNKF, FCCP, BCPS
Internal Medicine Clinical Pharmacist
Mercy Hospital St. Louis
St. Louis, Missouri, USA
Associate Professor and Vice Chair Education
Department of Pharmacy Practice
St. Louis College of Pharmacy at UHSP
St. Louis, Missouri, USA

Makeda Dawkins, MD
Internal Medicine Resident
Internal Medicine Residency Program
Westchester Medical Center, Valhalla
New York, USA

Jason Ehrlich, MD, FACP
Medical Director, Resident Clinic Director
Medicine Specialties at Glen Oaks
Long Island Jewish Medical Center
Northwell Health, Glen Oaks
New York, USA
Assistant Professor of Medicine
Associate Program Director
Medicine Residency
Zucker School of Medicine at Hofstra
  Northwell
Hempstead, New York, USA

Lev Ginzburg, MD
Clinical Assistant Professor
Department of Medicine
NYU Grossman School of Medicine,
  New York
New York, USA

Bruce E. Hirsch, MD, FACP, FIDSA, AAHIVM
Attending Physician Infectious Diseases
Assistant Professor of Medicine
Zucker School of Medicine at Hofstra/
  Northwell
Manhasset, New York, USA

Christopher W. Ho, PharmD, BCPS
Clinical Pharmacy Specialist - Internal
  Medicine
Department of Pharmacy
Long Island Jewish Medical Center -
  Northwell Health
New Hyde Park, New York, USA

Gregory J. Hughes, PharmD, BCPS, BCGP
Associate Clinical Professor
Department of Clinical Health Professions
St. John's University College of Pharmacy and
  Health Sciences
Queens, New York, USA
Assistant Professor
Department of Medicine
Donald and Barbara Zucker School of
  Medicine at Hofstra/Northwell
Hempstead, New York, USA

Jeannine Hummell, CNP
Instructor, Department of Medicine
University of Toledo College of Medicine and
  Life Sciences
Toledo, Ohio, USA

Annamaria Iakovou, MD
Assistant Professor of Medicine
Division of Pulmonary, Critical Care & Sleep
  Medicine
Zucker School of Medicine at Hofstra-
  Northwell
New Hyde Park, New York, USA

Shannon Jones, PharmD, BCPS
Clinical Lead Pharmacist
Truman Medical Center
Kansas City, Missouri, USA

Michael Kaplan, MD
Assistant Professor
Department of Medicine
Division of Rheumatology
Mount Sinai Hospital, New York
New York, USA

Lynn Eileen Kassel, PharmD, BCPS
Associate Professor of Clinical Sciences
Department of Clinical Sciences
Drake University College of Pharmacy &
  Health Sciences
Des Moines, Iowa, USA
Acute Care Pharmacist
Department of Pharmacy
MercyOne West Des Moines Medical Center
West Des Moines, Iowa, USA

Kyle C. Katona, MD, FACP
Assistant Professor of Medicine
Donald and Barbara Zucker School of
  Medicine at Hofstra/Northwell
Site Director, Associate Program Director
  Internal Medicine Residency Program
Attending Physician, Division of Hospital
  Medicine
North Shore University Hospital
Manhasset, New York, USA

Sameer Khanijo, MD, FACP, FCCP
Associate Professor of Medicine
Division of Pulmonary, Critical Care, and Sleep
  Medicine
Donald and Barbara Zucker School of
  Medicine at Hofstra/Northwell
New Hyde Park, New York, USA

Yuriy Khanin, MD
Nephrologist
Medical Diagnostic Associates
P.A., Atlantic Medical Group
Atlantic Health System, New Jersey, USA

Alan S. Lam, MD
Adjunct Instructor of Anesthesiology
Department of Anesthesia
University of Utah Health, Salt Lake City
Utah, USA

Chung-Shien Lee, PharmD, BCPS, BCOP
Associate Professor
Clinical Health Professions
St. John's University College of Pharmacy and
    Health Sciences
Queens, New York, USA
Clinical Coordinator, Monter Cancer Center
    of Northwell Health
Lake Success, New York, USA

Susan MK Lee, PharmD, BCPS, CDCES
Clinical Pharmacy Specialist
Division of Hepatology
Northwell Health - Sandra Atlas Bass Center
    for Liver Diseases
Manhasset, New York, USA

Devora Lichtman, MD, RDMS, RDCS, RVT
Internal Medicine Resident
Cleveland Clinic Foundation
Cleveland, Ohio, USA

Michelle T. Martin, PharmD, FCCP, BCPS, BCACP
Clinical Pharmacist, Liver Clinic
University of Illinois Hospital and Health
    Sciences System
Chicago, Illinois, USA
Clinical Associate Professor
Department of Pharmacy Practice
University of Illinois at Chicago College of
    Pharmacy
Chicago, Illinois, USA

Kimberly Means, PharmD, BCCCP
Clinical Pharmacist Surgical Services
Pharmacy Services
VCU Health, Richmond, Virginia, USA

Samantha Moore, PharmD, BCCCP
Assistant Professor, Industry Professional
Department of Clinical Health Professions
St. John's University College of Pharmacy and
    Health Sciences
Queens, New York, USA
Trauma/Surgical ICU Clinical Pharmacist
Bellevue Hospital, New York, New York

Julie A. Murphy, PharmD, FASHP, FCCP, BCPS
Associate Professor
Department of Pharmacy Practice
College of Pharmacy and Pharmaceutical
    Sciences
University of Toledo
Toledo, Ohio, USA

Alyson K. Myers, MD
Division of Endocrinology
Department of Medicine, Northwell Health
Great Neck, New York, USA
Medical Director, Inpatient Diabetes
North Shore University Hospital
Manhasset, New York, USA
Associate Professor
Donald and Barbara Zucker School of
    Medicine at Hofstra/Northwell
Hempstead, New York, USA

Kimberly E. Ng, PharmD, BCPS
Associate Professor
College of Pharmacy and Health Sciences
St. John's University
Queens, New York, USA

Neha Paralkar, MD
Assistant Professor
Division of General Internal Medicine
Donald and Barbara Zucker School of Medicine
    at Hofstra/Northwell, Northwell Health
Great Neck, New York, USA

Jamie M. Pitlick, PharmD, BCPS, BC-ADM
Associate Professor
Pharmacy Practice, Department of Clinical
    Sciences
Drake University College of Pharmacy and
    Health Sciences
Des Moines, Iowa, USA

Lubaina S. Presswala, DO
Attending Physician
Department of Medicine, Division of
    Endocrinology
North Shore University Hospital
Manhasset, New York, USA
Assistant Professor
Donald and Barbara Zucker School of
    Medicine at Hofstra/Northwell
Hempstead, New York, USA

Daniel Putterman, MD
Assistant Professor
Department of Radiology
Donald and Barbara Zucker School of
    Medicine at Hofstra/Northwell
Manhasset, New York, USA

Shuhao Qiu, MD, PhD
Assistant Professor
Department of Medicine
University of Toledo College of Medicine and
    Life Sciences
Toledo, Ohio, USA

Ali Seyar Rahyab, MD
Cardiologist, Department of Cardiology
Gagnon Cardiovascular Institute at
    Morristown Medical Center
Atlantic Health System, Morristown
New Jersey, USA

Joel Eugene Rand, PA-C, MPAS
Physician Assistant
General and Bariatric Surgery
MercyOne West Des Moines Medical Center
West Des Moines, Iowa, USA

**Joshua P. Rickard, PharmD, MPH, BCPS, BCACP,
CDCES**
Senior Director, Ambulatory Care (CDTM)
    Clinical Pharmacy
Office of Ambulatory Care and Population
    Health
New York City Health + Hospitals, New York
New York, USA

Jonathan S. Ruan, MD, FACC, RPVI
Noninvasive Cardiologist
Division of Cardiology, Department of
    Medicine
New York Presbyterian/Queens, Flushing
New York, USA

Maria Sedky Saad, PharmD
Pharmacy Practice Resident
NewYork-Presbyterian Hospital
New York, New York, USA

Fadi Safi, MD
Assistant Professor
University of Toledo College of Medicine and
    Life Sciences
Toledo, Ohio, USA

Nagashree Seetharamu, MD, MBBS
Associate Professor
Division of Hematology/Medical Oncology
Department of Medicine
Donald and Barbara Zucker School of
    Medicine at Hofstra/Northwell
Manhasset, New York, USA

Hira Shafeeq, PharmD, BCPS
Associate Professor
College of Pharmacy & Health Sciences
St. John's University
Queens, New York, USA
Clinical Specialist, Surgical/Trauma Intensive
    Care Unit
Department of Surgery, Nassau University
    Medical Center
East Meadow, New York, USA

Marcel Souffrant, MD
Resident Physician
Department of Internal Medicine
North Shore University Hospital
Long Island Jewish Medical Center
Manhasset, New York, USA

Tran H. Tran, PharmD, BCPS
Associate Professor
Department of Pharmacy Practice
Midwestern University Chicago College of
    Pharmacy
Downers Grove, Illinois, USA
Substance Use Intervention Team Clinical
    Pharmacist
Department of Psychiatry, Rush University
    Medical Center
Chicago, Illinois, USA

Shahab Ud Din, MD
Assistant Professor
Department of Medicine
University of Toledo College of Medicine and
    Life Sciences
Toledo, Ohio, USA

Nicholas W. Van Hise, PharmD, BCPS
Director of Clinical Research
Infectious Disease Clinical Specialist
Metro Infectious Disease Consultants
Burr Ridge, Illinois, USA

PREFACE

Repetition, repetition, repetition. All health care professionals in teaching facilities are familiar with repetition. The same topic discussions. The same journal club articles. The same case presentations. The same lectures on medication dosing and monitoring strategies. And at times, what seem like the same patients. There is obvious benefit to repetition in clinical medicine, a field where there is very little room for error. Repetition affords clinicians the opportunity to see, over and over again, so that they may refine their skills.

Repetition can also illuminate sources of waste. This is precisely what occurred in my experience in a quaternary care academic medical center. I have witnessed countless clinical learners fall into cyclic traps of preventable waste—wastes in time, resources, and human capital and energy. Thirty minutes spent by a medical resident scouring the literature on a particular therapeutic problem, for instance, may not seem like much of a burden. Calling one consultant to manage a minor clinical problem may not feel like an unsustainable taxation on the medical system, but multiplying these seemingly negligible devotions of time and action across institutions, across the nation, and across years unveils substantial direct and indirect costs. Perhaps, some clinical problems that drive waste could, and should, be easier to solve in the first place.

This book was born of the idea that some of the aforementioned repetition and waste is unnecessary and, in actuality, is avoidable. The goal herein is to curb this excess, as well as the resultant costs, particularly at the nexus where medications intersect with tests and procedures. That is, fewer tests and procedures will need to be repeated, canceled, or delayed if done correctly the first time. Clinicians will not need to search anew for the same practical information regarding medications and procedures over and over again. Adverse events, medical errors, and both financial and cognitive waste can be diminished through the utilization of this well-organized, informative guide to periprocedural medication management. The patient experience will ultimately benefit from this improved care, as well.

What follows is a repository of information in a logical, straight-to-the-point reference guide. It has been co-authored by physicians and clinical pharmacists in their respective specialties, writing with the goal of providing direct aid to the busy generalist clinician. These concise chapters are arranged by procedure and filled with high-yield practical pearls to ensure that clinicians are equipped to safely and expertly manage medications before, during, and after medical tests and procedures. Likewise, clinicians will be able to understand how the presence or absence of various medications affects the clinical interpretation of test results. Importantly, this book intends to minimize unnecessary consultations with specialists. Many of the chapters were written by such specialists with this precise goal in mind. In addition, some chapters address the treatment of common diagnoses following the described procedure and include links to additional helpful resources. At the time of publication, a resource such as this is non-existent.

This text was written and reviewed during the COVID-19 pandemic, which further highlighted the need for increased efficiency in health care settings. Indeed, the experiences of the co-authors of this very book illustrate this point, as they were forced to change their practices nearly overnight. Some switched entirely to working from home, while others devoted more time than ever to clinical responsibilities. Several in the latter group were even pulled from their specialties in order to care for COVID-19 patients when their workplaces required an all-hands-on-deck approach. Across the health care system, clinicians found their usual practices upended, allowing inefficiencies to abound. Meanwhile, the lack of scientific consensus on transmission, prophylaxis, and treatment led to false starts, missed opportunities, and clinical ambiguity across the world. One must wonder how much repetition and waste has occurred over the first year of the pandemic due to these events.

Hopefully, the worst of the COVID-19 pandemic is behind us. But it is a reminder that we must have accessible resources in place for when stresses are placed on our health care system and its individual workers. This reference intends to be one such resource. No, it will not prevent the next pandemic. But if it can prevent yet more repetition and waste, it just might allow clinicians more freedom and resources to tackle the problems of tomorrow. And that will be a success.

ACKNOWLEDGMENTS

This book would not have been realized and published without the support of a number of people in my life. First and foremost, thank you to my wife, Jen, for your unwavering support, critical eye, and in general just dealing with me through every phase of the writing and publication process. Your steadfast belief motivated me to accomplish my goal of helping colleagues and patients through the creation of this book. I would also like to thank my children for being such wonderful gifts and for sleeping through the night from a markedly early age. To you, you cannot yet appreciate how much you mean to me.

There were a number of colleagues from the University and hospital who were influential in the early phases of writing this book. Your guidance came in a variety of forms: some through lengthy conversations, some through brief interactions, and some were simply models to emulate. These interactions, even the briefest, played a significant role in the planning process, mentality, and inspiration to create this book. Your advice and cautionary tales helped create what I hope to be a meaningful contribution to the education of health care professionals. These colleagues include Mary Ann Howland, Judith Beizer, Liron Sinvani, Frank Barile, and many others. Thank you all.

I would also like to acknowledge Kevin Hughes, Roman Finkel, Michael Kaplan, as well as other family and friends for their astute critiques in reviewing a number of chapters and their guidance on general aspects of the book. I can always rely on my family, friends, and colleagues to remind me of how much there is to learn.

Then there is the large network of individuals from which the impetus for this book is derived. This is the nameless mass of physician and pharmacist trainees that I have worked with over the years in the general inpatient internal medicine setting, the College of Pharmacy, and the School of Medicine. Your curiosity and need for details about pharmacotherapy as it relates to tests and procedures was really the inspiration for this endeavor. I hope this book allows you, and future versions of you, to foster your individual growth, hone your skills, better care for your patients, and for the earliest of trainees, simply to follow what is happening on rounds.

I cannot overstate my gratitude to the 50 authors from around the country who produced the chapters that make up this book. Thank you for your hard work and for dealing with my onslaught of comments and particularities through the publication process. This text was created almost entirely during the COVID-19 pandemic, which was an unprecedented time of burden to our modern health care system. Many of the authors were pulled from their normal positions and responsibilities to directly or indirectly help with the pandemic efforts. I hope that simultaneously writing these chapters did not worsen any trauma that you endured.

EXPANDED TABLE OF CONTENTS

Many tests and procedures are commonly referred to using abbreviated terminology to avoid having to write and say lengthy phrases/terms. Some chapters of this text address multiple tests and procedures, each with their own abbreviations. To aid readers in locating content, this expanded table of contents includes such abbreviations and in what chapters they can be found. Additionally, the index at the end of the book further details how to locate specific topics.

Continued

Continued

CONTENTS

CHAPTER 1

Introduction

Gregory J. Hughes, PharmD, BCPS, BCGP

In the internal medicine setting, managing the large assortment of tests, procedures, and medications encountered on a daily basis can be a daunting task. For students and early trainees, the challenges can seem insurmountable. Tests, procedures, and medications are nearly ubiquitous parts of patients' histories and are heavily relied upon in modern medicine. These three types of interventions have roles in the diagnostic process and therapeutic management of patients. Each test, procedure, and medication carries with it a rich history, including indications for use as well as potential effectiveness, complications, and toxicities. As the field learns more about each, data accumulates and best practices evolve.

Effectively using tests, procedures, and medications is contingent upon understanding the nuances of each intervention. While some have clinical applications supported by robust evidence-based research, other applications are eminence-based or rely on inferred assumptions. Appreciating this distinction is an essential and challenging aspect of making patient-specific decisions. For ease of reading, throughout the remainder of this chapter, the term "procedure" will include both what are typically thought of as "tests" and things typically called "procedures."

The difficulty in making complex clinical decisions is inevitably compounded by interference, or the potential for interference, between procedures and medications. Some medications can be beneficial in the diagnostic and therapeutic process by increasing the yield of a procedure or reducing certain risks. Other combinations of medications and procedures can be harmful by causing complications, decreasing accuracy, or even requiring a procedure to be rescheduled. Awareness of these interactions has practical impacts on logistics, safety, and patient education. A key challenge for healthcare professionals is managing the multitude of scenarios that arise in a resourceful and timely manner.

Answers to clinical questions about the interactions between procedures and medications can be difficult to find. They vary in quality of evidence from randomized controlled trials to expert opinion. Prior to the publication of this text, healthcare professionals were left to their own research skills to scour a gamut of references, including primary literature, tertiary databases, professional guidelines, and generic internet queries. This text streamlines the process by helping healthcare professionals navigate the vast amount of information available.

The following chapters present healthcare professionals with an understanding of how procedures and medications interact with one another in a single compendium. While providing many details, the text should not be mistaken for a comprehensive instruction manual for performing procedures or the last and final word on a complex clinical question.

This book is organized in the following manner. Chapters 2 through 6 discuss and provide guidance on topics that are widely relevant to the diagnostic and therapeutic process and are therefore applicable to the remainder of the book. These include chapters on the diagnostic process itself (Chapters 2 and 3), chapters on anticoagulation and glycemic management in the periprocedural period (Chapters 4 and 5), and an introductory to anesthesia (Chapter 6). Chapters 7 through 60 each detail a procedure or group of procedures and are arranged alphabetically by procedure name.

Each procedure-based chapter follows the same organized, logical, and easy-to-follow format. Each chapter begins with a "Background" section, which provides a brief description of the procedure. Often, the etymology of the procedure is included, as it may help early trainees understand medical terminology and appreciate the importance of nomenclature. Then, the role of the procedure is described in the "How To Use It" section. This section details the circumstances in which the procedure is typically performed or its indications in addition to the type of information the procedure may garner. Next, in the "How It Is Done" section, the physical logistics of the procedure are described. While not intended to be a full instruction manual, this section includes enough information for a clinician to properly describe the procedure to a new practitioner, trainee, or patient (who may be nervous about undergoing a procedure for the first time). It also includes standard information such as the setting in which the procedure takes place (e.g., outpatient, at the bedside, in a radiology suite), whether the patient will be awake for the procedure, an approximation of the procedure duration, and how a "normal" result might be described. The focus of each chapter lies in the "Medication Implications" section. This section describes, as appropriate, which medications should be given or held before, during, or following the procedure. For example, certain procedures intrinsically involve a medication (e.g., dexamethasone in a dexamethasone suppression test). Some medications improve the yield of a procedure (e.g., iodinated contrast media in computed tomography). Others must be discontinued to avoid harm or invalidation of the results (e.g., caffeine before a stress test, opioids before a gastric emptying study). Some chapters, where appropriate, discuss pharmacotherapy for the most common diagnoses (e.g., antibiotics for pneumonia). The "Medication Implications" section includes rationales and specific logistics for timing and dosing, when reasonable, as well as discusses if the procedure can identify adverse medication effects. References are included throughout all chapters for readers seeking additional information or details.

CHAPTER 2

The Process of Diagnosing

Kyle Katona, MD ■ Neha Paralkar, MD

This text guides readers in the process of utilizing tests and procedures to reach a correct diagnosis for their patients. Intended for learning and practicing members of a patient's interdisciplinary care team, this guide provides information on how tests are performed, what results might be expected, and how medications can impact the diagnostic process. This chapter reviews the importance of the diagnostic process and how tests and procedures impact how medicine is practiced today. While the tests and procedures that are available are only increasing and providing more information, it is important to ensure that each medical procedure ordered is warranted and benefits the patient more than it causes harm.

So what is the diagnostic process? What does it entail?

A blank slate. That is how patients are considered early in a provider's training. That is how the diagnostic process starts. Often, the first patients encounters early in training consist of walking into an exam room without knowing anything about the person on the other side of the door. From those early, tepid introductions, clinicians begin to hone their interview skills, advancing from asking the patient every medical question by rote, regardless of potential usefulness, to developing the sense of when and to whom to ask what questions. From there, a physical exam is performed. Once again, early on, the skill is taught in its entirety, and it subsequently develops into a more customizable approach as one's experience grows. Only after the history and physical exam are complete does one dive into the realm of testing. Whether it is a screening blood test or confirmatory imaging, the diagnostic process seeks these tests as ancillary support to the gospel that is the history and physical exam.

That is how one is usually introduced to the idea of diagnostic testing and procedures: an adjunct to a complete history and physical exam, a tool or tools used to confirm or reject a list of potential diagnoses that one has developed on the basis of information gathered during a complete history and physical exam. In a patient with chest pain, radiographic imaging of the chest can confirm the diagnosis of suspected pneumonia, electrocardiogram changes can raise the suspicion of ischemia, or perhaps the absence of these changes can make gastroesophageal reflux more likely.

Once it is determined which appropriate tests or procedures the patient requires, the risks and benefits of completing the tests are discussed with the patient and consent is obtained. However, the clinician's job is still not complete. A study published in the *British Medical Journal* found that while diagnostic errors are made in 10%–20% of all cases, even when the correct diagnosis is made, up to 45% of patients did not receive recommended evidence-based care.[1] Additional considerations that might affect the potential tests the patient requires are a test's positive and negative likelihood ratios, sensitivity, specificity, and positive and negative predictive values. See Chapter 3: Nuances and Characteristics of Tests for more details. This knowledge will help determine whether proposed laboratory tests, physical tests, or procedures will provide valuable or equivocal information. Additionally, when ordering tests for patients, it is important to not only have thought about how the process of completing the test will impact the patient's life, but how the result may alter their future treatment plan as well. For example, if a biopsy may diagnose cancer, will the patient want treatment? If so, what treatment options are they eligible for? If the patient only wants to know the diagnosis and not receive treatment, is there a less invasive method to obtain the answer? Now, with the appropriate tests and procedures ordered, some of those blanks left over from the history and physical exam can be filled in, and that blank slate has emerged into a clearer picture of what the patient truly has.

The early years of training may be the last time that any practitioner sees a patient as a true blank slate. In this day and age of technology, informatics, and advancing testing, it is virtually unheard of to walk into a patient's room knowing nothing. The electrocardiogram or chest X-ray is often performed and interpreted before any clinician says a word to a patient. Technology and electronic medical records help ensure that this information is available to any provider who sees a patient at a later date. Preemptively, this information can make practitioners susceptible to bias. For example, patients are often admitted from the emergency room with a diagnosis that does not later change despite availability of new information. This is often due to anchoring bias, as practitioners may become biased by the first diagnosis they hear. When test results are interpreted in such a way as to confirm one particular diagnosis, there is danger of making the wrong diagnosis due to framing bias. For example, a patient with anemia who recently traveled to Africa may be assumed to have malaria, and tests may only be ordered to confirm this suspicion while not ruling out other causes. If a test supports that anemia is present and the diagnosis is finalized, then it is likely to commit a type of bias known as premature closure.[2] A systematic review found that autopsy results demonstrated the median misdiagnosis rate to be 23.5%.[3] It is important to recognize the potential biases that can detract from obtaining the correct diagnosis and treatment plan.

In addition to the abundance of information available via advances in diagnostic testing, pharmaceutical treatments have developed drastically. Some days, it seems that polypharmacy, or use of five or more prescription medications, has become the rule rather than the exception. A study utilizing data from the National Social Life, Health, and Aging Project found that older patients were at most risk for polypharmacy. The prevalence of prescription medication use in older patients in the United States increased from 84.1% to 87.7% from 2005-2006 to 2010-2011. Polypharmacy also increased by almost 6% in the same time frame.[4] A study utilizing the Canadian National Population Health Survey found that over 50% of older adults living in healthcare institutions are also affected by polypharmacy.[5] The World Health Organization reported that 1/9 of the population is age 60 or older and this will likely increase to 1/5 in 2050, which suggests that the issue of polypharmacy will only become more relevant.[6] To classify increasing polypharmacy as a positive or negative trend is not helpful, nor is the issue that simple, but what cannot be argued with is that polypharmacy is ever present.

Whether it is the ideal approach to our patients or not, clinicians often never see a blank slate. Polypharmacy and over-testing are ubiquitous in the current healthcare environment. Medicare expenditure on tests increased by 96%, other procedures by 82%, and imaging by 75% from 2000 to 2017, making these the largest portions of Medicare expenditure and the greatest growing areas of expenditure.[7] Seeing patients deal with the effects of polypharmacy means seeing patients. Seeing patients with a handful of tests and procedures already ordered and performed means seeing patients.

As diagnostic tests and pharmaceutical treatments grow ever more complex, it behooves the astute clinician to become aware of how these areas influence one another. While the history and physical exam remain the most critical components of the diagnostic process, rarely are they enough. Part of applying the concept of the right test for the right patient means being aware of the impact of medications on these tests. Whether it is the rather obvious question of safety of blood thinners in invasive testing to the more nuanced questions of how steroids can affect a basic complete blood count and how one interprets a gastric emptying study in the setting of opioid use, it is essential to be aware of these questions and the impact medications have on various tests.

While this book serves as a guide for how medications can affect common tests, procedures, and the overall diagnostic process, nothing can replace what the provider adds to the care of the patient. Patients place great trust in healthcare professionals to study the information available, discuss the options with them, and help them make the best decisions. This book provides information to guide clinicians in making informed decisions. Importantly, it highlights the value of considering the diagnostic process as outlined above in efforts to best care for patients.

References

1. Scott Ian A. Errors in clinical reasoning: causes and remedial strategies. *BMJ*. 2009;338:b1860.
2. Wellbery C. Flaws in clinical reasoning: a common cause of diagnostic error. *Am Fam Physician*. 2011;84:1042–1048.
3. Shojania KG, Burton EC, McDonald KM, et al. Changes in rates of autopsy-detected diagnostic errors over time: a systematic review. *JAMA*. 2003;289:2849–2856.
4. Qato DM, Wilder J, Schumm LP, et al. Changes in prescription and over-the-counter medication and dietary supplement use among older adults in the United States, 2005 vs 2011. *JAMA Intern Med*. 2016;176:473–482.
5. Kwan D, Farrell B. Polypharmacy: optimizing medication use in elderly patients. *Can Geriatr J*. 2014;4:21–27.
6. Dagli RJ, Sharma A. Polypharmacy: a global risk factor for elderly people. *J Int Oral Health*. 2014;6:i–ii.
7. Medicare Payment Advisory Commission. *A Data Book: Healthcare Spending and the Medicare Program*; 2019. http://www.medpac.gov/docs/default-source/data-book/jun18_databookentirereport_sec.pdf. Published July 19, 2019. Accessed March 2, 2020.

CHAPTER 3

Nuances and Characteristics of Tests

Frank Cacace, MD ▪ Jason Ehrlich, MD

This book embarks on medical tests and procedures and how they interface with pharmacologic interventions. In general, testing can include:
- The questions asked of patients with chief concerns at their histories
- Physical exam maneuvers performed on the patient
- Laboratory, imaging tests, and procedures performed to elucidate further information

With each diagnostic intervention, a positive or negative observation is elicited and funneled into the diagnostic process. On a case-by-case basis, clinicians apply the power of tests to discriminate presence vs absence of disease to the pre-testing sense of probability that a disease process is present. For example, before applying a D-dimer or computed tomography (CT) angiogram to a patient with pleuritic shortness of breath in the emergency department or on the wards, clinicians generate a sense of probability of a pulmonary embolism (PE). Clinical reasoning then directs clinicians as to what individualized testing to apply to further increase or decrease the sense of PE probability in that patient. Clinicians work toward the highest or lowest post-test probability to rule in or rule out a diagnosis, respectively.

Tests and their accuracy characteristics, therefore, are inextricably intertwined with clinical reasoning. From the start of a patient assessment, the spinning wheels of clinical reasoning move in real time with every visual observation, concern-based question, hypothesis-driven bedside exam, laboratory test, and image ordered. Through history and exam, the initial pre-testing sense of diagnostic probabilities is made and tests are then applied.

The rest of this introductory chapter will discuss the knowledge of a test's accuracy measures and how that knowledge is fundamental to making correct diagnoses.

Sensitivity

No doubt the reader has come across a number of definitions or ways to think about a test's sensitivity. These may include the following:
- A test's ability to identify a disease state
- The probability of testing positive if the patient has the disease state
- True positive (TP)/(TP + false negative [FN])
- An accuracy measure of a test best suited to rule out disease

Each of the above conceptual definitions of sensitivity is useful. Most of the understanding of sensitivity can be achieved by laying out the famous 2 × 2 table. Table 3.1 crosses the test in question's positive and negative findings on the vertical left column with a comparator gold standard's positive and negative findings in the upper row.

Using the 2 × 2 visually, one has **TP** for the test in question in the upper-left quadrant (a), **false positive (FP)** for the test in the upper-right quadrant (b), **FN** in the lower-left quadrant (c), and **true negative (TN)** in the lower-right quadrant (d). For the sensitivity calculation, this comes to sensitivity = a/(a + c).

Notice where the statement that sensitivity best rules out disease comes from. If a test has a sensitivity of 97%, there is only a 3/100 FN rate. This means that when this test produces a negative result, with a gold standard used as a comparator, the patient testing negative is without disease 97% of the time. A negative test, when the test is highly sensitive like this one, nearly assures absence of disease.

Examples would include a Lyme ELISA for Lyme disease, an antinuclear antibody (ANA) for lupus, or adding nuclear material to stress testing for coronary ischemia.[1–3]

The issue that clinicians must deal with, however, is that highly sensitive tests often suffer from specificity that is not nearly as good. There is a compromise in the ability of such a test to discriminate true disease from lack thereof because of an over-labeling of disease, a tendency to ascribe disease to too many. This is further examined through specificity.

Specificity

The following defines the accuracy measure of a clinical test called specificity. The reader has likely come across one or all of the following:

- A test's ability to identify the absence of a disease state
- The probability of testing negative if the patient does not have a disease state
- TN/(TN + FP)
- An accuracy measure of a test best suited to rule in disease

Again, each of these conceptual definitions is correct and by looking at Table 3.1, which crosses the test in question's positive and negative findings in the left-side column with a gold standard's positive and negative findings in the upper row, specificity is derived as d/(d + b).

Notice again where the statement specificity rules in disease comes from. If a test has a specificity of 95%, there is only a 5/100 FP rate. This means when the test produces a positive result, with a gold standard used as a comparator, the patient testing positive is truly with disease 95% of the time. A positive test, when the test is highly specific like this one, nearly assures presence of disease.

Examples of specificity's ability to discriminate the presence of disease are dsDNA or anti-Smith antibody in lupus, anti-cyclic citrullinated peptide antibodies in rheumatoid arthritis, a drop test for full-thickness rotator cuff tear, or 4/5 affirmative answers on a POUND (pulsatile, one-day duration or 4–72 hours, unilateral, nausea, disabling nature) series for migraine.[4–7]

Again, clinicians have to consider that highly specific tests can suffer from suboptimal sensitivity. They can over-label an absence of disease and contribute to missed diagnoses.

The definitions of sensitivity and specificity, their strengths and weaknesses in terms of discrimination of disease vs absence of disease, and their typical dual relationship are the first level of thinking in clinical reasoning that builds on the first clinical impressions. The next level of accuracy measure understanding that contributes to the diagnostic thought process is positive predictive value (PPV) and negative predictive value (NPV).

Positive Predictive Value

With each patient response to a question in development of the chief concern each part of the exam, and each laboratory test or image, a positive finding is associated with a PPV for a target diagnosis being considered.

The reader may have heard of these two definitions of PPV:

- The probability a patient testing positive has disease
- TP/(TP + FP), or TP/all positive tests

Each of these conceptual definitions is useful, and by referring to Table 3.1, PPV can be derived as a/(a + b).

TABLE 3.1 ■ **Contingency Table Used in Analyzing Sensitivity, Specificity, and Positive and Negative Predictive Values**

Test in Question	Gold Standard	
	+	−
+	a [true positive (TP)]	b [false positive (FP)]
−	c [false negative (FN)]	d [true negative (TN)]

Negative Predictive Value

Similarly, every time a patient answers a historical question in the negative, an exam maneuver is unremarkable, or a laboratory test or image is negative, such negative findings are associated with a NPV for a target diagnosis being considered.

The reader may have come across the following two definitions of NPV:
- The probability a patient testing negative does not have disease
- TN/(TN + FN), or TN/all negative tests

These conceptual definitions are correct, and by referring to Table 3.1, NPV can be derived as d/(d + c).

For clinicians on a quest for testing information that helps confirm or deny a pre-test sense of a diagnostic probability, predictive values are inherently problematic. They have an essential flaw. Consider applying ANA to diagnose lupus in a large group of younger patients with synovitis and rash (common manifestations of lupus at an age when lupus tends to present). There will be a certain PPV and NPV for diagnosing lupus achieved by the application of the ANA. Now consider applying that same ANA test to a large group of older patients with morning stiffness and spurs on their hands on X-ray (an uncommon manifestation of lupus at an age less likely to be presenting with lupus for the first time). ANA is a highly sensitive test but will inevitably produce some false positivity in the latter group. That false positivity will compromise the test's PPV in this subgroup of patients.

What is the difference between these two tested populations? As with a population of patients with diabetes with symptoms of coronary disease vs a population with low pre-test probability of coronary disease, the difference is *prevalence* of disease. Predictive value performance, both positive and negative, will be different for populations tested based on prevalence. The answer to this short-coming, for the clinician preferring a prevalence-free accuracy measure that links pre- to post-test probability of disease, is the concept of a likelihood ratio (LR). Before moving to LR, just a word on the overall accuracy of any test.

Accuracy of a Test

The reader has likely heard this term used in a myriad of ways, such as:
- A test's ability to reliably identify both presence and absence of disease
- A test's probability of relaying a correct discrimination of positive from negative disease
- (TP + TN)/(TP + FP + TN + FN) or true tests/all tests done

Likelihood Ratio

LRs can be defined as follows: they are an accuracy measure of a question series, exam technique, laboratory result, or image that links pre-test probability to post-test probability independent of the prevalence of the target condition.

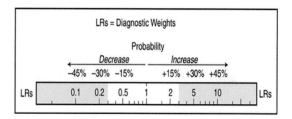

Fig. 3.1   Effect of likelihood ratio on post-test probability following a negative or positive result. (Reprinted with permission from McGee S. *Evidence-Based Physical Diagnosis*. 4th ed. Elsevier; 2017:13.)

The reader will be reminded that LRs can be expressed in the following terms:
- LR+ = sensitivity/(1 – specificity)
- LR– = (1 – sensitivity)/specificity

When presented with the raw 2 × 2 table data in an article presenting a new diagnostic technique, readers can calculate these LRs from the TP/FP rates and TN/FN rates. It is important to carry some basic realizations about the effect of LRs on clinical thinking.
- LRs for a positive test that are >10 are significant in that the test's discriminatory power can have an impressive effect on pre- to post-test thinking.
- LRs for a negative test that are <0.1 are similarly significant in that the test's discriminatory power can have an impressive effect on pre- to post-test thinking.

LRs for a positive test of 2, 5, and 10 increase the considered pre-test probability of disease by 15%, 30%, and 45%, respectively. Similarly, LRs for a negative test of 0.5, 0.2, and 0.1 decrease the considered pre-test probability of disease by 15%, 30%, and 45%, respectively. In a schematic, this is represented in Fig. 3.1.

Also worth remembering is that a test that produces a LR+ or LR– of 1 produces no change in pre- to post-test thinking, often leading to the need for further testing.

The LR, then, is a fulcrum of inflection between pre-clinical probabilistic assessment of, for example, PE in a patient with chest pain and shortness of breath, to the post-testing probabilistic assessment. This test property and utilization is at the heart of Bayesian thinking in the diagnostic process, that the diagnostic belief is rooted in a probability of an event, which is then adjusted further for the associative odds of other observed events.

To link clinical evaluation for a target condition to a post-test probability, and for how a test can further favor or disfavor the initial thought process, clinicians can rely on the visual connect-the-dot exercise seen in Fig. 3.2. The Fagan nomogram presents an algorithmic link to plot a test's positive and negative LR between the connected pre- to post-test probabilities. Use of the nomogram is an excellent visual reminder that choosing the test with LRs of the most discerning power to confirm or eliminate a diagnosis is the highest value test choice to make. For example, the 25-year-old weight lifter with pleuritic pain, and without tachycardia or hypoxemia, who just added a large amount of weight to his lifting routine would be best served with a D-dimer, while the negative LR is particularly suited to help confirm absence of PE without exposing the patient to an excess risk of over-diagnosis secondary to incidental findings on a CT angiogram (in addition to risks and costs of the test such as those associated with contrast media, radiation, or stressful hospital charges to the patient). Conversely, a CT angiogram with its superior positive LR should be used on an older patient with the same symptoms who has cancer (a population with a much higher pre-test probability). See Chapter 17: Computed Tomography for more details about this test.

Another advantage of LR is that they can be reported for different levels of positivity. When original data on a new diagnostic technique is reported by level of positivity, positive LRs can be determined for each level of positivity. This was demonstrated in the PIOPED study, in which

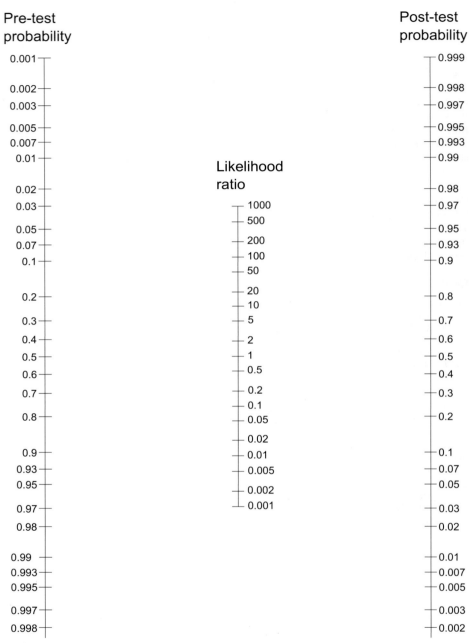

Fig. 3.2 The Fagan nomogram allows clinicians to use the pre-test probability and likelihood ratio to determine post-test probability and assists with determining which tests perform in a given scenario.

ventilation/perfusion (V/Q) scanning in the diagnosis of PE was represented as negative, low-, intermediate-, and high-probability scan.[8] Building on the pre-test probability arrived upon with the initial clinical assessment, this test was used in the pre-CT angiogram era to decide whether treatment should be initiated or further testing with traditional angiogram was needed. LRs of 0, 0.25, 1, and 17 would be applied on the Fagan nomogram to estimate post-test probability of PE for negative, low-, intermediate-, and high-probability tests, respectively. These data, generated by comparing V/Q scan results to pulmonary angiogram results, the gold standard at the time, were foundational for clinicians. Intermediate-probability tests produced no change in pre- to post-test thinking, so further testing was required if suspicion was high enough, and high-probability tests led to an immediate decision to treat. See Chapter 60: Ventilation-Perfusion Scan for more details about this test.

In conclusion, evaluations of patient presentations consist of formulating a sense of pre-test probability for multiple conditions at once. Clinicians meet the challenge of confirming or rejecting diagnostic hypotheses with targeted testing that can take the form of history taking, physical exam, and various laboratory and imaging modalities. Each diagnostic intervention possesses accuracy measures consisting of sensitivity, specificity, PPVs, NPVs, and LRs. Appreciation of these concepts is foundational to judicious and ultimately successful leveraging of tests to reach correct diagnoses.

References

1. Solomon DH, Kavanaugh AJ, Schur PH, et al. Evidence-based guidelines for the use of immunologic tests: antinuclear antibody testing. *Arthritis Rheum.* 2002;47:434.
2. Branda JA, Aguero-Rosenfeld ME, Ferraro MJ, et al. 2-tiered antibody testing for early and late Lyme disease using only an immunoglobulin G blot with the addition of a VlsE band as the second-tier test. *Clin Infect Dis.* 2010;50:20.
3. Lee TH, Boucher CA. Clinical practice: noninvasive tests in patients with stable coronary artery disease. *N Engl J Med.* 2001;344:1840.
4. Kavanaugh AJ, Solomon DH, American College of Rheumatology Ad Hoc Committee on Immunologic Testing Guidelines. Guidelines for immunologic laboratory testing in the rheumatic diseases: anti-DNA antibody tests. *Arthritis Rheum.* 2002;47:546.
5. Lee DM, Schur PH. Clinical utility of the anti-CCP assay in patients with rheumatic diseases. *Ann Rheum Dis.* 2003;62:870.
6. Park HB, Yokota A, Gill HS, et al. Diagnostic accuracy of clinical tests for the different degrees of subacromial impingement syndrome. *J Bone Joint Surg Am.* 2005;87:1446.
7. Michel P, Henry P, Letteneur P, et al. Diagnostic screen for assessment of the HIS criteria for migraine by general practitioners. *Cephalalgia.* 1993;13:54–59.
8. PIOPED Investigators. Value of the ventilation/perfusion scan in acute pulmonary embolism: results of the prospective investigation of pulmonary embolism diagnosis (PIOPED). *JAMA.* 1990;263:2753.

CHAPTER 4

Anticoagulation Management in the Periprocedural Period

Christopher W. Ho, PharmD

General Considerations for Periprocedural Anticoagulation

When evaluating a patient on anticoagulation during the periprocedural period, it is important to review the bleeding risk, both for the procedure and the individual patient, and the thromboembolic risk of the patient. The bleeding risk guides how early to hold anticoagulants prior to the procedure and how long to wait after the procedure to restart anticoagulation. The same patient at high thrombotic risk may require the use of bridging anticoagulation prior to the procedure and, in certain instances, early resumption of anticoagulation after the procedure. The anticoagulant the patient is using may also affect the timing of the procedure to allow for bleeding risk to reach a safe margin. For example, due to the short half-life of heparin IV infusion, using this anticoagulant may decrease the time needed to wait prior to the procedure, whereas using direct oral anticoagulants (DOACs) requires a much longer delay. Lastly, the nature of the procedure, emergent vs elective, should also be considered to weigh the benefits of the procedure against the risk of bleeding and thrombosis.[1]

The exact management of anticoagulation during this period is a balance between the risk of bleeding and the risk of thrombosis. It is important to remind the reader that most of the research and the recommendations found in the ACC Expert Consensus Decision Pathway for Periprocedural Management of Anticoagulation in Patients with Nonvalvular Atrial Fibrillation guideline are directed toward the management of patients on anticoagulation for atrial fibrillation (AF).[1] In this chapter, the anticoagulant management strategies certainly apply to patients with AF and may apply or may be modified to apply to expanded patient groups as well. Lastly, use of these anticoagulant management strategies will play a significant role in the outcomes during the periprocedural period.

Evaluating Bleeding Risks

Procedure bleeding risks are categorized as low, intermediate, or high and are affected by intricacies such as the level of vascularization at the area of manipulation and the implications of bleeds in that space (e.g., intraspinal/epidural spaces). These bleeding risks are largely driven by expert opinion, as there is a lack of large observational data for most procedures. Nevertheless, common procedures along with their bleeding risk category are available on the online appendix copublished with the ACC Expert Consensus Decision Pathway for Periprocedural Management of Anticoagulation in Patients with Nonvalvular Atrial Fibrillation.[1] Patient-specific bleeding risks assess the likelihood of bleeding with patient-specific risk factors such as advanced age, hypertension, history of bleeding (increased risk if <3 months from last bleed or bleeding from similar procedure or bridging), liver or renal disease, thrombocytopenia or platelet dysfunction (e.g., uremia), history of stroke, labile or supratherapeutic international normalized ratio (INR), antiplatelet or nonsteroidal anti-inflammatory drug use, or alcohol use. Several risk scores have been studied and developed to assist in quantifying patient-specific bleeding risks, including the HAS-BLED, ATRIA, HEMORR2HAGES, and SAMe-TT2R2 scores.[1-5] However, a high bleeding risk based on these scores does not directly affect the management of periprocedural anticoagulation because these risk scores may better serve to aid in identifying reversible risk factors that can be attenuated to reduce the patient-specific bleeding risk.[1]

Although major bleeding risks between prophylactic- and therapeutic-dose parenteral anticoagulants are not as different as one would expect, the clinically relevant nonmajor bleeding risks are not well documented.[6] When evaluating a patient's anticoagulant regimen for bleeding risk, it would still be prudent to consider therapeutic-dose anticoagulation to be a higher risk of a bleed compared with prophylactic-dose anticoagulation.

EVALUATION AND MANAGEMENT OF ANTIPLATELET AGENTS

When caring for patients entering the periprocedural period, careful medication reconciliation must be performed, and any antiplatelet use should be identified because these agents may contribute to the patient's overall bleeding risk. However, there remains a relative lack of rigorous guidance regarding management of antiplatelet therapy in the periprocedural period, mainly due to the paucity of good clinical trial data.[7] The limited data that is available suggests continuing aspirin for secondary prevention of cardiovascular diseases for most common procedures performed during a modern-day medicine service, such as[8,9]:

- Arthrocentesis
- Lumbar punctures
- Paracentesis
- Thoracentesis
- Central venous catheter placements
- Diagnostic gastrointestinal procedures
- Endoscopic retrograde cholangiopancreatography (ERCP) with stent placement
- Percutaneous endoscopic gastrostomy (PEG) placement
- Endoscopic ultrasound (EUS) with fine-needle aspiration (FNA)

Dual antiplatelet therapy confers higher bleeding risk. Therefore, procedures with higher risk of bleeding or risk of a life-threatening bleed will generally require the $P2Y_{12}$ inhibitor to be held and potentially substituted with aspirin, if the patient is not already on aspirin.[8,9] Ultimately, the decision to continue or withhold antiplatelet therapy is made after carefully assessing important bleeding risk factors such as tissue injury during the procedure, proximity of the procedure to vital organs or vascular structures, whether bleeding can be readily detected and controlled, and the associated morbidity of a bleed (e.g., small bleed in a noncompressible space vs small bleed in an open space). In the event $P2Y_{12}$ inhibitors need to be held, ticagrelor and clopidogrel should be held 5 days and prasugrel 7 days prior to a procedure with major bleeding risks.[8] Because of the irreversible nature of most $P2Y_{12}$ inhibitors, the lengthier hold period for these agents are to allow time for regeneration of enough unaffected platelets to support a high bleeding risk procedure.[8]

HALF-LIFE AND TIMING OF ANTICOAGULANTS

Another point to consider when evaluating a patient's procedural bleed risk is the half-life of the anticoagulant and timing of the last dose. The half-life of each anticoagulant dictates the time period that should elapse prior to the procedure. Warfarin is an exception, as the regeneration of thrombin is the rate-limiting step in limiting procedural bleed risk. Nevertheless, the passing of each half-life allows for the elimination of 50% of the anticoagulant. Therefore, only 12.5% of the

TABLE 4.1 ■ Half-Life of Direct Oral Anticoagulants in Patients With Normal Renal Function[11-14]

Medication	Half-Life (Hours)
Dabigatran	13
Apixaban	12
Rivaroxaban	5–9
Edoxaban	10–14

anticoagulant remains after 3 half-lives, while only 3.125% of the anticoagulant remains after 5 half-lives. This strategy is particularly important when managing DOACs in the preprocedural period, when 2–3 half-lives should elapse prior to low–bleed risk procedures and 4–5 half-lives for intermediate– and high–bleed risk procedures, an approach that was adopted by the PAUSE trial, which studied the periprocedural management of DOACs.[1,10] See Table 4.1 for DOAC half-lives.[11-14]

Knowledge of when the last dose was administered allows the practitioner to determine whether the patient is approaching peak anticoagulant activity or the end of the duration of action of the anticoagulant. This approach has been incorporated into the design of the PAUSE trial and is particularly important for subcutaneous anticoagulants with short half-lives such as unfractionated heparin (UFH) and low–molecular weight heparins (LMWH).[10] The concept is used in the ASRA Regional Anesthesia in the Patient Receiving Antithrombotic or Thrombolytic Therapy guidelines, which suggest performing neuraxial procedures at the end of the dosing period for patients administered prophylactic doses of heparin and avoiding such procedures near the peak effect of prophylactic doses of LMWH.[15]

LABORATORY MEASUREMENT OF ANTICOAGULANT ACTIVITY

When the timing of the last dose of the anticoagulant is unclear, as commonly happens in the emergency department, anticoagulant activity may be measured to guide the decision-making process for emergency procedures. INR remains the standard for which warfarin activity is measured, and an INR of <1.5 is generally accepted as the threshold for procedures, whereas LMWH activity is measured using an anti-Xa assay.[16] The measurement of DOAC activity is less straightforward because it is dependent on whether specialized assays are available at each institution. When specialized assays with rapid turnaround times are available, dilute thrombin time, ecarin clotting time, or ecarin chromogenic assay should be used to measure dabigatran, and chromogenic anti-Xa assay calibrated for apixaban, rivaroxaban, and edoxaban should be used to measure these DOACs prior to an emergent procedure. When only the standard anti-Xa assay (calibrated to LMWH) is available, it may be used to exclude clinically relevant levels of apixaban, rivaroxaban, and edoxaban. Normal levels or the absence of activity of these specialized assays suggests that the concentration of DOAC is not a clinically relevant contributor to surgical bleed risk, whereas patients with high bleeding risk and a DOAC level of >30 ng/mL may require appropriate reversal.[17]

When specialized assays are not available, normal thrombin time or activated partial thromboplastin time (aPTT) will usually exclude clinically relevant levels of dabigatran, whereas normal prothrombin time (PT) or aPTT are unreliable in excluding clinically relevant levels of apixaban, rivaroxaban, or edoxaban. Patients with prolonged aPTT on dabigatran or prolonged PT on the remaining DOACs are considered to have at least on-therapy levels of DOACs affecting the clotting cascade.[17] These suggestions are summarized in Table 4.2.

TABLE 4.2 ■ Suggested Laboratory Measurements When Specialized Assays Are Not Available

Anticoagulant	Exclude Clinically Relevant Levels	Does Not Exclude Clinically Relevant Levels	Includes Clinically Relevant Levels
Dabigatran	Normal TT or aPTT	N/A	Prolonged aPTT
Other DOACs[a]	N/A	Normal PT or aPTT	Prolonged PT

[a]Includes apixaban, rivaroxaban, and edoxaban.
aPTT, activated partial thromboplastin time; DOACs, direct oral anticoagulants; PT, prothrombin time; TT, thromboplastin time.

REVERSIBILITY OF ANTICOAGULANTS

In the event a patient requires reversal of an anticoagulant to facilitate an emergency procedure with a high bleeding risk, knowledge of the availability and reliability of the reversal agent is of utmost importance. This is described in Table 4.3. The reversal of therapeutic doses of UFH and LMWH may be achieved using protamine.[18] Given the incomplete reversal of anticoagulant effects of LMWH with protamine, therapeutic UFH may be a better option in situations in which an emergency procedure is likely.[18]

The reversal of warfarin for emergent procedures entails using a four-factor prothrombin complex concentrate (4FPCC) with IV vitamin K. Substitution of 4FPCC with other prothrombin complex concentrates (PCCs) or plasma should only occur when 4FPCC is unavailable.[17] Of note, the Food and Drug Administration-labeled dosing for 4FPCC (brand name Kcentra) is weight-based and dependent on pre-treatment INR, while many institutions have evaluated a fixed-dose approach in an effort to hasten the ordering and administration of this reversal agent during emergencies.[19,20] In general, 4FPCC with IV vitamin K has shown favorable and significant INR reductions prior to urgent procedures with a phase IIIb trial demonstrating effective hemostasis in nearly 90% of cases.[20,21] Given the good reversibility of warfarin, there should be limited hesitation on reversibility for urgent procedures in those appropriately reversed using 4FPCC and IV vitamin K.

Since the first DOAC (dabigatran) has entered the market, DOAC use has been favored by practitioners and patients alike. Given the increased usage, the likelihood of caring for a patient who requires reversal of a DOAC will continue to increase. Dabigatran is a direct thrombin

TABLE 4.3 ■ Reversal Agents for Emergent Procedures[17]

Anticoagulant	First Line	Second Line
Apixaban	4FPCC	aPCC
Rivaroxaban	4FPCC	aPCC
Edoxaban	4FPCC	aPCC
Dabigatran	Idarucizumab	aPCC or 4FPCC
Warfarin	4FPCC	Plasma
IV UFH	Protamine	N/A
LMWH	Protamine	N/A

4FPCC, four-factor prothrombin complex concentrate; aPCC, activated prothrombin complex concentrate; LMWH, low–molecular weight heparin; UFH, unfractionated heparin.

inhibitor and is reversed with idarucizumab, which is labeled for this indication.[11,22] In the event idarucizumab is unavailable, an activated PCC (aPCC) may be used in its place.[17] The REVERSE-AD trial studied idarucizumab for two indications, reversal for bleeding and reversal for emergency surgery or urgent procedures, and demonstrated normal periprocedural hemostasis in over 93% of patients requiring emergency surgery or urgent procedures.[23] As with warfarin, there should be limited hesitation on reversibility when preparing a patient for urgent procedures after idarucizumab is administered.

The remaining DOACs are factor-Xa (FXa) inhibitors that include rivaroxaban and apixaban. DOACs may be pharmacodynamically reversed using the FXa decoy protein, andexanet, or by replenishing clotting factors with 4FPCC.[17,24] The 4FPCCs have been recommended by the American College of Emergency Physicians (ACEP) and have retrospective data suggesting effective hemostasis, which makes this an acceptable reversal strategy.[25,26] However, there is significant controversy regarding the use of andexanet during the periprocedural period. While ACEP endorses the use of andexanet for periprocedural use, the landmark trial studying andexanet, ANNEXA-4, only enrolled patients with acute major bleeds.[25,27] Combined with the short half-life of andexanet and lack of data in the periprocedural population, practitioners must use extreme caution when considering andexanet over 4FPCC in the setting of urgent procedures. In the meantime, ANNEXA-S is actively recruiting patients to study the role of andexanet in reversing FXa inhibitors in those requiring urgent surgical procedures.[28]

Evaluating Thrombotic Risks

After thoroughly evaluating for bleeding risk, thrombotic risk evaluation should follow. The risk of thrombosis may be estimated using the suggested criteria in Table 4.4 for patients with AF, mechanical heart valves, or venous thromboembolism. When both bleeding and thrombotic risk have been determined, the decision to continue or to interrupt anticoagulation, with or without bridging, can be made weighing the risks of bleeding with the risk of thrombosis.

Management of Periprocedural Anticoagulation

PREPROCEDURAL MANAGEMENT OF DIRECT ORAL ANTICOAGULANTS

When evaluating a patient procedure, it is important to first identify and optimize any patient-specific risk factors for bleeding, such as uncontrolled blood pressure, antiplatelet use, or any abnormal liver or renal function. Once these are optimized, the procedural bleed risk should be identified as not clinically important, low, or high/uncertain. The next step would be to evaluate the patient's thrombotic risk. However, since DOACs have short half-lives and are held for shorter times than warfarin even with high thrombotic risk, bridging anticoagulants offer few benefits and are rarely needed. In fact, a practical hold-and-restart strategy for low– and high–bleeding risk procedures was studied in the PAUSE trial, and demonstrated an average rate of major bleeding of <2% and an arterial thromboemboli rate of <1.5%.[10] Therefore, based on the procedural bleeding risk, the following anticoagulant management may be considered:

- No clinically important bleed risk[1]:
  - Conservative approach: hold the dose prior to the procedure.
  - Proceed **without** DOAC treatment interruption but with the procedure timed to coincide with the predicted nadir of the DOAC.
- Low– and high–bleeding risk procedures[1,10]:
  - DOACs should be held based on bleeding risk and renal function as detailed in Table 4.5.

TABLE 4.4 ■ **Thrombotic Risk Estimates for MHV, AF, and VTE**[7,30,31]

Risk Category	MHV	AF	VTE
High risk (>10%/year risk of ATE or >10%/month risk of VTE)	Any mechanical mitral valve	CHADS$_2$ score of 5–6 or CHA$_2$DS$_2$VASc score of 6–9	Recent (within 3 months) VTE
	Caged-ball or tilting disc valve in mitral/aortic position	Recent (within 3 months) stroke or TIA	Severe thrombophilia
			Deficiency of protein C, protein S, or antithrombin
	Recent (within 6 month) stroke or TIA	Rheumatic valvular heart disease	Multiple thrombophilias
			Antiphospholipid syndrome
Moderate risk (5%–10%/year risk of ATE or 5%–10%/month risk of VTE)	Bileaflet AVR with major risk factors for stroke	CHADS$_2$ score of 3–4 or CHA$_2$DS$_2$VASc score of 4–5	VTE within past 3–12 months
			Recurrent VTE
			Nonsevere thrombophilia
			Active cancer
Low risk (<5%/year risk of ATE or <2%/month risk of VTE)	Bileaflet AVR without major risk factors for stroke	CHADS$_2$ score of 0–2 or CHA$_2$DS$_2$VASc score of 0–3 (and no risk of stroke or TIA)	VTE more than 12 months ago

MHV, mechanical heart valve; *AF,* atrial fibrillation; *ATE,* arterial thromboembolism; *VTE,* venous thromboembolism; *AVR,* aortic valve replacement; *TIA,* transient ischemic attack.

TABLE 4.5 ■ **Direct Oral Anticoagulant Interruption Period Based on Bleeding Risk and Renal Function**[1,10]

	Estimated CrCl (mL/min)				
Low Bleeding Risk	≥80	50–79	30–49	15–29	<15
Dabigatran	≥24 hrs	≥36 hrs	≥48 hrs	≥72 hrs	Consider ≥96 hrs
Apixaban					
Rivaroxaban	≥24 hrs			≥36 hrs	Consider ≥48 hrs
Edoxaban					
Intermediate to High[a] **Bleeding Risk**	≥80	50–79	30–49	15–29	<15
Dabigatran	≥48 hrs	≥72 hrs	≥96 hrs	≥120 hrs	Unknown
Apixaban					
Rivaroxaban	≥48 hrs			Consider ≥72 hrs	
Edoxaban					

[a]Uncertain bleeding risk.
CrCl, creatinine clearance; *hrs,* hours.

TABLE 4.6 ■ Warfarin Interruption Based on Procedural Bleeding Risk and Patient-Specific Risk Factors For Bleeding[1]

	Bleeding Risk	
	With Patient-Specific Risk Factors for Bleeding	Without Patient-Specific Risk Factors for Bleeding
No clinically important or low bleed risk	Consider interruption of warfarin	Do not interrupt warfarin therapy
Intermediate or high bleed risk	Interrupt warfarin therapy	Interrupt warfarin therapy
Uncertain bleed risk	Interrupt warfarin therapy	Consider interruption of warfarin

Patients undergoing neuraxial procedures are at risk of bleeding into a high-risk space—spinal or epidural hematoma, which are catastrophic bleeds. Therefore, the ASRA guidelines recommend DOACs be held for 3–5 days prior to procedures, depending on renal function.[15]

PREPROCEDURAL MANAGEMENT OF WARFARIN

Similarly to DOAC management, when evaluating patients on warfarin for a procedure, patient-specific risk factors for bleeding should be optimized and procedural bleed risk should be stratified. Based on the factors found in Table 4.6, the corresponding warfarin interruption plan should be considered. The following approach may be used to plan preprocedural management of warfarin based on preprocedural INR:

- Preprocedural INR of 1.5–1.9[1]:
    - Warfarin should be held for 3–4 days prior to the procedure if normal INR (i.e., ~1.0) is required.
    - Check INR 24 hours prior to the procedure if normal INR is required.
    - Shorter periods may be considered if normal INR is not required.
- Preprocedural INR of 2–3[1]:
    - Warfarin should be held for 5 days prior to the procedure if normal INR is required.
    - Check INR 24 hours prior to the procedure if normal INR is required.
    - Shorter periods may be considered if normal INR is not required.
- Preprocedural INR of >3[1]:
    - Warfarin should be held for ≥5 days prior to the procedure and INR rechecked as the procedure date nears.
    - Check INR 24 hours prior to the procedure if normal INR is required.

Based on the BRIDGE trial, which was a randomized, double-blinded, placebo-controlled trial studying the need for bridging in patients with AF undergoing an invasive procedure, there was no difference in arterial thromboemboli with or without bridging, but there were more major bleeding events in the bridging group.[29] Therefore, only patients at high thrombotic risk or with a recent stroke or arterial thromboembolism should be considered for bridging if their bleeding risk is not high. When bridging is indicated, LMWH should be discontinued 24 hours prior to the procedure and IV UFH should be discontinued at least 4 hours prior to the procedure.[1]

POSTPROCEDURAL ANTICOAGULANT MANAGEMENT

The timing of postprocedural resumption of anticoagulation is dependent on the procedure bleed risk, procedure site hemostasis, patient-specific bleeding risk factors, type of anticoagulant to be restarted, and the consequences of bleeding, should it occur. For example, anticoagulants may be restarted earlier with low–bleed risk procedures, whereas high–bleed risk procedures may warrant

TABLE 4.7 ■ Resumption of Anticoagulant After Procedures[1]

Anticoagulant to Be Restarted	Timing of Resumption After Procedure	
	High bleeding risk	Low bleeding risk
IV UFH	48–72 hours	≤24 hours
LMWH (therapeutic dose)		
Warfarin	≤24 hours	
DOACs	48–72 hours	≤24 hours (suggest day after procedure)

DOACs, direct oral anticoagulants; IV, intravenous; LMWH, low-molecular-weight heparin; UFH, unfractionated heparin.

a delayed resumption, with an exception for warfarin since the anticoagulant effect of warfarin is typically delayed.[1] The timing for resumption of specific anticoagulants based on procedural bleeding risk is described in Table 4.7. In the event both postprocedural bleeding risks and thrombotic risks are concomitantly high, suggested management strategies include using IV UFH without bolus dosing, utilizing prophylactic doses of parenteral anticoagulants, or if warfarin is chosen, initiating or restarting warfarin without bridging.[1]

Periprocedural anticoagulation management may be complicated, but with an evidence-based and thoughtful approach, thrombotic risk can be controlled and periprocedural bleeding minimized.

References

1. Doherty JU, Gluckman TJ, Hucker WJ, et al. ACC Expert consensus decision pathway for periprocedural management of anticoagulation in patients with nonvalvular atrial fibrillation: a report of the American College of Cardiology Clinical Expert Consensus Document Task Force. *J Am Coll Cardiol.* 2017;69:871–878.
2. Fang MC, Go AS, Chang Y, et al. A new risk scheme to predict warfarin-associated hemorrhage: the ATRIA (Anticoagulation and Risk Factors in Atrial Fibrillation) study. *J Am Coll Cardiol.* 2011;58: 395–401.
3. Gage BF, Yan Y, Milligan PE, et al. Clinical classification schemes for predicting hemorrhage: results from the National Registry of Atrial Fibrillation (NRAF). *Am Heart J.* 2006;151:713–719.
4. Gallego P, Roldán V, Marin F, et al. SAMe-TT$_2$R$_2$ score, time in therapeutic range, and outcomes in anticoagulated patients with atrial fibrillation. *Am J Med.* 2014;127:1083–1088.
5. Pisters R, Lane DA, Nieuwlaat R, et al. A novel user-friendly score (HAS-BLED) to assess 1-year risk of major bleeding in patients with atrial fibrillation: the Euro Heart Survey. *Chest.* 2010;138:1093–1100.
6. Crowther MA, Warkentin TE. Bleeding risk and the management of bleeding complications in patients undergoing anticoagulant therapy: focus on new anticoagulant agents. *Blood.* 2008;111:4871–4879.
7. Douketis JD, Spyropoulos AC, Spencer FA, et al. Perioperative management of antithrombotic therapy: antithrombotic therapy and prevention of thrombosis, 9th ed American College of Chest Physicians Evidence-Based Clinical Practice Guidelines. *Chest.* 2012;141:e326S–e350S.
8. Feinbloom D. Periprocedural management of antithrombotic therapy in hospitalized patients. *J Hosp Med.* 2014;9:337–346.
9. Acosta RD, Abraham NS, Chandrasekhara V, et al. The management of antithrombotic agents for patients undergoing GI endoscopy. *Gastrointest Endosc.* 2016;83:3–16.
10. Douketis JD, Spyropoulos AC, Duncan J, et al. Perioperative management of patients with atrial fibrillation receiving a direct oral anticoagulant. *JAMA Intern Med.* 2019;179:1469–1478.
11. Pradaxa Package Insert. Boehringer Ingelheim Pharmaceuticals Inc; 2019.

12. Eliquis Package Insert. Bristol-Myers Squibb Co; 2019.
13. Xarelto Package Insert. Janssen Pharmaceuticals Inc; 2020.
14. Savaysa Package Insert. Daiichi Sankyo Inc; 2020.
15. Horlocker TT, Vandermeuelen E, Kopp SL, et al. Regional anesthesia in the patient receiving antithrombotic or thrombolytic therapy: American Society of Regional Anesthesia and Pain Medicine Evidence-Based Guidelines (Fourth Edition). *Reg Anesth Pain Med*. 2018;43:263–309.
16. Scott R, Kersten B, Basior J, et al. Evaluation of fixed-dose four-factor prothrombin complex concentrate for emergent warfarin reversal in patients with intracranial hemorrhage. *J Emerg Med*. 2018;54:861–866.
17. Tomaselli GF, Mahaffey KW, Cuker A, et al. ACC Expert consensus decision pathway on management of bleeding in patients on oral anticoagulants. *J Am Coll Cardiol*. 2017;70:3042–3067.
18. Dhakal P, Rayamajhi S, Verma V, et al. Reversal of anticoagulation and management of bleeding in patients on anticoagulants. *Clin Appl Thromb Hemost*. 2017;23:410–415.
19. Kcentra Package Insert. CSL Behring LLC; 2018.
20. Schwebach AA, Waybright RA, Johnson TJ. Fixed-dose four-factor prothrombin complex concentrate for vitamin K antagonist reversal: does one dose fit all? *Pharmacotherapy*. 2019;39:599–608.
21. Goldstein JN, Refaai MA, Jr Milling TJ, et al. Four-factor prothrombin complex concentrate versus plasma for rapid vitamin K antagonist reversal in patients needing urgent surgical or invasive interventions: a phase 3b, open-label, non-inferiority, randomised trial. *Lancet*. 2015;385:2077–2087.
22. Praxbind Package Insert. Boehringer Ingelheim Pharmaceuticals, Inc; 2018.
23. Pollack CV Jr, Reilly PA, van Ryn J, et al. Idarucizumab for dabigatran reversal—full cohort analysis. *N Engl J Med*. 2017;377:431–441.
24. Andexxa Package Insert. Portola Pharmaceuticals Inc; 2020.
25. Baugh CW, Levine M, Cornutt D, et al. Anticoagulant reversal strategies in the emergency department setting: recommendations of a multidisciplinary expert panel. *Ann Emerg Med*. 2020;76:470–485.
26. Piran S, Gabriel C, Schulman S. Prothrombin complex concentrate for reversal of direct factor Xa inhibitors prior to emergency surgery or invasive procedure: a retrospective study. *J Thromb Thrombolysis*. 2018;45:486–495.
27. Connolly SJ, Crowther M, Eikelboom JW, et al. Full study report of andexanet alfa for bleeding associated with factor Xa inhibitors. *N Engl J Med*. 2019;380:1326–1335.
28. Trial of andexanet in patients receiving an oral FXa inhibitor who require urgent surgery (ANNEXA-S). ClinicalTrials.gov identifier: NCT04233073. Updated March 25, 2020. Accessed April 21, 2020. https://clinicaltrials.gov/ct2/show/NCT04233073.
29. Douketis JD, Spyropoulos AC, Kaatz S, et al. Perioperative bridging anticoagulation in patients with atrial fibrillation. *N Engl J Med*. 2015;373:823–833.
30. Friberg L, Rosenqvist M, Lip GYH. Evaluation of risk stratification schemes for ischaemic stroke and bleeding in 182 678 patients with atrial fibrillation: the Swedish Atrial Fibrillation cohort study. *Eur Heart J*. 2012;33:1500–1510.
31. Spyropoulos AC, Al-Bardi A, Sherwood MW, et al. Periprocedural management of patients receiving a vitamin K antagonist or a direct oral anticoagulant requiring an elective procedure or surgery. *J Thromb Haemost*. 2016;14(5):875–885.

Glycemic Considerations for Tests and Procedures

Makeda Dawkins, BS ■ Marcel Souffrant, BS ■ Alyson K. Myers, MD

Background

Achieving glycemic control is imperative for patients with diabetes undergoing tests and procedures, many of which require dietary restrictions. For these patients, mismanagement of diabetes medications during fasting periods can have dangerous consequences including hypo- or hyperglycemia. This chapter will review glycemic management and guidelines for patients with type 1 diabetes (T1D) and type 2 diabetes (T2D) undergoing tests and procedures in both the inpatient and outpatient settings.

General Approach to Glycemic Management While NPO

The glycemic management of patients who are *nil per os* (NPO or "nothing by mouth") should begin with plasma blood glucose checks every 4–6 hours. Basal insulin should still be administered, but with a 20%–40% reduction.[1] Patients with T1D require daily basal insulin to avoid diabetic ketoacidosis, a life-threatening complication of hyperglycemia.[2] Basal insulin products are intermediate or long-acting which include insulin glargine, insulin detemir, and insulin degludec. While bolus premeal insulin should be held to avoid potential hypoglycemic episodes, correctional bolus insulin should be made available in the instance of hyperglycemia. Bolus insulin for before meals or as a correctional is rapid-acting and included insulin aspart, insulin lispro, and insulin glulisine.

An Overview of Inpatient Diabetes

INPATIENT GLYCEMIC TARGETS

Persistent hyperglycemia is associated with a range of adverse outcomes in hospitalized patients. According to the American Diabetes Association, all patients with diabetes or hyperglycemia (blood glucose ≥140 mg/dL or 7.8 mmol/L) should have a hemoglobin A1c (HbA1c) test upon admission if one was not performed within 3 months preceding admission.[3] Injectable insulin, not oral or noninsulin subcutaneous (SQ) agents, should be prescribed in patients with pre-existing diagnoses or those with a HbA1c ≥6.5%, allowing for dosage adjustments based on blood glucose fluctuations. Once insulin therapy has been initiated, an inpatient glycemic target of 140–180 mg/dL or 7.8–10 mmol/L should be maintained.[1] Tighter glycemic control, maintaining a target of 110–140 mg/dL or 6.1–7.8 mmol/L, is recommended only for critically ill postsurgical patients and those undergoing cardiac surgery, taking care to avoid hypoglycemia.[3] Tight glycemic control in patients outside of these categories has been linked to increased mortality and should be avoided. Bedside glucose monitoring should occur before meals and at bedtime in patients who are eating, and every 4–6 hours in NPO patients.

INPATIENT INSULIN MANAGEMENT

In hospital settings, basal insulin or basal-bolus insulin regimens with corrective sliding scales are preferred for management of diabetes and hyperglycemia. If previous oral agents were discontinued during admission, they should be restarted 1–2 days prior to discharge, as home oral antihyperglycemic agents have been shown to exacerbate medical comorbidities in the hospital setting.[1,3] Basal insulin in conjunction with rapid-acting insulin allows for meal coverage and correction for hyperglycemic episodes unrelated to nutrition. This balance of basal-bolus insulin is designed to mimic physiologic insulin release. Long-acting basal insulin should provide up to 24 hours of constant insulin supply, effectively suppressing liver and renal gluconeogenesis between meals, while bolus insulin provides insulin coverage for meals and prevents postprandial glucose elevations, reaching its peak effect within an hour. Rapid-acting insulin should be given up to 15 minutes prior to a meal, sooner than regular insulin, which should be given 30 minutes prior to a meal as it has a slower onset of action. However, in the case of preprandial hypoglycemia below 70 mg/dL, bolus insulin should not be administered until hypoglycemia is corrected and the patient is eating.[4] The amount of total insulin administered daily will depend on the patient's weight, renal function, and nutritional intake but will generally be divided equally between the basal and total bolus doses.

Presurgical Targets and Medication Adjustments

According to the American Diabetes Association, presurgical glycemic targets should be maintained at 80–180 mg/dL or 4.4–10 mmol/L, although higher levels may be preferred per anesthesia guidelines.[1] All oral antihyperglycemic agents should be discontinued the day of surgery, whereas sulfonylureas and sodium-glucose cotransporter-2 (SGLT2) inhibitors need to be held longer. The Food and Drug Administration (FDA) has recommended that SGLT2 inhibitors should be held 3 (canagliflozin, dapagliflozin, empagliflozin) or 4 days (ertugliflozin) prior to surgery in order to avoid diabetic ketoacidosis.[4] Sulfonylureas cause the pancreas to produce more insulin, with effects lasting 1–2 days, but the effect can be even longer in those with renal disease. Therefore, they should be discontinued 1–2 days prior to the procedure. If prescribed on the day of surgery, half the dosage of NPH (an intermediate-acting insulin) should be administered and 60%–80% of other basal insulins should be given preceding surgery.[1] Patients should be monitored for 4–6 hours prior to surgery if NPO, and levels should be adjusted using a corrective scale.

Surgical NPO Management

CARDIAC PROCEDURES

Coronary artery bypass grafting (CABG): Insulin infusions are often used in the perioperative care of patients undergoing a CABG, as patients will often have increased insulin requirements during surgery due to the stress of the procedure and increased insulin resistance from their NPO status. Proper glycemic control allows for improved outcomes. A glycemic target of 125–200 mg/dL results in greater survival and improved wound healing compared with the more lenient target of <250 mg/dL.[5] Evidence suggests that trying to impose tighter glycemic control (90–120 mg/dL) leads to more hypoglycemia as opposed to those with a goal of 120–180 mg/dL, with no improvements in morbidity or mortality.[6] See Chapter 20: Coronary Artery Bypass Grafting for more details about this procedure.

Transcatheter aortic valve replacement (TAVR): A TAVR is a much shorter procedure (about 1 hour). Insulin infusion is less likely to be used. See Chapter 56: Transcatheter Aortic Valve Replacement for more details about this procedure.

GASTROINTESTINAL PROCEDURES

Esophagogastroduodenoscopy (EGD)/colonoscopy: In preparation for gastrointestinal proce-dures, patients should not eat for 8 hours prior. Clear liquids are permitted until 2 hours before-hand.[7] In some cases, patients are required to have a full day of clear liquids or bowel prep the day before their procedure, in which case they will need to adjust their medications both the day before and day of the procedure. See Chapter 32: Gastrointestinal Endoscopy, Upper and Chapter 31: Gastrointestinal Endoscopy, Lower for more details about these procedures.

Percutaneous endoscopic gastrostomy (PEG) placement: In patients with newly established PEG tubes, feedings should not be initiated until 24 hours after placement. Both before tube place-ment and following initiation of diabetic-specified formula feedings, these patients should receive SQ premeal bolus insulin every 4–6 hours to correct hyperglycemia.[3] All regimens should include basal, bolus, and correctional requirements. Patients with T1D and those with T2D should still receive SQ basal-bolus insulin even if feedings are discontinued. Each patient's basal insulin require-ment can be estimated using their preadmission long- or intermediate-acting dosages, or, alterna-tively, weight-based dosing can be used at 0.4–0.6 units/kg, with half given as a basal dosage and the other half divided over three meals daily as short-acting nutritional doses.[8] See Chapter 47: Percutaneous Endoscopic Gastrostomy Tube for more details about this procedure.

Enhanced recovery procedure (ERP): ERP has been used to decrease surgical stress and decrease length of stay for several types of surgery, including colorectal and hepatic surgeries.[5,6] It allows patients to drink clear liquids up until 2 hours prior to anesthesia. According to the American Society of Anesthesiologists, clear liquids include but are not limited to water, fruit juices without pulp, carbonated beverages, carbohydrate (CHO)-rich nutritional drinks, clear tea, and black coffee. Following consumption, patients are specifically required to drink 45 g CHO 2 hours prior to the surgery, decreasing insulin resistance via increasing endogenous insulin pro-duction, leading to less perioperative hyperglycemia.[9] As a result, patients with T1D and those with T2D who use bolus insulin will require a bolus dose for the CHO load. The bolus dosage to account for this load can be calculated by dividing 45 by the patient's insulin-to-CHO ratio (ICR) (which is determined by dividing 450 by their usual total daily insulin dose).[10]

TRANSPLANT

Postoperative corticosteroid regimens have been noted to induce consistent hyperglycemia until discontinuation. Likewise, transplant medications, specifically tacrolimus, sirolimus, and cyclo-sporine, have been shown to induce hyperglycemia via increased jejunal glucose absorption and/or increased insulin resistance.[11] As steroids preferentially affect postprandial glycemic control, adjustments to premeal insulin should be made first. Rather than a 50:50 basal:bolus regimen, a bolus-heavy regimen should be used in a 40:60 or 30:70 basal:bolus ratio.[12]

An Overview of Outpatient Diabetes

GLYCEMIC TARGETS

The management of blood glucose levels begins with two techniques—self-monitoring of blood glucose (SMBG) and continuous glucose monitoring (CGM). Regular use of these tools may reduce complications and provide insight into the efficacy of glycemic control for patients and providers.[2] With the information provided by SMBG and CGM, individualized guidance with regard to medication, nutrition, and physical activity can be better achieved. For nonpregnant adults, HbA1c of <7% is within the parameters of the goal, but this value may range from 6.5% to 8% depending on the patient's clinical scenario. An acceptable glycemic status is considered to be 80–130 mg/dL preprandially and can reach up to 180 mg/dL postprandially. As with HbA1c, these targets may fluctuate depending on the individual. See Chapter 18: Continuous Glucose Monitoring for details about these devices and practices.

Medication Management for Same-Day NPO Procedures

Oral antihyperglycemic agents should be held the day of any NPO-requiring procedures, and some agents, such as sulfonylureas and SGLT2 inhibitors, should be held for a longer period of time. Sulfonylureas are a class of medications that cause the pancreas to release insulin with an effect that lasts 1–2 days, or longer in those with renal disease, which can lead to hypoglycemia, especially if a patient is not eating.[13] It is suggested that these agents (e.g., glipizide, glyburide, glimepiride) be held 1–2 days prior to the same-day procedure. SGLT2 inhibitors can induce euglycemic ketoacidosis or diabetic ketoacidosis in the perioperative period and need to be held for 3–4 days prior to procedures, and not restarted until the patient resumes oral intake.[4,14]

Patients who use metformin should hold this medication the day of the procedure. However, if the procedure requires intravenous contrast such as that used with computed tomography scanning or cardiac catheterizations and has acute kidney injury (AKI), metformin should be held for 48 hours after the use of the intravenous contrast.[15] Those without AKI and with an estimated glomerular filtration rate (eGFR) $\geq$30 mL/min/1.73m^2 can resume metformin when they resume eating even if earlier than 48 hours postcontrast. Metformin does not cause an increase in the risk of AKI but can accumulate in the setting of AKI, causing a higher risk of adverse effects (e.g., lactate accumulation). There are no interactions when gadolinium contrast is used. See Chapter 17: Computed Tomography for more details about the effects of contrast.

For patients using insulin, the recommendations given for inpatients would apply—reduce the basal dose of insulin by 20%–40% the night before. The same dose reduction should be applied for persons who take their basal insulin twice daily. The dose the night before and the morning of the procedure should be both reduced by 20%–40%.

Conclusion

Diabetes medication management in NPO patients requires that the provider be aware of the type of diabetes, renal function, diabetes medications, and procedure. All patients with T1D and some of those with T2D require basal-bolus insulin, with dosage reductions of 20%–40% the night before the procedure if their basal insulin is once daily and both the night before and the morning of the procedure if their basal insulin is twice daily. In the case of some gastrointestinal procedures in which the patient drinks only clear liquids the day before, insulin adjustments may have to be made starting 2 days before the procedure. For those with T2D who use oral or SQ noninsulin agents, the medication should be held the day of the procedure. Patients on SGLT2 inhibitors should hold these medications for 3–4 days, and patients on sulfonylureas should consider holding their medications for 1–2 days, depending on their renal function, in an effort to avoid hypoglycemia.[4]

References

1. American Diabetes Association. Diabetes care in the hospital: standards of medical care in diabetes—2020. *Diabetes Care.* 2020;43:S193–S202.
2. Rushakoff RJ. Inpatient Diabetes Management. In: Feingold KR, Anawalt B, Boyce A, et al., eds. *Endotext* *MDText.com, Inc.*; 2000.
3. Magaji V, Johnston JM. Inpatient management of hyperglycemia and diabetes. *Clinical Diabetes.* 2011;29:3–9.

4. U.S. Food and Drug Administration. FDA revises labels of SGLT2 inhibitors for diabetes to include warnings about too much acid in the blood and serious urinary tract infections. https://www.fda.gov/drugs/drug-safety-and-availability/fda-revises-labels-sglt2-inhibitors-diabetes-include-warnings-about-too-much-acid-blood-and-serious. Last accessed September 27, 2020.
5. Lazar HL, Chipkin SR, Fitzgerald CA, et al. Tight glycemic control in diabetic coronary artery bypass graft patients improves perioperative outcomes and decreases recurrent ischemic events. *Circulation.* 2004;109:1497–1502.
6. Lazar HL, McDonnell MM, Chipkin S, et al. Effects of aggressive versus moderate glycemic control on clinical outcomes in diabetic coronary artery bypass graft patients. *Ann Surg.* 2011;254:458–464.
7. The American Society of Anesthesiologists Task Force. Practice guidelines for preoperative fasting and the use of pharmacologic agents to reduce the risk of pulmonary aspiration: application to healthy patients undergoing elective procedures: an updated report by the American Society of Anesthesiologists Task Force on Preoperative Fasting and the Use of Pharmacologic Agents to Reduce the Risk of Pulmonary Aspiration*. *Anesthesiology.* 2017;216:376–393.
8. Nau KC, Lorenzetti RC, Cucuzzella M, et al. Glycemic control in hospitalized patients not in intensive care: beyond sliding scale. *Am Fam Physician.* 2010;81:1130–1135.
9. Gustafsson UO, Scott MJ, Schwenk W, et al. Guidelines for perioperative care in elective colonic surgery: Enhanced Recovery After Surgery (ERAS(R)) Society recommendations. *World J Surg.* 2013;37:259–284.
10. Gillespie SJ, Kulkarni KA, Daly AE. Using carbohydrate counting in diabetes clinical practice. *J Am Diet Assoc.* 1998;98:897–905.
11. Li Z, Sun F, Zhang Y, et al. Tacrolimus induces insulin resistance and increases the glucose absorption in the jejunum: a potential mechanism of the diabetogenic effects. *PLoS One.* 2015;10:e0143405.
12. Tamez-Pérez HE, Quintanilla-Flores DL, Rodríguez-Gutiérrez R, et al. Steroid hyperglycemia: prevalence, early detection and therapeutic recommendations: a narrative review. *World J Diabetes.* 2015;6:1073.
13. Deusenberry CM, Coley KC, Korytkowski MT, et al. Hypoglycemia in hospitalized patients treated with sulfonylureas. *Pharmacotherapy.* 2012;32:613–617.
14. Handelsman Y, Henry RR, Bloomgarden ZT, et al. American Association of Clinical Endocrinologists and American College of Endocrinology position statement on the association of SGLT-2 inhibitors and diabetic ketoacidosis. *Endocr Pract.* 2016;22:753–762.
15. American College of Radiology Committee on Drugs and Contrast Media. *Manual on Contrast Media.* American College of Radiology; 2020.

CHAPTER 6

Introduction to Anesthesia

Alan S. Lam, MD

An anesthesiologist takes care of patients in the periods immediately before, during, and immediately after surgery, which are known as the preoperative, perioperative, and postoperative periods, respectively. In the perioperative period, the goals of an anesthesiologist can be broadly broken down into three components:

1. Keeping the patient safe, above all else. This includes monitoring the patient's vital signs and responding to changes that may be harmful to the patient, as well as anticipating any changes that may be brought about because of the specific stage of surgery.
2. Ensuring patient comfort, which includes providing analgesia (a state of minimal pain) and amnesia (a state of minimal recall).
3. Creating a favorable surgical environment for the procedurist (within reason). This typically involves ensuring immobility of the patient during the operation.

General Anesthesia vs Sedation

Anesthesia can be thought of as existing on a continuum, ranging from light sedation to general anesthesia, separated according to the patient's ability to maintain respirations and responsiveness to verbal, tactile, and painful stimulation (Table 6.1).

GENERAL ANESTHESIA

General anesthesia is the deepest level of anesthesia that can be provided, and it involves putting the patient to sleep (known as "induction") using a combination of medications. Propofol is most commonly used for patients who are expected to have the ability to increase their cardiac output to handle some myocardial suppression and vasodilation caused by this agent. Patients who would not fit into this category include any patient in extremis (e.g., actively exsanguinating, cardiac tamponade or experiencing large pulmonary embolism) and patients with severe heart failure, severe cardiac valvular disorders (particularly stenotic lesions), severe pulmonary hypertension, severe sepsis, or shock of any etiology. Following induction, an advanced airway device, such as an endotracheal tube (ETT) or a laryngeal mask airway (LMA), is placed to assist the patient's respirations. An ETT sits in the patient's trachea below the epiglottis, and an LMA sits above the patient's epiglottis. To facilitate the placement of an ETT, the patient is almost always paralyzed, usually with succinylcholine (which acts and wears off quickly but has several contraindications, the most serious being hyperkalemia and subsequent hyperkalemic cardiac arrest in certain patient populations) or with rocuronium. Paralysis is not typically needed for placement of an LMA. Placement of an ETT vs an LMA is dependent on a variety of factors, such as risk of gastric regurgitation entering the lungs, known as aspiration, and the need for paralysis. An ETT has a tracheal cuff that minimizes the chance that gastric contents can enter the trachea, whereas the LMA does not. In patients receiving paralytics during the procedure, the risk of aspiration is higher if using LMA due to positive pressure ventilation insufflating the stomach (this is more of a concern when using higher inspiratory pressures), whereas nearly all of the inspiratory gases given through an ETT will be entering the patient's lungs instead of the stomach. In contrast, the LMA results

TABLE 6.1 ■ **Differing Depths of Anesthesia**

	Minimal Sedation	Moderate Sedation	Deep Sedation	General Anesthesia
Responsiveness	Unaffected	Intentional movements with verbal/tactile stimulation	Intentional movements with repeated tactile or noxious stimulation only	No intentional movements to repeated noxious stimulation
Ability to maintain airway	Yes	Yes	May require assistance (jaw thrust maneuver, inserting OPA or NPA)	Usually requires advanced airway (LMA vs ETT)
Spontaneous ventilation	Yes	Yes	May not be insufficient	Usually insufficient

Differences among various depths of anesthesia, from light and moderate sedation to deep sedation and general anesthesia. *ETT*, endotracheal tube; *LMA*, laryngeal mask airway; *NPA*, nasopharyngeal airway; *OPA*, oropharyngeal airway. (Modified from Continuum of Depth of Sedation: Definition of General Anesthesia and Levels of Sedation/Analgesia, American Society of Anesthesiologists, 2019. Available at: https://www.asahq.org/standards-and-guidelines/continuum-of-depth-of-sedation-definition-of-general-anesthesia-and-levels-of-sedationanalgesia.)

in improved hemodynamic stability during placement, a lower incidence of postoperative hoarse voice, and decreased rates of coughing and laryngospasm (resulting in obstruction of the airway) as the patient wakes up.[1,2] Patients are usually kept asleep with an inhalational anesthetic (desflurane, sevoflurane, isoflurane, and nitrous oxide are most commonly used) but can be kept asleep with the use of only IV anesthetics, called total IV anesthesia (TIVA), which is often employed as well. The agents chosen for TIVA can include, but are not limited to, propofol and a fentanyl analogue (e.g., sufentanil, alfentanil, remifentanil). As the procedure nears its conclusion, the inhaled anesthetic or TIVA is weaned off and any residual paralysis can be reversed with sugammadex (if rocuronium was used) or neostigmine with glycopyrrolate.

SEDATION

Procedures done under sedation, in contrast, would not require an advanced airway device and would not require paralysis. The medications used in these cases include, but are not limited to, opioids (e.g., fentanyl, hydromorphone), propofol, dexmedetomidine, ketamine, and midazolam.

The appropriate depth of anesthesia to administer is based on a combination of factors including the patient's past medical history, the patient's preference, the procedure itself, and the procedurist's individual preference. The anesthesiologist will take all of this into consideration and develop a plan that will keep the patient safe and comfortable while providing a favorable surgical environment for the procedurist (which involves a state of minimal movement from the patient when under sedation and possibly relaxing muscles with paralytics when under general anesthesia).

LOCAL AND REGIONAL ANESTHESIA

Some procedures can be performed under either sedation (with a component of local or regional anesthesia) or general anesthesia. Local anesthesia, otherwise known as a field block, is the injection of a local anesthetic (e.g., lidocaine, bupivacaine) around the incision site. In contrast, in regional anesthesia (also known as a nerve block), local anesthetic is deposited around the specific nerve or bundle of nerves that is responsible for the sensation of the surgical area, often with the help of ultrasound imaging. Take, for example, a surgical procedure in the forearm, as would be performed for the creation of an arteriovenous fistula for hemodialysis. Such a procedure can be performed with local anesthetic deposited in the forearm around the expected incision site, with a targeted nerve block of the brachial plexus (the nerve bundle that is responsible for sensation in the arm) under ultrasound guidance, or with general anesthesia. Since inducing light or moderate sedation will require less medication than inducing general anesthesia and because the most common agents used to induce general anesthesia can all cause some degree of hypotension (via myocardial depression and/or vasodilation), moderate sedation can be expected to cause fewer perturbations in vital signs than inducing general anesthesia in the majority of cases.[3] However, other factors to consider include:

- Can the patient remain motionless in the required position for the entirety of the procedure? Patients with conditions such as anxiety, back pain, or heart failure may be unable to lay supine for prolonged periods.
- Does the patient look potentially difficult to intubate? Under all circumstances, an anesthesiologist should be prepared to convert to general anesthesia within 1 or 2 minutes. If the patient has risk factors for being potentially difficult to intubate, such as a history of sleep apnea, morbid obesity, retrognathia, a small mouth opening, a large tongue, or a history of neck radiation, then the anesthesiologist may opt to induce general anesthesia from the beginning of the procedure. In these patients, inserting an ETT in a controlled environment with optimal positioning, adequate preoxygenation (having the patient breathe 100% oxygen until their expired oxygen concentrations are >80%), nearby emergency intubation equipment (such as a video laryngoscope, fiberoptic scope, or bougie), and perhaps a second anesthesiologist in the room for assistance may be desirable compared with suddenly needing to intubate in the middle of a procedure when a patient becomes compromised. If a patient is already desaturating (meaning that oxygen levels in the blood are decreasing), repositioning and lack of emergency equipment and personnel can waste precious seconds, which can lead to an adverse outcome. It is for this reason that an anesthesiologist may elect to administer a general anesthetic for the excision of a small back lipoma (to be done with prone positioning), even though the surgery may only last a few minutes.

Anesthetic Complications and the Inpatient

There are a number of anesthetic-related complications that can be influenced or encountered by inpatient practitioners. A few common scenarios are listed below. It is recommended to check local institution-specific guidelines that may exist regarding any of these medications/situations.

- Generally speaking, oral antihypertensives should not be held prior to surgery. For some antihypertensives, such as alpha-2 agonists, withdrawal may precipitate an intraoperative reflex hypertensive event.[4] Withholding preoperative beta blockers may result in ischemia in patients who have coronary artery disease and has been associated with increased morbidity and mortality.[5] One possible exception to this rule is suspending angiotensin-converting enzyme inhibitors (ACEIs) and angiotensin II receptor blockers (ARBs) on the day of the procedure (some centers may hold them beginning 24 hours prior to surgery), as some studies have found that these medications are associated with increased rates of hypotension when continued into the perioperative period.[6] There is no general consensus as the data is conflicted with regard to 30-day mortality, so it is reasonable to consider holding ACEIs and ARBs prior to surgery.

- Administering opioids and/or benzodiazepines prior to transporting the patient to the procedure area may hinder the ability of the patient to consent to both the procedure and to being anesthetized if they cannot verbalize their understanding of the risks and benefits of undergoing anesthesia. In addition, one must also be wary of these medications and any others that have a potential for sedation in the immediate postoperative hours, particularly if the patient is obese and/or has obstructive sleep apnea (OSA) and was placed under general anesthesia. These include the aforementioned benzodiazepines and opioids, in addition to barbiturates, antipsychotics, and common sleep medications. The reasoning for this is as follows:

- The most common method of administering general anesthetic is via the inhaled route. The termination of action of these anesthetics requires sufficient gas exchange at the level of the alveoli (the most downstream segment of the lung). Therefore, when a patient with OSA, or presumed to have OSA because of obesity, has an episode of airway obstruction and hypoventilation during sleep, accumulation of the inhaled anesthetic can occur in the alveoli and can reanesthetize the patient.[7] In addition, benzodiazepines and opioids also decrease the ventilatory response (which can be thought of as the desire to breathe) to hypoxia and hypercarbia. Further compounding this is the lethargy and sedation that occurs with hypercapnia. All of these factors can result in a positive feedback loop that can ultimately cause hypercapnic respiratory failure requiring reintubation. Unfortunately, this desaturation is often not acutely detected and there have been instances in which floor nurses have discovered patients expired overnight or having suffered irreparable brain injury with this as a contributing factor. Some methods that can interrupt this cycle are the use of continuous positive airway pressure (CPAP) in the postoperative period, which can minimize the episodes of airway obstruction and help the patient maintain ventilation; use of continuous pulse oximetry to alert medical personnel of desaturations under 90%; encouraging patients to sleep in a nonsupine position, as lateral or semi-recumbent positioning is associated with less pharyngeal collapse and subsequently less airway obstruction; and use of patient-controlled (instead of provider-controlled) analgesia, in which the patient can deliver their own small doses of opioids with a set minimum time limit between doses in addition to a set limit of doses in a given time period, with the caveat of avoiding background basal infusions.[8] See Chapter 44: Oxygen Supplementation for details about continuous positive airway pressure. See Chapter 45: Patient-Controlled Analgesia for more details about this practice. In summary, one should exercise caution when administering sedating medications, particularly benzodiazepines and opioids, in patients with morbid obesity and/or OSA in the immediate postoperative day/night after having received general anesthesia and should consider giving these medications only on an as-needed basis instead of prophylactically.[9]

- For a patient requiring a surgery in which a regional nerve block may be used as either the primary anesthetic or as an adjunct for postoperative pain control, the risk and benefit of suspending pharmacologic venous thromboembolism prophylaxis must be weighed. Surgical procedures involving the extremities and/or hips or those requiring large abdominal incisions are primary examples for which suspending the anticoagulant is considered. The basis of using nerve blocks is the principle that with better pain control, there are fewer intraoperative hemodynamic changes and less postoperative opioid use. This has been shown to result in less constipation, less delirium, less nausea and vomiting,[10] increased tidal volumes (the size of a particular breath) resulting in less postoperative atelectasis and fewer pulmonary complications,[11] and faster hospital discharge.[12]

- Patients are made *nil per os* (NPO), Latin for nothing by mouth, prior to surgery as a protective measure against aspiration. Aspiration occurs when food or gastric contents enter the trachea and lungs, possibly resulting in chemical pneumonitis, pneumonia, acute respiratory distress syndrome, and even death. This can occur with anesthesia because as patients lose consciousness, there is a loss of the cough reflex that would otherwise protect the airway from aspiration as well as a decline in the tone of both the upper and lower esophageal sphincter (the bundle of muscles that prevent gastric contents from entering the oropharynx and esophagus, respectively).[13] The exact recommended duration of NPO status prior to surgery depends on the fluid/food ingested. The American Society of Anesthesiologists recommends at least 2 hours for clear liquids (which include water, coffee, tea, carbonated beverages, and pulpless fruit juice); 4 hours for breast milk; 6 hours for light meals (those with minimal amounts of fat and/or meat), nonhuman milk, formula, and other liquids not classified under clear liquids; and 8 hours for heavy meals.[14]

- Patients with diabetes who are to be NPO have their own specific needs with regard to dosing of their basal insulin. Assuming a daytime surgery, patients taking twice-daily NPH should take their regular bedtime dose of NPH the night before surgery and a daytime dose of NPH reduced by 50%. For patients using once-daily basal insulin such as insulin glargine or insulin detemir, their dose prior to surgery should be reduced by 25%. Those who are taking twice-daily insulin glargine or insulin detemir should reduce both the dose the morning of surgery and the dose the evening prior to surgery by 25%. Patients who take >80 units/day of insulin, have >60% of their total daily insulin as basal, or are otherwise at high risk for hypoglycemia (those with kidney or liver impairment, a history of hypoglycemia, or advanced age) should have their doses decreased by 50% to 75%.[15] Regardless, blood glucose should still be checked every 4 to 6 hours throughout the day of surgery in these patients. Nutritional insulin (mealtime standing bolus doses) should be held as the patient will not be eating a meal, but correctional bolus insulin should still be administered. Consider consulting with an endocrinologist if the patient is particularly sensitive to changes in their diabetes regimen. See Chapter 5: Glycemic Considerations for Tests and Procedures for details.

- Patients who undergo cardiac catheterization and have a stent placed in their coronary artery are usually started on dual antiplatelet therapy (DAPT), such as aspirin with a $P2Y_{12}$ inhibitor (e.g., clopidogrel), to prevent stent thrombosis and myocardial infarction. When these patients are to have a procedure, the necessity of the procedure, the risk of bleeding if continued on DAPT, and the risk of stent thrombosis if discontinuing DAPT must be taken into consideration. Suspending DAPT after a recent stent placement when superimposed on the general prothrombotic/proinflammatory state that is associated with surgery puts the patient at a very high risk for stent thrombosis. The current recommendations from American College of Cardiology/American Heart Association (AHA) are as follows: completely elective surgeries should be delayed for at least 30 days after bare metal stent placement and 6 months following drug-eluting stent placement.[16] For patients with drug-eluting stents who require a time-sensitive surgical procedure, the procedure should be delayed for at least 3 months following stent placement, if possible. However, if the risk of delaying the surgery is greater than the risk of stent thrombosis, then the surgery should be performed. Ideally, DAPT would be continued in these patients, but for procedures in which bleeding would have catastrophic consequences—such as in intracranial or intraocular surgeries—it may be necessary to hold one (typically the $P2Y_{12}$ inhibitor) or both medications[16,17] (Fig. 6.1). This decision should be made on a case-by-case basis and only after a discussion with the surgeon and cardiologist. See Chapter 4: Anticoagulation Management in the Periprocedural Period and Chapter 46: Percutaneous Coronary Intervention.

- For a patient who has an elevated risk for major adverse cardiac events (MACE > 1%) and who has poor exercise tolerance (defined as <4 metabolic equivalents; e.g., being unable to walk at 3 mph, vacuum, sweep floors, carry groceries), obtaining cardiac imaging and/or consulting with a cardiologist may be warranted.[16,18] There are several online calculators

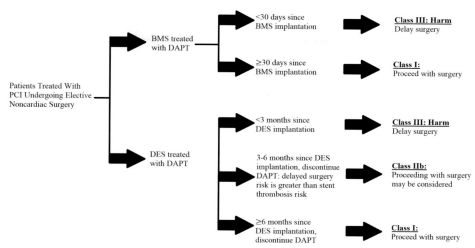

Fig. 6.1 Decision algorithm for timing elective noncardiac surgery following PCI. (Modified from Levine GH, et al.)[16]

that have been devised to calculate a patient's risk for MACE, two of which highlighted by the AHA are the Revised Cardiac Risk Index and the American College of Surgeons NSQIP Surgical Risk Calculator. Obtaining imaging such as an echocardiogram or a stress test may uncover hitherto unknown cardiac diseases. For example, aortic stenosis or severe coronary artery disease may require intervention with an aortic valve replacement or a coronary artery bypass graft, respectively, prior to the originally planned surgical procedure.

References

1. Lamb K, James MF, Janicki K. The laryngeal mask airway for intraocular surgery: effects on intraocular pressure and stress responses. *Br J Anaesth*. 1992;69:143–147.
2. Yu SH, Beirne OR. Laryngeal mask airways have a lower risk of airway complications compared with endotracheal intubation: a systematic review. *J Oral Maxillofac Surg*. 2010;68:2359–2376.
3. Fairfield JE, Dritsas A, Beale RJ. Haemodynamic effects of propofol: induction with 2.5 mg kg-1. *Br J Anaesth*. 1991;67:618–620.
4. Hart GR, Anderson RJ. Withdrawal syndromes and the cessation of antihypertensive therapy. *Arch Intern Med*. 1981;141:1125–1127.
5. Kertai MD, Cooter M, Pollard RJ, et al. Is compliance with Surgical Care Improvement Project Cardiac (SCIP-Card-2) measures for perioperative beta-blockers associated with reduced incidence of mortality and cardiovascular-related critical quality indicators after noncardiac surgery? *Anesth Analg*. 2018;126:1829–1838.
6. Shiffermiller JF, Monson BJ, Vokoun CW, et al. Prospective randomized evaluation of preoperative angiotensin-converting enzyme inhibition (PREOP-ACEI). *J Hosp Med*. 2018;13:661–667.
7. Leeson S, Roberson RS, Philip JH. Hypoventilation after inhaled anesthesia results in reanesthetization. *Anesth Analg*. 2014;119:829–835 Erratum in: *Anesth Analg* 2015;121:578.
8. Practice guidelines for the perioperative management of patients with obstructive sleep apnea: an updated report by the American Society of Anesthesiologists Task Force on Perioperative Management of Patients with Obstructive Sleep Apnea. *Anesthesiology*. 2014;120:268–286.
9. Wolfe RM, Pomerantz J, Miller DE, et al. Obstructive sleep apnea: preoperative screening and postoperative care. *J Am Board Fam Med*. 2016;29:263–275.
10. Kettner SC, Willschke H, Marhofer P. Does regional anaesthesia really improve outcome? *Br J Anaesth*. 2011;107:i90–i95.

11. Vukosavljevic S, Randjelovic T, Pavlovic D. Thoracal epidural analgesia in upper abdominal surgery. *Crit Care*. 2008;12:271.

12. Bulka CM, Shotwell MS, Gupta RK, et al. Regional anesthesia, time to hospital discharge, and in-hospital mortality: a propensity score matched analysis. *Reg Anesth Pain Med*. 2014;39:381–386. Erratum in: *Reg Anesth Pain Med*. 2015;40:297.

13. Adnet F, Baud F. Relation between Glasgow Coma Scale and aspiration pneumonia. *Lancet*. 1996;348:123–124.

14. American Society of Anesthesiologists Committee. Practice guidelines for preoperative fasting and the use of pharmacologic agents to reduce the risk of pulmonary aspiration: Application to healthy patients undergoing elective procedures: an updated report by the American Society of Anesthesiologists Task Force on Preoperative Fasting and the Use of Pharmacologic Agents to Reduce the Risk of Pulmonary Aspiration*. *Anesthesiology*. 2017;216:376–393.

15. Dogra P, Jialal I. Diabetic perioperative management. In: *StatPearls*. StatPearls Publishing; 2020. https://www.ncbi.nlm.nih.gov/books/NBK540965.

16. Levine GN, Bates ER, Bittl JA, et al. 2016 ACC/AHA guideline focused update on duration of dual antiplatelet therapy in patients with coronary artery disease: a report of the American College of Cardiology/American Heart Association Task Force on Clinical Practice Guidelines: an update of the 2011 ACCF/AHA/SCAI guideline for percutaneous coronary intervention, 2011 ACCF/AHA guideline for coronary artery bypass graft surgery, 2012 ACC/AHA/ACP/AATS/PCNA/SCAI/STS guideline for the diagnosis and management of patients with stable ischemic heart disease, 2013 ACCF/AHA guideline for the management of ST-elevation myocardial infarction, 2014 ACC/AHA guideline for the management of patients with non–ST-elevation acute coronary syndromes, and 2014 ACC/AHA guideline on perioperative cardiovascular evaluation and management of patients undergoing noncardiac surgery. *J Am Coll Cardiol*. 2016;68:1082–1115.

17. Rossini R, Musumeci G, Capodanno D, et al. Perioperative management of oral antiplatelet therapy and clinical outcomes in coronary stent patients undergoing surgery. Results of a multicentre registry. *Thromb Haemost*. 2015;113:272–282.

18. Fleisher LA, Fleischmann KE, Auerbach AD, et al. 2014 ACC/AHA guideline on perioperative cardiovascular evaluation and management of patients undergoing noncardiac surgery: a report of the American College of Cardiology/American Heart Association Task Force on Practice Guidelines. *Circulation*. 2014;130:2215–2245.

CHAPTER 7

Abdominal Ultrasound

Devora Lichtman, MD, RDMS, RDCS, RVT

Background

An abdominal ultrasound is a test that utilizes pulsed high-frequency sound waves (2–5 MHz) to create images of the abdominal organs without ionizing radiation. It creates real-time two-dimensional images of the various abdominal organs that can be displayed in either the longitudinal or transverse planes. There are a few different versions of the abdominal ultrasound. The right upper quadrant ultrasound, a foreshortened test, only includes the organs in the right upper quadrant of the abdomen (e.g., liver, gallbladder, right kidney). An abdominal Doppler is another version that adds Doppler imaging to evaluate the major abdominal arteries for stenosis (e.g., celiac axis, renal arteries, main mesenteric arteries).[1]

How to Use It

Abdominal ultrasound is an inexpensive and readily portable tool that is useful in interrogating the abdominal organs including the liver, gallbladder, pancreas, spleen, and kidneys. In some institutions, it is used to evaluate the appendix as well. It is extremely useful in differentiating between solid and cystic lesions and gathering information regarding the global structural anatomy of the organ being visualized. It is used to find masses, thrombosis, stenosis, cholecystitis, cholelithiasis, cirrhosis, and nephrolithiasis, and as a guide for biopsies. Fluid-filled structures appear black/dark on imaging, with a posterior enhancement, that means that the structures are brighter. Solid masses may be many shades of gray. Calcified lesions or gallstones will appear echogenic or bright with a posterior shadowing. The test is typically ordered as a complete abdominal ultrasound, and if a limited right upper quadrant is warranted, it can be specified in the order.[1]

How It Is Done

The patient is positioned in both a supine and left-lateral decubitus position for this test. It is typically performed by a sonographer but may be performed by physician, nurse practitioner, or physician assistant. It is utilized in the emergency department, radiology department, or intensive care unit and can be used in the inpatient and outpatient settings. The operator uses ultrasound gel and a high-frequency ultrasound probe to obtain images of the abdominal organs. The images are obtained in the sagittal/long axis and in the transverse/short axis. Pulsed high-frequency sound waves are emitted from an ultrasound probe, and the echoes from those pulsed sound waves are sent back to the probe. The echoes are displayed as pictures based on the speed of the waves when they hit the probe and the time it takes for the echoes to return to the probe. See Chapter 50: Renal Ultrasound, Fig. 50.1, for an example of an ultrasound image. Ideally, patients fast for 8 hours before the exam to optimize image acquisition and minimize bowel gas, which obstructs the clarity of the images by casting a shadow over the target organs. In an emergent situation, an abdominal ultrasound can be performed on a patient who has not fasted, but the image quality will likely be compromised due to increased bowel gas, and the gallbladder may be contracted and difficult to fully assess. The organs are interrogated with color Doppler and pulsed-wave Doppler to evaluate blood flow velocity. The test takes approximately 30 minutes to complete. A normal test result is typically a homogeneous liver texture without masses or cysts; a gallbladder without cholelithiasis, polyps, or masses; a common bile duct (CBD) <6 mm; normal renal parenchyma without hydronephrosis; and homogeneous splenic parenchyma without masses.[1]

Medication Implications

- Routine medications do not need to be held prior to the exam.[1]
- The abdominal ultrasound is noninvasive, and no medications are administered prior to the test, including sedation or pain control medications.[1]
- Ultrasound contrast administered intravenously (e.g., brand names Lumason, Definity, Optison, or Sonazoid) may be utilized to enhance visualization of masses with vascular components. This contrast is composed of encapsulated microbubbles in suspension. A thin shell of albumin or lipids contain the gas core, which is made up of perflutrens or sulfur hexafluoride. The bubbles persist in circulation for several minutes. It does not contain any iodine and therefore can be utilized in patients with renal and liver impairment or failure.[2-5]
  - Ultrasound contrast products share some common warnings and precautions. All products include a boxed warning in the prescribing information for serious cardiopulmonary reactions including fatalities. These reactions tend to occur within 30 minutes of administration, so resuscitation equipment and trained personnel should be available when using these agents. Patients with unstable cardiac conditions are at higher risk of cardiopulmonary events. These events include cardiac and pulmonary arrest, shock, syncope, arrhythmias, and others.
  - Patients with cardiac shunts are at risk of arterial embolization by the contrast microbubbles as they may not be filtered by the lungs. Known or suspected cardiac shunts are contraindications to some of these agents, and all patients should be assessed for embolic phenomena after administration. For this same reason, contrast agents should never be given by intra-articular injection.
  - Some contrast agents include albumin, a human blood product that carries its own risks of administration and may be refused by certain populations (e.g., Jehovah's Witnesses).
- Biopsies of solid organs, such as liver or renal biopsies, are commonly performed under ultrasound guidance.
  - There are no medications that need to be given prior to the biopsy, but it is common practice that lidocaine 1% is injected locally along the path that the biopsy needle will take.[6]
  - Bleeding is one of the more common and serious complications of a renal biopsy, and at times, desmopressin is used prior to biopsy in patients who are at high risk of bleeding. It can decrease the risk of bleeding and the size of the hematoma in the instance that postbiopsy bleeding occurs.[7] See Chapter 34: Hemodialysis Access for more details.
  - Bleeding after a liver biopsy may be secondary to an intraperitoneal hemorrhage, hematoma, or hemobilia. Intraperitoneal hemorrhage can be diagnosed by visualizing free fluid in the peritoneal cavity. The fluid is visible with ultrasound and is seen as hypoechoic (dark) fluid surrounding the abdominal organs in the most dependent portion of the abdominal cavity.[8]
  - Warfarin is held prior to a renal or liver biopsy. Typically, the international normalized ratio (INR) is allowed to drift below 1.5 to minimize the risk of bleeding; however, this is a general recommendation and may differ based on individual patient bleeding risk and procedurist preference. If a patient is taking warfarin and requires an urgent biopsy, then

warfarin's effect can be reversed.[9] See Chapter 4: Anticoagulation Management in the Periprocedural Period for details about bleeding risks and reversal strategies.

- Heparin should be held 6 hours prior to biopsy, and the activated partial thromboplastin time (aPTT) should be allowed to normalize prior to the procedure. Heparin should be held for at least 12–24 hours postprocedure. In some instances, it is preferred to hold heparin for up to 1 week postbiopsy as bleeding can occur up to 1 week after the procedure.[10]
- Direct oral anticoagulants (e.g., dabigatran, rivaroxaban, apixaban, edoxaban) should be held 2–4 days prior to the biopsy depending on renal function and other patient-specific factors. See Chapter 4: Anticoagulation Management in the Periprocedural Period for details about holding and resuming these medications.[11,12]

References

1. Hertzberg BS, Middleton WD. Chapter 2: Gallbladder, Chapter 3: Liver, Chapter 5: Kidney. In: *Ultrasound: The Requisites*. 3rd ed. Elsevier; 2016.
2. Chong WK, Papadopoulou V, Dayton PA. Imaging with ultrasound contrast agents: current status and future. *Abdom Radiol*. 2018;43:762–772.
3. Lumason Package Insert. BRACCO Suisse SA; 2016.
4. Definity Package Insert. Lantheus; 2018.
5. Optison Package Insert. GE Healthcare AS; 2016.
6. Korbet SM. Percutaneous renal biopsy. *Semin Nephrol*. 2002;22:254–267.
7. Manno C, Bonifati C, Torres DD, et al. Desmopressin acetate in percutaneous ultrasound-guided kidney biopsy: a randomized controlled trial. *Am J Kidney Dis*. 2011;57:850–855.
8. Hederström E, Forsberg L, Florén CH, Prytz H. Liver biopsy complications monitored by ultrasound. *J Hepatol*. 1989;8(1):94–98. doi:10.1016/0168-8278(89)90167-0.
9. Kearon C, Hirsh J. Management of anticoagulation before and after elective surgery. *N Engl J Med*. 1997;336:1506–1511.
10. Whittier WL, Korbet SM. Timing of complications in percutaneous renal biopsy. *J Am Soc Nephrol*. 2004;15:142–147.
11. Schulman S, Carrier M, Lee AY, et al. Perioperative management of dabigatran: a prospective cohort study. *Circulation*. 2015;132:167–173.
12. Sunkara T, Ofori E, Zarubin V, et al. Perioperative management of direct oral anticoagulants (DOACs): a systemic review. *Health Serv Insights*. 2016;9:25–36.

CHAPTER 8

Adrenocorticotropic Hormone Stimulation Test

Shannon M. Jones, PharmD　■　Andrew J. Crannage, PharmD

Background

The adrenocorticotropic hormone (ACTH) stimulation test is a relatively noninvasive laboratory assessment that involves the administration of a medication followed by the collection of blood samples. ACTH is a naturally occurring hormone released from the pituitary gland that stimulates the secretion of cortisol from the adrenal glands. Cortisol is a glucocorticoid that is responsible for the regulation of fat, carbohydrate, and protein metabolism. The test is extremely valuable, as it is safe and reliable in the diagnosis and assessment of adrenal insufficiency. Other names for this test include corticotropin or cosyntropin stimulation test, or short Synacthen test.[1-3]

How to Use It

Adrenal insufficiency, either from a primary or secondary origin, is a condition in which the adrenal cortex of the adrenal gland does not produce adequate amounts of cortisol, aldosterone, and/or various androgens. In primary adrenal insufficiency (PAI), or Addison's disease, the adrenal cortex is destroyed through various mechanisms, with the majority of cases (80%–90%) in developed countries due to autoimmune dysfunction. Other causes of PAI include medications that can either inhibit cortisol synthesis or increase cortisol metabolism. Secondary adrenal insufficiency (SAI) results in low concentrations of cortisol and ACTH, and it is commonly associated with long-term and/or high-dose exogenous glucocorticoid use. Chronic use of glucocorticoids may potentially result in atrophy of the anterior pituitary and hypothalamus, consequently leading to impaired recovery and function of these organs and prolonging cortisol insufficiency. Other causes of SAI are tumors, surgery, or radiation in the hypothalamic-pituitary region. To distinguish between these causes, comprehensive patient history and laboratory work are required, including the ACTH stimulation test. The ACTH stimulation test is currently regarded as the diagnostic gold standard for diagnosis of PAI and may potentially be used in determining the presence or resolution of SAI.[1-3]

How It Is Done

PAI is first suspected with a low morning cortisol concentration from a blood draw and then confirmed by the ACTH stimulation test. The ACTH stimulation test is generally performed in an outpatient setting under the expertise of an endocrinologist. Although ACTH is lowest around midnight, the test is performed without concern for a specific time of day.[4,5] The standard or "high-dose" test begins with intravenous administration of 250 mcg of synthetic ACTH (cosyntropin) for adults, 125 mcg for children <2 years of age, or 15 mcg/kg for infants. After administration, a rise in cortisol is expected in about 30 minutes, with plasma cortisol concentrations peaking between 45 and 60 minutes. Blood samples are obtained to measure serum cortisol concentrations at the time of cosyntropin administration, then again 30 and/or 60 minutes after the injection. Peak cortisol concentrations <18 mcg/dL (500 nmol/L) indicate PAI.[2,3,5,6] These results are diagnostic; however, a normal concentration (>18 mcg/dL) could still be present in patients with SAI. Therefore, other testing is required to determine the presence of SAI and could include a corticotropin-releasing hormone stimulation test or insulin-induced hypoglycemia test. Changes in stress response should be considered for the management of patients in the setting of critical illness, since these factors greatly affect the sensitivity of the ACTH stimulation test.[3,5]

Medication Implications

- The ACTH stimulation test is only performed at the initial diagnosis of PAI, and only symptomatic monitoring is required following diagnosis.[2,6]
- Cosyntropin is a synthetic derivative of ACTH that is used for evaluation and diagnosis of adrenocortical insufficiency.[5,7]
  - Cosyntropin stimulates adrenal activity to the same extent of natural ACTH and may be referred to as tetracosactide outside of the United States.[5]
  - Side effects are rare, since it is only used for diagnostic purposes, but may include anaphylactic reaction, bradycardia, tachycardia, hypertension, peripheral edema, and rash; it may also accentuate electrolyte loss associated with diuretic therapy.[7]
  - Since there is potential for anaphylactic reactions, healthcare professionals should be prepared to treat an acute reaction prior to administering cosyntropin injection.[7]
  - Cosyntropin is considered as Pregnancy Category C; administration to pregnant women should only be done if the benefits outweigh the risks, and caution should be used during breastfeeding.[7]
- The reference limit ranges for serum cortisol in correspondence with diagnosis should be based on assay-specific normative data.[2]
- The ACTH stimulation test results may be severely affected by conditions such as cortisol-binding globulin (CBG) deficiency, glucocorticoid resistance, and hypersensitivity.[2]
- Factors that will affect interpretation of test results include:
  - CBG and albumin concentrations: Plasma cortisol is 80%–90% protein bound to CBG and 6%–10% bound to albumin. Therefore, only about 4% of cortisol is considered unbound or free. Medications that increase CBG concentrations (e.g., estrogen-containing oral contraceptives, mitotane) or albumin concentrations need to be considered when interpreting cortisol concentrations.[2,5]
  - Conditions such as nephrotic syndrome, cirrhosis, hyperthyroidism, immediate postoperative period, and patients requiring intensive care may have lower CBG and albumin concentrations, therefore lowering initial cortisol measurements.[5,8]
  - Medications that should be held prior to testing on test day: cortisone, hydrocortisone, and spironolactone; estrogen-containing drugs should be held 4–6 weeks prior to testing.[7]
- An accurate medication history is vital to determine a potential cause of adrenal insufficiency. Drug-induced PAI may be caused by the following: adrenal hemorrhage (e.g., anticoagulants), inhibiting cortisol synthesis (e.g., ketoconazole, aminoglutethimide, mitotane, metyrapone, or etomidate), activation of glucocorticoid metabolism by anticonvulsants (e.g., phenytoin or phenobarbital), increased cortisol metabolism (e.g., levothyroxine), or antibiotics (e.g., rifampin).[2,5]
- Exogenous glucocorticoid administration via any route (e.g., oral, intravenous, inhaled) may lead to adrenal suppression in patients taking supraphysiological doses, which is >20–30 mg prednisolone or equivalent for >3 weeks (see Table 8.1 for glucocorticoid equivalency).[3] Formulations with longer half-lives have a higher risk of inducing adrenal insufficiency and include prednisolone, dexamethasone, and methylprednisolone. Glucocorticoids administered

TABLE 8.1 ■ Equivalent Doses and Approximate Half-Lives of Common Glucocorticoids

Glucocorticoid Equivalency Table		
Glucocorticoid	Equivalent Dose (mg)	Approximate Half-Life (hour)
Cortisone	25	0.5
Hydrocortisone	20	1.5
Prednisone	5	1
Prednisolone	5	3.33
Methylprednisolone	4	3
Dexamethasone	0.75	1.7–5

(Adapted from Dipiro JT, Talbert JT, Yee GC, et al., eds. *Pharmacotherapy: A Pathophysiologic Approach.* 10th ed. New York, NY: McGraw-Hill; 2017; Table 76.13.)

at doses as low as 5 mg/day prednisolone or equivalent have been shown to result in inadequate cortisol concentrations when undergoing ACTH stimulation testing. Thus, screening for use of these medications before testing is of utmost importance. Prior to discontinuing glucocorticoid therapy, a slow taper is required so that the hypothalamic-pituitary-adrenal (HPA) axis can regain its ability to respond to appropriate stimulation. Slowly reducing the dose every 3–4 days over a few weeks allows recovery of the HPA axis. After approximately 2–3 months of being on the same reduced dose of glucocorticoid, the ACTH stimulation test may be used to assess function of the HPA axis. Full recovery of the axis could take a total of 9–12 months. Once there is an adequate response to the test, ultimately signifying return of adrenal function, glucocorticoids may be safely discontinued.[5,8,9]

■ The Pharmacogenomics of Adrenal Suppression with Inhaled Steroids (PASS) study found that children between 5 and 18 years of age who use inhaled corticosteroids (ICS) for asthma may be tested via the ACTH stimulation test to identify if adrenal suppression is present. The study was performed in the United Kingdom and used a "low-dose" test that was 0.5 mcg of cosyntropin. The results identified that children may have impaired cortisol response to the ACTH stimulation test when taking various doses of ICS as well as when regularly taking oral corticosteroids. Clinical consequences of the potential adrenal suppression require further investigation.[9]

■ The "low-dose" ACTH stimulation test is available using 1 mcg of cosyntropin; however, it is reserved to be used only when the standard dose is not available or in short supply due to the fact that the high dose has been validated against other tests, whereas the low dose has yet to be validated.[2,3,5]

■ Utility of the ACTH stimulation test is limited in patients who are acutely ill or pregnant, since alteration of cortisol concentrations may interfere with interpretation.[2,3]

 ■ Critical illness-related cortisol insufficiency (CIRCI) represents patients with inadequate glucocorticoid production as well as tissue resistance to corticosteroids. This state of adrenal insufficiency is estimated to affect 20% of critically ill patients and as many as 60% of patients with severe sepsis or septic shock. In patients admitted to intensive care units, adrenal insufficiency may be diagnosed with the use of the ACTH stimulation test. The response to signify adrenal insufficiency will differ from noncritically ill patients with a peak serum cortisol concentration <9 mcg/dL, rather than <18 mcg/dL, therefore accommodating for the presence of CIRCI. ACTH stimulation testing should not be used in patients with septic shock or acute respiratory distress syndrome (ARDS) as a basis of determining if glucocorticoid therapy (i.e., stress-dose steroids) is indicated.[3,5,8,10]

- Etomidate is an induction agent used for rapid sequence intubation with well-established risk of adrenal suppression. A single dose has been demonstrated to inhibit cortisol production for up to 48 hours. An alternative induction medication should be used if the patient is at risk of developing CIRCI.[5]
- If the ACTH stimulation test reveals PAI, treatment includes[2,6]:
  - Corticosteroids with the following agents of choice: prednisone 5 mg/day, hydrocortisone 20 mg/day, or cortisone 25 mg/day given in two to three divided doses in the morning and afternoon.
  - Additional mineralocorticoid replacement (e.g., fludrocortisone acetate 0.05–2.0 mg/day) may be recommended if there is associated reduction in aldosterone production.
  - Treatment should continue until signs and symptoms of adrenal insufficiency are diminished (e.g., hyperpigmentation of skin) without restriction of salt intake.
  - Follow-up monitoring should take place annually and predominantly includes evaluation of signs or symptoms of adrenal insufficiency or overtreatment.

References

1. Jameson JL, Kasper DL, Longo DL, et al. *Harrison's Principles of Internal Medicine.* 20th ed. New York, NY: McGraw-Hill; 2018.
2. Bornstein SR, Allolio B, Arlt W, et al. Diagnosis and treatment of primary adrenal insufficiency: an endocrine society clinical practice guideline. *J Clin Endocrinol Metab.* 2016;101:364–389.
3. Dipiro JT, Talbert JT, Yee GC, et al. *Pharmacotherapy: A Pathophysiologic Approach.* 10th ed. New York, NY: McGraw-Hill; 2017.
4. Munro V, Elnenaei M, Doucette S, et al. The effect of time of day testing and utility of 30- and 60-minute cortisol values in the 250 mcg ACTH stimulation test. *Clin Biochem.* 2018;54:37–41.
5. Hamilton DD, Cotton BA. Cosyntropin as a diagnostic agent in the screening of patients for adrenocortical insufficiency. *Clin Pharmacol.* 2010;2:77–82.
6. Lee M. *Basic Skills in Interpreting Laboratory Data.* 6th ed. Bethesda, MD: American Society of Health-System Pharmacists; 2017.
7. Cosyntropin [package insert]. Princeton, NJ: Sandoz Canada Inc; 2018.
8. Wallace I, Cunningham S, Lindsay J. The diagnosis and investigation of adrenal insufficiency in adults. *Ann Clin Biochem.* 2009;46:351–367.
9. Hawcutt DB, Jorgensen AL, Wallin N, eds. Adrenal responses to a low-dose short synacthen test in children with asthma. *Clin Endocrinol.* 2015;82:648–656.
10. Nicolaides NC, Pavlaki AN, Maria Alexandra MA, et al. Glucocorticoid therapy and adrenal suppression. In: Feingold KR, Anawalt B, Boyce A, et al., eds. *Endotext.* South Dartmouth, MA: MDText.com, Inc; 2000.

CHAPTER 9

Ankle-Brachial Index Test

Jonathan S. Ruan, MD, FACC, RPVI ▪ Kimberly E. Ng, PharmD, BCPS

Background

The ankle-brachial index (ABI) is a common noninvasive test used to determine if there is occlusive disease of the peripheral vasculature. It uses the brachial arterial systolic blood pressure as the control, assuming it to be nonocclusive, and compares it to either that of the posterior tibial (PT) or dorsalis pedis (DP) arteries. The ABI is calculated in each foot by dividing the higher systolic blood pressure reading of either of the PT or DP arteries by the higher systolic blood pressure reading of either the left or right brachial artery. This index suggests occlusive peripheral artery disease (PAD) when it is ≤0.9.[1] Furthermore, the location of the occlusion may be inferred by using segmental blood pressure readings and supportive data such as pulse volume recordings (PVRs).

How to Use It

This test is ordered when there is a suspicion of obstructive vascular pathology, most commonly due to obstructive atherosclerosis of the lower extremities, but may also include obstruction due to vasculitis or thromboembolic disease. It is indicated in patients who are asymptomatic but have risk factors for atherosclerotic cardiovascular disease (ASCVD), who have symptoms of occlusive PAD (such as claudication or erectile dysfunction), or who have physical signs of limb ischemia such as poor wound healing.[2]

How It Is Done

This test can be performed as either an inpatient or outpatient test, but is most commonly performed in the outpatient setting. A plethysmographic cuff is placed around the left and right arms, and the left and right lower calves just above the ankle. Segmental pressure readings require additional plethysmographic cuffs to be placed around the upper thighs, lower thighs, and upper calves. PVRs are used to help interpret the results of ABIs and may be obtained by the use of pneumoplethysmographic cuffs or alternatively obtained using continuous-wave Doppler. Testing is usually performed at rest but can also be performed post exercise using a standardized exercise protocol if there is clinical suspicion of obstructive PAD despite a normal resting ABI.[1] In this case, the patient is exercised according to an institution's protocol and, shortly after, ABIs are obtained at regular intervals. When there is suspicion of obstructive PAD in patients with calcified vessels (which often produces an ABI >1.4), a toe-brachial index may be performed by placing a small plethysmographic cuff usually around the great toe.[1]

HOW IT IS INTERPRETED

Compared with the brachial artery, systolic arterial pressure should be similar or slightly higher in the more distal arteries. As such, the normal ABI is 1.0–1.4. An abnormal ABI is ≤0.9 and is suggestive of occlusive PAD. Borderline normal ABI is 0.91–0.99. An ABI >1.4 suggests non-compressible calcified vessels that may or may not be obstructed. An ABI >1.4 is an abnormal finding and is associated with an increased risk of stroke, heart failure, and a higher incidence of occlusive PAD compared with normal ABI.

Further testing in patients with ABI >1.4 using a toe-brachial index is indicated, as the small arterial vessels in the toes are rarely calcified. A normal toe-brachial index is >0.7. If the toe-brachial index is ≤0.7, it is abnormal and diagnostic of occlusive PAD. In addition, when there is further clinical suspicion of occlusive PAD in the setting of a normal or borderline normal ABI, an exercise ABI is indicated.[1]

Segmental plethysmographic readings may help localize disease to various areas of the lower extremity such as the aortoiliac, femoropopliteal, or infrapopliteal regions. If blood pressure decreases from one contiguous segment to the next by more than 20 mmHg, it can be inferred that there is a focal arterial occlusion between those two segments.[3]

FOLLOW-UP TESTS

Once occlusive PAD is diagnosed with an abnormal ABI, follow-up imaging may be indicated if the patient is symptomatic despite medical therapy and there is a goal for revascularization. Lower extremity arterial duplex ultrasound is a cost-effective and risk-free way of assessing the degree and level of occlusive PAD by using two-dimensional ultrasound and color Doppler ultrasound. Computed tomographic angiography (CTA) and magnetic resonance angiography (MRA) may also be used, but carry their specific risks. These tests have the benefit of evaluating the vasculature of the lower extremities in greater detail than lower extremity arterial duplex ultrasound. Finally, in symptomatic patients on goal-directed medical therapy who still have symptoms and whose quality of life may benefit from revascularization, invasive angiography is indicated.[2]

Medication Implications

ASPIRIN

Multiple double-blinded, randomized controlled trials have found that patients with occlusive, symptomatic PAD benefit from aspirin.[4-7] In these patients, aspirin 75–325 mg orally once daily results in a reduction in the incidence of cerebral vascular accident (CVA), myocardial infarction (MI), and vascular-related deaths. This is because occlusive PAD is a regional manifestation of ASCVD and has significant overlap with coronary atherosclerosis and cerebral atherosclerosis. However, while aspirin has shown dramatic reduction in ASCVD-related events in patients with symptomatic PAD, no reductions have been demonstrated in asymptomatic patients with PAD. Even so, the American College of Cardiology and the American Heart Association, in collaboration with many other organizations, recommend the use of aspirin in asymptomatic patients with PAD, based on expert opinion.[2]

CLOPIDOGREL

In patients who had a recent CVA, recent MI, or have evidence of limb ischemia, the use of clopidogrel 75 mg orally once daily as monotherapy has been shown to reduce CVA, MI, or cardiovascular-related deaths compared with the use of aspirin 325 mg orally once daily.[7] This benefit comes at no additional risk of bleeding. Current guidelines recommend the use of either aspirin or clopidogrel in patients with symptomatic PAD.[2]

DUAL ANTIPLATELET THERAPY

Dual antiplatelet therapy with aspirin and clopidogrel, while beneficial to cardiovascular patients following an MI, has not been soundly proven to be as beneficial in patients with symptomatic PAD. In addition, there has not been strong evidence balancing the benefits of dual antiplatelet therapy with its risks of bleeding in patients with symptomatic PAD. Current guidelines state that it may be reasonable to consider its use in select high-risk populations with low bleeding risks. However, after revascularization, it is reasonable to use antiplatelet therapy with aspirin and clopidogrel to prevent limb ischemia.[2]

VORAPAXAR

Vorapaxar is a protease-activated receptor-1 antagonist that prevents platelet activation. Clinically, vorapaxar 2.08 mg orally once daily compared with placebo has been shown to reduce the incidence of acute limb ischemia and the need for peripheral revascularization in patients with stable coronary artery disease, CVA, or PAD.[8] However, it did not reduce the incidence of MI, CVA, or cardiovascular-related deaths. In addition, vorapaxar is associated with increased moderate-severe bleeding compared with placebo, and its product labeling contains a boxed warning against use in patients with a history of CVA, transient ischemic attack, intracranial hemorrhage, or pathological bleeding.[9] Currently, the use of vorapaxar has not been strongly recommended in guidelines by major professional organizations.[2]

HMG-COA REDUCTASE INHIBITORS (STATINS)

High-intensity statins are indicated in patients with clinical ASCVD including claudication or chronic limb ischemia. It is recommended that low-density lipoprotein cholesterol (LDL-C) goals are reduced to <50% of baseline LDL-C. In very high-risk patients, high-intensity statins should also be initiated and the goal LDL-C should be <50% of the baseline LDL-C. If LDL-C cannot be lowered to <70 mg/dL by using statins alone, ezetimibe or proprotein convertase subtilisin/kexin type 9 (PCSK9) inhibitors may be added.[10]

CILOSTAZOL

Cilostazol is a specific cyclic adenosine monophosphate phosphodiesterase inhibitor in platelets and vascular smooth muscle cells. It inhibits platelet aggregation, causes vasodilatation, and lowers lipids. It is used for the treatment of claudication in patients with stable PAD and may improve walking distances. Cilostazol 100 mg orally twice daily is the only medication that has been shown to decrease claudication. Its mechanism of action is multifactorial. Cilostazol is contraindicated in heart failure. Although it inhibits platelet aggregation, concurrent use with aspirin does not cause additional risk of bleeding.[2]

PENTOXIFYLLINE

Although approved to treat intermittent claudication in the United States, pentoxifylline is no longer recommended to treat claudication, as it has not been effective in prolonging maximal walking distances.[2]

References

1. Aboyans V, Criqui MH, Abraham P, et al. Measurement and interpretation of the ankle-brachial index: a scientific statement from the American Heart Association. *Circulation*. 2012;126:2890–2909.

2. Gerhard-Herman MD, Gornik HL, Barrett C, et al. 2016 AHA/ACC guideline on the management of patients with lower extremity peripheral artery disease: a report of the American College of Cardiology/American Heart Association Task Force on Clinical Practice Guidelines. *J Am Coll Cardiol*. 2017;69: e71–e126.

3. Hirsch AT, Haskal ZJ, Hertzer NR, et al. ACC/AHA 2005 practice guidelines for the management of patients with peripheral arterial disease. *Circulation*. 2006;113:e463–e654.

4. Antithrombotic Trialists' Collaboration Collaborative meta-analysis of randomised trials of antiplatelet therapy for prevention of death, myocardial infarction, and stroke in high risk patients. *BMJ*. 2002;324:71–86.

5. Catalano M, Born G, Peto R. Prevention of serious vascular events by aspirin amongst patients with peripheral arterial disease: randomized, double-blind trial. *J Intern Med*. 2007;261:276–284.

6. Berger JS, Krantz MJ, Kittelson JM, et al. Aspirin for the prevention of cardiovascular events in patients with peripheral artery disease: a meta-analysis of randomized trials. *JAMA*. 2009;301:1909–1919.

7. CAPRIE Steering Committee. A randomised, blinded, trial of clopidogrel versus aspirin in patients at risk of ischaemic events (CAPRIE). *Lancet*. 1996;348:1329–1339.

8. Morrow DA, Braunwald E, Bonaca MP, et al. Vorapaxar in the secondary prevention of atherothrombotic events. *N Engl J Med*. 2012;366:1404–1413.

9. Zontivity [package insert]. Whitehouse Station, NJ: Merck & CO, Inc; 2014.

10. Grundy SM, Stone NJ, Bailey AL, et al. 2018 AHA/ACC/AACVPR/AAPA/ABC/ACPM/ADA/AGS/APhA/ASPC/NLA/PCNA guideline on the management of blood cholesterol: a report of the American College of Cardiology/American Heart Association Task Force on Clinical Practice Guidelines. *J Am Coll Cardiol*. 2019;73:e285–e350.

CHAPTER 10

Atrial Fibrillation Ablation

Amit Alam, MD   ■   Ali Seyar Rahyab, MD

Background

An atrial fibrillation (AF) ablation is an invasive procedure that is intended to treat AF. AF is the most common cardiac arrhythmia and is caused by disorganized and rapid electrical impulses in the atria of the heart. In an untreated patient, the ventricular rate also tends to be rapid and variable, between 120 and 160 beats/minute, but in some patients it may exceed 200 beats/minute. This is visualized on the 12-lead electrocardiogram (EKG) as a lack of discernable normal P waves, many small atrial waves preceding the QRS complex, and an irregularly irregular ventricular heart rate that varies due to the chaotic impulses from the atria.[1] See Chapter 26: Electrocardiography for more details about EKG.

The word "ablation" comes from the Latin word *ablatio*, which means to take away. Ablation can be used in the medical lexicon for a procedure that causes the destruction of tissue via various techniques. In the case of AF ablation, the tissue that is targeted is located in the left atrium of the heart. This tissue predisposes patients to the arrhythmia.[1]

How to Use It

An AF ablation may be considered for patients with AF in the following clinical scenarios[2,3]:
1. Symptomatic paroxysmal or persistent AF that is either refractory to treatment with an antiarrhythmic medication or the patient is intolerant of the medication due to side effects.
2. Recurrent episodes of symptomatic paroxysmal AF or symptomatic persistent AF before trying antiarrhythmic medication.
3. Symptomatic AF and heart failure with reduced ejection fraction.

An AF ablation should <u>not</u> be performed in any patient who cannot be treated with anticoagulation during and after the procedure.[2,3]

How It Is Done

An AF ablation is performed by an electrophysiologist who is a cardiologist with additional training in electrophysiology. Electrophysiology is the field of cardiology that specializes in electrical disorders of the heart, including arrhythmias. The procedure is performed in the electrophysiology laboratory in an inpatient setting. The electrophysiology laboratory is similar to an operating room or cardiac catheterization laboratory and contains specialized cardiac monitoring and treatment equipment.[4]

During the procedure, the patient is required to be motionless while lying on the table for several hours. The ablation can be painful. Therefore, conscious sedation or general anesthesia is utilized for the procedure. Patients are typically informed not to eat or drink anything starting at midnight the day of the procedure.[4]

Physically, the procedure entails[4]:

1. Right heart cardiac catheterization, which involves the introduction of catheters into the right atrium of the heart via the large veins (usually femoral vein) and passing the catheter across the interatrial septum (transatrial septal puncture) into the left atrium.[4]
2. Ablation of the regions of the left atrium that are known to initiate AF, which most commonly includes the regions of the left atrium around the pulmonary veins.[4]

An extensive area of the left atrium is usually ablated. Over time, new areas can develop that trigger AF. This can be due to de novo trigger sites in the atria or areas that were not treated during the ablation procedure.[4]

The expected outcome is that normal sinus rhythm is restored after one ablation procedure in approximately 60% of patients. For patients who undergo multiple ablation procedures, approximately 70% remain in normal sinus rhythm. Recurrence of AF in the first 3 months after the procedure is common and does not mean the procedure was not successful. Recurrence of AF after 3 months may require antiarrhythmic medication or consideration for a repeat ablation procedure.[2-4]

There is a 4.5% incidence of a major complication from the procedure which includes[2-4]:

1. Cardiac tamponade: 1.3% incidence.
2. Stroke or transient ischemic attack: 0.94% incidence.
3. Atrial-esophageal fistula: 0.04% incidence.
4. Death: 0.15% incidence.

Medication Implications

BEFORE THE PROCEDURE

- Some electrophysiologists may stop antiarrhythmic medications prior to the procedure, as they may interfere with the ability to locate foci of the arrhythmia and will typically resume the medication post procedure.
- The choice of antiarrhythmic medication depends on the presence of any underlying cardiac disease and is not influenced by whether or not the patient will be undergoing an ablation[3]:
  - For patients with no structural heart disease, the first-line agents are:
    - Flecainide, propafenone, dronedarone, sotalol, dofetilide
  - For patients with coronary artery disease, the first-line agents are:
    - Sotalol, amiodarone, dronedarone, dofetilide
  - For patients with heart failure, the first-line agents are:
    - Amiodarone, dofetilide
  - For patients with severe ventricular hypertrophy, the first-line agent is:
    - Amiodarone
  - Characteristics of the antiarrhythmics including mechanism, metabolism, adverse effects, and dosing are listed in Table 10.1.[5]
- Current guidelines recommend the continuation of oral anticoagulants for at least 3 weeks prior to the procedure, with direct oral anticoagulants (DOACs) being preferred over vitamin K antagonists for most patients. The most commonly utilized medications are[2,4]:
  - DOACs: apixaban, rivaroxaban, edoxaban, dabigatran
  - Vitamin K antagonist: warfarin
  - For patients with moderate to severe mitral stenosis or a mechanical heart valve, the recommended medication is warfarin.[2]
  - For further anticoagulant details including mechanism, clinical considerations, and dosing, see Table 10.2.[1,6]

TABLE 10.1 ■ Antiarrhythmic Medications[5]

Medication	Cardiac Channels Blocked	Metabolism	Cardiac Adverse Effects	Non-Cardiac Adverse Effects	Dosing
Flecainide	Sodium	Renal/hepatic CYP2D6	Atrial flutter, ventricular tachycardia, contraindicated with coronary artery disease	Dizziness, headache, blurred vision	50–100 mg bid, max dose 300–400 mg/day
Propafenone	Sodium, Beta	Hepatic	Atrial flutter, ventricular tachycardia, contraindicated with coronary artery disease	Metallic taste, dizziness	150–300 mg every 8 hours
Dronedarone	Potassium, Sodium, Calcium, Beta, Alpha, Acetylcholine	Renal, hepatic, gastrointestinal	Bradycardia	Anorexia, nausea, hepatotoxicity	400 mg bid
Amiodarone	Potassium, Sodium, Calcium, Beta, Alpha, Acetylcholine	Hepatic	Bradycardia	Pulmonary disease, hepatotoxicity, thyroid disease, photosensitivity, blue-gray skin discoloration, nausea, ataxia, tremor, alopecia	Oral load: 10 g over 7–10 days and then 400 mg daily for 3 weeks, maintenance: 200 mg daily
Sotalol	Potassium, Beta	Renal	Bradycardia, torsades de pointes	Bronchospasm	80–120 mg bid, max dose 240 mg bid
Dofetilide	Potassium	Renal/hepatic CYP3A4	Torsades de pointes	None	CrCl > 60: 500 mcg bid, CrCl 40–60: 250 mcg bid, CrCl 20–39: 125 mcg bid

bid, twice daily; *CrCl*, creatinine clearance (in mL/min); *CYP*, cytochrome P450.

TABLE 10.2 ■ Anticoagulant Medications[1,6]

Medication	Mechanism	Clinical Considerations	Dosing
Apixaban	Direct inhibitor of factor Xa	Preferred in moderate renal dysfunction and in patients with higher risk of bleeding.	5 mg bid If 2 of 3 criteria (serum creatinine ≥1.5 mg/dL, age ≥80 years or weight ≤60 kg), then 2.5 mg bid
Rivaroxaban	Direct inhibitor of factor Xa	Preferred in moderate renal dysfunction. Once-daily dosing.	CrCl >50: 20 mg daily with evening meal CrCl ≤50: 15 mg daily with evening meal
Edoxaban	Direct inhibitor of factor Xa	Preferred in moderate renal dysfunction and in patients with higher risk of bleeding. Once-daily dosing. Requires 5–10 days of pretreatment with parenteral anticoagulation prior to initiation if used for the treatment of venous thromboembolism.	CrCl 50–95: 60 mg daily, do not use if CrCl >95 CrCl 15–50: 30 mg daily
Dabigatran	Direct inhibitor of thrombin	Significant reduction in ischemic stroke risk compared to warfarin. Requires 5–10 days of pretreatment with parenteral anticoagulation prior to initiation if used for the treatment of venous thromboembolism.	CrCl >30: 150 mg bid CrCl 15–30: 75 mg bid
Warfarin	Vitamin K antagonist	Variable metabolism and effect, therefore blood INR levels must be monitored. Multiple dietary and drug interactions.	Dose is adjusted by individual patient to maintain INR between 2 and 3

bid, twice daily, *CrCl,* creatinine clearance (in mL/min); *INR,* international normalized ratio; *LMWH,* low-molecular-weight heparin.

DURING THE PROCEDURE

■ Heparin is used intravenously to reduce the risk of stroke.
  ■ Heparin potentiates the action of antithrombin III, inducing the inactivation of Xa and IIa (thrombin).
■ Oral anticoagulants, including DOACs and vitamin K antagonists, are continued uninterrupted during the procedure. Randomized controlled trials have demonstrated comparable major bleeding rates using uninterrupted DOACs or vitamin K antagonists for AF ablation procedures.[7,8]
■ Adenosine may be used to evaluate the effectiveness of the ablation during the procedure.
  ■ Adenosine inhibits the atrioventricular node to slow conduction and leads to a decreased heart rate.
■ Isoproterenol may be used to stimulate areas that may need to be targeted.
  ■ Isoproterenol is a beta agonist that leads to cardiac stimulation and an increased heart rate.[4]

AFTER THE PROCEDURE

■ Proton pump inhibitors (PPIs) are started post procedure to reduce the risk of esophageal complications.[4]

- There is a lack of data on the effectiveness of PPI therapy to reduce the risk of esophageal complications.[9]
  - A typical regimen is omeprazole or pantoprazole 40 mg orally twice a day for 30 days[10]
- Sucralfate or H2 antihistamine medications may also be used in conjunction with PPI therapy.[4]
- The decision to start a new antiarrhythmic medication after the procedure (in patients who are not already taking an antiarrhythmic prior) or to continue an antiarrhythmic medication is determined on a case-by-case basis, with the two most important considerations being whether a patient is maintaining normal sinus rhythm balanced with the presence of any adverse events from the medications. A patient who is unable to maintain normal sinus rhythm is more likely to continue or start the antiarrhythmic medication, and a patient who has developed adverse events from a medication will have that antiarrhythmic stopped or changed to a different agent.[4]
- The decision to continue anticoagulation 2 months post procedure is based on the patient's risk of stroke and not whether the procedure was successful or not.[4]
  - The recommended stroke risk assessment model for patients with AF (except with moderate-severe mitral stenosis or a mechanical heart valve) is the CHA_2DS_2-VASc score[1,2,4]
    - C: Congestive heart failure: 1 point
    - H: Hypertension: 1 point
    - A: Age ≥ 75: 2 points
    - D: Diabetes mellitus: 1 point
    - S: Prior stroke or transient ischemic attack: 2 points
    - V: Vascular disease (such as coronary artery disease or peripheral arterial disease): 1 point
    - A: Age 65–74: 1 point
    - Sc: Sex Female: 1 point
  - It is recommended that men with a score of ≥ 2 or women with a score of ≥ 3 continue anticoagulation even if normal sinus rhythm is achieved with the combination of ablation and/or antiarrhythmic therapy.[2]
  - For men with a score of 1 or women with a score of 2, an oral anticoagulant may be considered.[2]
  - For men with a score of 0 or women with a score of 1, it is reasonable to omit anticoagulant therapy (unless the patient has moderate-severe mitral stenosis or a mechanical heart valve).[2]
  - The use of aspirin monotherapy in patients with a score of 0–1 point has not been well established.[10]

References

1. Michaud GF, Stevenson WG. Atrial Fibrillation. In: Jameson J, Fauci AS, Kasper DL, Hauser SL, Longo DL, Loscalzo J. eds. *Harrison's Principles of Internal Medicine*. 20th ed. New York, NY: McGraw-Hill; http://accessmedicine.mhmedical.com/content.aspx?bookid=2129&sectionid=192028757. Accessed February 08, 2020.
2. January CT, Wann LS, Calkins H, et al. 2019 AHA/ACC/HRS focused update of the 2014 AHA/ACC/HRS guideline for the management of patients with atrial fibrillation: A Report of the American College of Cardiology/American Heart Association Task Force on Clinical Practice Guidelines and the Heart Rhythm Society. *Heart Rhythm*. 2019;16:e66–e93.
3. January CT, Wann LS, Alpert JS, et al. 2014 AHA/ACC/HRS guideline for the management of patients with atrial fibrillation: a report of the American College of Cardiology/American Heart Association Task Force on Practice Guidelines and the Heart Rhythm Society. *J Am Coll Cardiol*. 2014;64:e1–e76.
4. Calkins H, Hindricks G, Cappato R, et al. 2017 HRS/EHRA/ECAS/APHRS/SOLAECE expert consensus statement on catheter and surgical ablation of atrial fibrillation. *Europace*. 2018;20:e1–e160.

5. Zimetbaum P. Antiarrhythmic drug therapy for atrial fibrillation. *Circulation*. 2012;125:381–389.
6. Barnes GD, Kurtz B. Direct oral anticoagulants: unique properties and practical approaches to management. *Heart*. 2016;102:1620–1626.
7. Hohnloser SH, Camm J, Cappato R, et al. Uninterrupted edoxaban vs. vitamin K antagonists for ablation of atrial fibrillation: the ELIMINATE-AF trial. *Eur Heart J*. 2019;40:3013–3021.
8. Cappato R, Marchlinski FE, Hohnloser SH, et al. Uninterrupted rivaroxaban vs. uninterrupted vitamin K antagonists for catheter ablation in non-valvular atrial fibrillation. *Eur Heart J*. 2015;36:1805–1811.
9. Zellerhoff S, Lenze F, Eckardt L. Prophylactic proton pump inhibition after atrial fibrillation ablation: is there any evidence? *Europace*. 2011;13:1219–1221.
10. Kirchhof P, Benussi S, Kotecha D, et al. 2016 ESC Guidelines for the management of atrial fibrillation developed in collaboration with EACTS. *Eur Heart J*. 2016;37:2893–2962.

CHAPTER 11

Bariatric Surgery

Lynn Eileen Kassel, PharmD, BCPS ■ Joel Eugene Rand, PA-C, MPAS

Background

Bariatric surgery, or weight loss surgery, is any procedure intended to reduce weight in patients with morbid obesity. Bariatric, translated from Greek, literally means "weight medicine." Bariatric surgery procedures are classified as restrictive (reduced stomach size; limiting the amount a patient may comfortably eat at any given time) or malabsorptive (alterations to the small intestine length to inhibit caloric absorption). Procedures may be restrictive (e.g., adjustable gastric band [or LAP-BAND®] or vertical sleeve gastrectomy [VSG]), malabsorptive (e.g., biliopancreatic diversion/duodenal switch [BPD-DS]), or both (e.g., Roux-en-Y gastric bypass [RYGB]).

Bariatric surgery centers utilize an interdisciplinary team to evaluate patients for suitability and educate them on the lifelong changes that must be implemented to be successful following surgery; patients must comply with strict dietary and exercise recommendations.

How to Use It

It is well established that surgery is often the only definitive treatment for patients with morbid obesity and is particularly effective for those patients who are 100 or more pounds overweight with comorbidities such as obstructive sleep apnea, diabetes mellitus, hypertension, and hyperlipidemia.[1] Bariatric surgery is recommended in the American Diabetes Association guidelines for management of obesity in the treatment of type 2 diabetes mellitus (T2D).[2]

How It Is Done

All bariatric surgeries are performed under general anesthesia using laparoscopic techniques. The VSG uses a linear stapling device along an esophageal dilator to remove and discard approximately 80% of the stomach. The remaining tubular gastric conduit is just slightly wider than the esophagus. The RYGB uses a linear stapler over a sizing balloon to create a small gastric pouch, approximately the size of an egg, that is separated from the remainder of the stomach. The remnant stomach remains in place. The duodenum is bypassed by creating an end-to-side jejunojejunostomy, and a Roux limb is anastomosed to the gastric pouch. This leaves a common channel of small bowel where food mixes with digestive juices and is absorbed into the blood circulation. Following either a VSG or RYGB, a 1- or 2-night stay is expected in the hospital. Fluoroscopic imaging using water-soluble contrast, rather than barium, may be performed during the hospitalization. Fig. 11.1 illustrates the major types of bariatric surgery.

EXPECTED RESULTS

Patients with morbid obesity are afflicted with high recidivism rates following medical weight loss and diet programs. Bariatric surgery is highly effective at attaining substantial weight loss over the first 1–2 years postoperatively, but many studies have also proven that its effects are sustainable over a decade or longer. The measurement of percentage of excess body weight lost

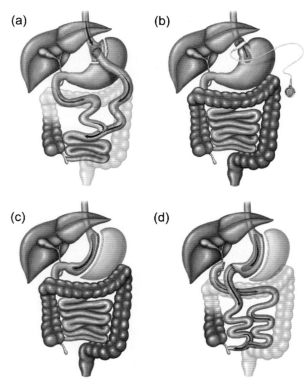

Fig. 11.1 Major types of bariatric surgery. (A) Roux-en-Y gastric bypass. (B) Adjustable gastric band. (C) Sleeve gastrectomy. (D) Biliopancreatic diversion. (Reprinted with permission from Neff KJ, Olbers T, le Roux CW. Bariatric surgery: the challenges with candidate selection, individualizing treatment and clinical outcomes. *BMC Med* 2013;11:8.)

(%EBWL) is a standard metric monitored in multiple randomized controlled trials. RYGB patients average 59% EBWL and VSG patients average 53% EBWL at 10 years. Remission of T2D may occur within days of RYGB, and in both RYGB and VSG patients, a T2D remission rate of approximately 80% is common more than 10 years postoperatively. A substantial body of evidence has shown that surgery achieves superior glycemic control compared with lifestyle or medical interventions.[3]

AVAILABLE SURGERIES

The VSG and RYGB are the most popular bariatric surgeries performed in the United States. The American Society of Metabolic and Bariatric Surgery estimates the number of procedures performed annually by using quality assurance data.[4] In 2011, 158,000 surgeries were performed (17.8% VSG and 36.7% RYGB). The total number of surgeries continues to grow, with 252,000 performed in 2018 (61.4% VSG, 17.8% RYGB, 15.4% revision). The use of adjustable gastric bands continues to decrease, which has consistently been less than 5% since 2016, and the BPD-DS has been less than 1% since 2014. Some of the undesirable features of adjustable gastric bands are that patients may require surgery for removal in the event of band slip, dysphagia with or without distal esophageal dilation, or esophageal motility disorders.

Medication Implications

PREOPERATIVE

- Patients are often required to follow a liquid diet for approximately 2 weeks to shrink the liver for better intraoperative exposure.[5] This may result in patients being dehydrated the day of surgery.
- Prophylaxis for venous thromboembolism (VTE) is recommended for all patients and typically consists of unfractionated heparin (UFH) or low-molecular-weight heparin (LMWH).[6] Individual bariatric centers create specific protocols based on provider preferences and surgical training.

SMOKING CESSATION

- Patients should refrain from use of tobacco. Cessation of smoking is encouraged at least 6 weeks prior to surgery; however, some insurance companies may require cessation before that point.[5] Cessation is important due to tobacco's deleterious effects on wound healing, anastomotic ulcer development, and overall poor health.[5]

MULTIDISCIPLINARY CARE

- The Metabolic and Bariatric Surgery Accreditation and Quality Improvement Program (MBSAQIP) is the accrediting body for bariatric surgery centers. Each level of accredited centers performs within a certain facility volume, patient age range, and with specific required standards.
- A multidisciplinary care team is essential to the care of patients receiving bariatric surgery, and this multidisciplinary team works with the program director to guide therapy and monitoring of patients within the center.[7]
- In addition to surgical teams, these may consist of mental health professionals, exercise physiologists, dietitians, bariatricians, internists, pharmacists, and nurses.

ENHANCED RECOVERY AFTER SURGERY (ERAS)

- Many bariatric surgery programs have implemented Enhanced Recovery After Surgery (ERAS) protocols that include oral intake of a high-carbohydrate liquid the night before surgery and 2–4 hours prior to surgery. Antiemetics and multimodal pain medication regimens, including acetaminophen, gabapentin, celecoxib, scopolamine, and aprepitant, among other agents, are used to limit postoperative nausea and vomiting (PONV) and narcotic usage.[8-10]
- Use of ERAS has also been associated with decreased length of stay, with no difference in adverse effects.

POSTOPERATIVE

Patients' medication regimens may change drastically or very minimally

- Medications for mental illness, seizures, thyroid conditions, and others where abrupt withdrawal will cause issues (e.g., beta blockers) are continued immediately postoperatively.
- Medications that impact blood glucose, such as insulin or sulfonylureas, may be held with appropriate monitoring. Short-acting insulin is used commonly in the immediate postoperative period to control blood glucose, though at discharge from the surgical encounter, insulin may only be necessary for patients with insulin-dependent diabetes mellitus.
- Some blood pressure agents (i.e., diuretics, angiotensin-converting enzyme inhibitors) are typically withheld to avoid dehydration or acute kidney injury immediately following surgery.

NECESSARY MEDICATIONS

- Patients are at increased risk of VTE following surgery and should receive VTE chemo-prophylaxis for a short period of time following surgery in addition to early ambulation and sequential compression devices.[5] Risk calculators, such as one from the Cleveland Clinic, are available to assess the risk of VTE using patient-specific factors.[11] As with preoperative VTE prophylaxis, dosing strategy following surgery is not universally recognized; provider discretion in collaboration with the patient's primary care provider is common practice.
- Patients require acid-suppression therapy, such as proton pump inhibitors, for at least 3 months following surgery to protect the anastomoses and staple line.[5] Continuation of these after the 3-month period is dependent upon patient-specific factors, such as reflux.
- Use of vitamins is critical to obtaining adequate vitamin and mineral levels following surgery. Vitamin and mineral levels should be monitored every 3, 6, or 12 months to ensure adequate nutrition and vitamin supplementation.[5]

MEDICATIONS TO AVOID

- Some medications may increase the risk of complications in the postoperative period.
- As examples, use of medications that decrease blood glucose levels should be avoided or have the dose reduced to avoid hypoglycemia; estrogen-containing medications may increase the risk of VTE and should be avoided, particularly in patients who have additional risk factors.[5]
- Nonsteroidal anti-inflammatory drugs (NSAIDs) should be completely avoided after bariatric surgery, if possible, because they have been implicated in the development of anastomotic ulcerations/perforations.[5] Use of alternative medication classes, such as corticosteroids, may be substituted for NSAIDs if future diagnoses require, such as pericarditis or arthritis.[12]

VITAMIN DEFICIENCIES

- Vitamin deficiencies occur in bariatric surgery patients due to inherently low-caloric intake, alterations in gastric acid production and gastrointestinal (GI) transit time, bypassed portions of small bowel, and small intestinal bacterial overgrowth.[13]
- The most commonly deficient nutrients are fat-soluble vitamins or those normally absorbed by the bypassed duodenum. Patients must take supplemental folate, iron, calcium, in addition to vitamins B1 (thiamine), B12 (cyanocobalamin), A, and D.
- There are commercially available over-the-counter preparations in doses appropriate for bariatric patients, or usual over-the-counter sources may be used in amounts greater than standard recommendations. For example, RYGB patients require a multivitamin with 200% of the recommended daily dose of nutrients.[14]

DOSAGE AND/OR DOSAGE FORM ISSUES

- Special attention to dosage forms is required following bariatric surgery. Alterations in gastric pH, time spent within the stomach, and specific location of absorption from the GI tract are critical elements that may alter how much of an oral medication is absorbed.
- Surgeries that alter the length of the GI tract, such as RYGB, are likely to have a bigger impact upon the dosage forms used to deliver medication compared with restrictive procedures.
- Patients requiring oral contrast following bariatric surgery require a lower volume with imaging performed more quickly than in nonbariatric surgery patients.

Examples

- Oral birth control pills with estrogens require activation, via glucuronidation, through portal vein uptake before being returned to the GI tract via the bile duct. Nonoral forms, such as patches or intravaginal rings, may provide more consistent effects for patients following RYGB. Patches may not be as effective at weights greater than 90 kg, indicating that selection of an appropriate dosage form requires patient-specific considerations.[15]

- Extended-release (ER) or controlled-release (CD) diltiazem may not provide adequate rate, rhythm, or blood pressure coverage for patients following bariatric surgery due to the release point in the GI tract. Changes to GI tract length, such as with RYGB, may decrease absorption of ER diltiazem products, whereas an immediate-release (IR) product may provide optimal coverage, although it must be taken multiple times per day.

- ER venlafaxine is available as a capsule that may be opened up and sprinkled onto a soft food, which is then swallowed whole, to increase the likelihood of absorption of the full dosage. Venlafaxine is also available as an IR tablet, but this must be taken multiple times per day to exert an effect similar to that of the ER tablet.

- Opioids are available in multiple formulations; however, changing to a liquid may allow for a dose reduction and better pain control for a patient. The change to a liquid allows the medication to be more readily available for absorption, thus providing better pain relief. Caution should be used when changing opioids to a liquid formulation, as an unquantifiable increase in absorption has the risk of unexpected respiratory suppression; dose reductions should occur when changing formulations.

References

1. Sjostrom L, Narbro K, Sjostrom CD, et al. Effects of bariatric surgery on mortality in Swedish obese subjects. *N Engl J Med.* 2007;357:741–752.
2. American Diabetes Association 8. Obesity management for the treatment of type 2 diabetes: Standards of Medical Care in Diabetes – 2020. *Diabetes Care.* 2020;43(Suppl 1):S89–S97.
3. Azagury D, Papasavas P, Hamdallah I, et al. ASMBS Position Statement on medium- and long-term durability of weight loss and diabetic outcomes after conventional stapled bariatric procedures. *Surg Obes Relat Dis.* 2018;14:1425–1441.
4. American Society of Metabolic and Bariatric Surgery (ASMBS). Estimate of Bariatric Surgery Numbers, 2011-2018. https://asmbs.org/resources/estimate-of-bariatric-surgery-numbers. Accessed on Feb 4, 2020.
5. Mechanick JI, Youdim A, Jones DB, et al. Clinical practice guidelines for the perioperative nutritional, metabolic, and nonsurgical support of the bariatric surgery patient –2013 update: cosponsored by American Association of Clinical Endocrinologists, The Obesity Society, and American Society for Metabolic and Bariatric Surgery. *Surg Obes Relat Dis.* 2013;9:159–191.
6. Bariatric Surgery Clinical Issues Committee. ASMBS updated position statement on prophylactic measures to reduce the risk of venous thromboembolism in bariatric surgery patients. *Surg Obes Relat Dis.* 2013;9:493–497.
7. Saber AA, Bashah MM, Zarabi S. Chapter 63. Metabolic and Bariatric Surgery Accreditation and Quality Improvement Program (MBSAQIP) by American Society of Metabolic and Bariatric Surgery (ASMBS) and American College of Surgery (ACS). In: Agrawal S, ed. *Obesity, Bariatric and Metabolic Surgery: A Practical Guide*; 2016. doi:10.1007/978-3-319-04343-2_63.
8. Malczak P, Pisarska M, Piotr M, et al. Enhanced recovery after bariatric surgery: systematic review and meta-analysis. *Obes Surg.* 2017;27:226–235.
9. Lam J, Suzuki T, Bernstein D, et al. An ERAS protocol for bariatric surgery: is it safe to discharge on post-operative day 1? *Surg Endosc.* 2019;33:580–586.
10. Ahmed OS, Rogers AC, Bolger JC, et al. Meta-analysis of enhanced recovery protocols in bariatric surgery. *J Gastrointest Surg.* 2018;22:964–972.
11. The Cleveland Clinic Foundation. Bariatric Surgery Calculator. Cleveland Clinic Innovations app. *Copyright Cleveland Clinic.* 2017. https://apps.apple.com/us/app/bariatric-surgery-calculator /id1296342971?ign-mpt=uo%3D4.

12. Kassel LE, Hutton A, Zumach G, et al. Systematic review of perioperative use of immunosuppressive agents in patients undergoing bariatric surgery. *Surg Obes Relat Dis*. 2019:1–14.

13. Carpenter M, Pisano M, Bland C. Implications of bariatric surgery on absorption of nutrients and medications. *US Pharm*. 2016;41:HS2–HS8.

14. Stein J, Steir C, Raab H, et al. Review article: The Nutritional and Pharmacological Consequences of Obesity Surgery. *Aliment Pharmacol Ther*. 2014;40:582–609.

15. Ortho-Evra® (Norelgestromin/Ethinyl Estradiol Transdermal system) prescribing information. Available at https://www.accessdata.fda.gov/drugsatfda_docs/label/2008/021180s026lbl.pdf. Accessed on March 11, 2020.

CHAPTER 12

Bladder Scan

Devora Lichtman, MD ▪ Gregory J. Hughes, PharmD, BCPS, BCGP

Background

A bladder scan is a portable noninvasive ultrasound device that measures the volume of urine in the bladder by using ultrasound waves measured in three dimensions. The machine calculates a volume measurement of urine in the bladder without displaying an image on the screen. Bladder scans are used mostly during inpatient encounters to evaluate patients for urinary retention. Acute urinary retention (AUR) is defined as the inability to voluntarily pass urine, can cause severe pain, and is considered a medical emergency.[1] Without prompt diagnosis and treatment, AUR can result in permanent damage to the kidneys and genitourinary system. AUR is more common in men than in women and is usually due to underlying benign prostatic hypertrophy (BPH). In women, urinary retention is usually due to pelvic organ prolapse or masses in the pelvis.[2] The diagnosis of urinary retention is suspected when greater than 200 mL of urine is retained in the urinary bladder after the patient voluntarily voids. When the volume of urine in the bladder is greater than 100 mL, the bladder scan is 90% accurate compared with urinary bladder catheterization.[3]

How to Use It

A bladder scan displays approximately how much urine is in the bladder at a given time. When the urine volume is measured after a patient voluntarily voids, it is called a postvoid residual (PVR), which is a marker for urinary retention. In addition to being used to diagnose urinary retention, it can be used to monitor urine volumes after an indwelling urethral catheter (i.e., Foley catheter) is removed for several hours to evaluate if the patient needs the catheter to be reinserted. It is also used in patients with decreased urine output to evaluate if the etiology is due to bladder outlet obstruction. Bladder scan has helped to minimize unnecessary catheterization and associated urinary tract infections. See Chapter 59: Urinary Catheters for more details about types and risks of catheters. See Chapter 23: Cultures – Urine for details about urinary tract infections. Bladder scans can be falsely elevated in patients with obesity, abdominal ascites, and anasarca; therefore, bladder volume in these patients may need to be confirmed with an ultrasound image of the urinary bladder.[4]

How It Is Done

A handheld ultrasound device is used to measure the volume of urine remaining in the urinary bladder approximately 10 minutes after the patient voids. The machine scans the bladder in three dimensions and calculates a volume. The patient is positioned in the supine position. A small amount of ultrasound gel is applied to the ultrasound probe, and the probe scanner head is placed on the abdomen in the suprapubic area. No discomfort is usually experienced, and no sedation or anesthesia is required. The scan is initiated by pushing the button on the handle of the probe and the volume will be displayed on the screen in under a minute. Many facilities practice measuring the volume two to three times and then average the measurements to increase accuracy. There is no specific preparation needed prior to performing the exam in terms of diet or activity.[5] A normal bladder scan PVR in a patient without urinary retention should be 50 mL or less.

Medication Implications

- The bladder scan is noninvasive and there are no medications that need to be given prior or during the test.
- There are no medications that need to be held prior to exam.
- If the bladder scan reveals urinary retention, an indwelling urethral (i.e., Foley) catheter will likely need to be placed. Once the obstruction is alleviated with a catheter, the patient's medications should be reviewed, as many medications can cause urinary retention.
- The most common medications that cause urinary retention are anticholinergic medications and sympathomimetics (medications that stimulate the sympathetic nervous system).[6] Anticholinergic medications cause urinary retention by reducing the contractility of the detrusor muscle, which is the main muscle in the wall of the bladder that causes voiding. It should be noted that many of these are available as over-the-counter (OTC) medications, so a thorough medication history that includes OTC medications should be performed.
- Anticholinergic medications and opioids cause urinary retention by decreasing bladder sensation.[1]
- Categories of offending medications and some examples (not all inclusive) include:
  - Sympathomimetics (alpha adrenergic agents)—ephedrine, phenylephrine, pseudoephedrine
  - Tricyclic antidepressants—imipramine, nortriptyline, amitriptyline, doxepin
  - Antiarrhythmics (class 1a)—quinidine, procainamide, disopyramide
  - Anticholinergics—atropine, scopolamine, glycopyrrolate, oxybutynin, hyoscyamine, dicyclomine
  - Antiparkinsonian agents—trihexyphenidyl, benztropine, amantadine, levodopa, bromocriptine mesylate
  - Hormonal agents—progesterone, estrogen, testosterone
  - Antipsychotics—haloperidol, thiothixene, chlorpromazine, fluphenazine, prochlorperazine
  - Antihistamines—diphenhydramine, cyproheptadine, hydroxyzine, dimenhydrinate
  - Antihypertensive—hydralazine, nifedipine
  - Muscle relaxants—diazepam, baclofen, cyclobenzaprine[7]
- Urinary retention in men is most commonly caused by BPH and can result in significant symptoms (known as lower urinary tract symptoms [LUTS]), AUR, impairments to quality of life, and the need for surgical intervention. For decades, the pharmacologic management of LUTS included alpha-1 adrenergic antagonists and 5-alpha-reductase inhibitors but now also includes muscarinic receptor antagonists (anticholinergic) and phosphodiesterase-5 inhibitors. A systematic review and meta-analysis revealed that alpha-1 adrenergic antagonists, 5-alpha-reductase inhibitors, and phosphodiesterase-5 inhibitors all improve LUTS scores. Effects on maximum urinary flow, obstructive symptoms, and irritative symptoms were more varied among classes and combinations.[8]
  - Alpha-1 adrenergic antagonists work by relaxing prostatic smooth muscle and improve symptoms by 3 months of daily use. Examples include tamsulosin, doxazosin, and terazosin[9]
  - 5-alpha-reductase inhibitors work by inhibiting the production of dihydrotestosterone (which causes prostate growth) and can take 6 months to years to demonstrate benefit on LUTS scores or AUR rates. Examples include finasteride and dutasteride[9]

- Muscarinic receptor antagonists (anticholinergics) improve storage-related symptoms in BPH (e.g., frequency, urgency) but have the concern of increasing the PVR or AUR rate based directly on their anticholinergic mechanism. Because of this concern, muscarinic receptor antagonists should be avoided in patients with a significantly elevated PVR, though the specific threshold varies by agent and study. Also, during treatment with these agents, it is reasonable to perform a bladder scan to monitor the medication's effect on the PVR and assess risk for AUR. Examples include oxybutynin, tolterodine, and solifenacin[10]
- Phosphodiesterase-5 inhibitors are the newest treatment options for BPH, as they were originally used to treat erectile dysfunction. They work by regulating smooth muscle in the prostate. Examples include sildenafil, tadalafil, vardenafil, and avanafil[8]

References

1. Marshall JR, Haber J, Josephson EB. An evidence-based approach to emergency department management of acute urinary retention. *Emerg Med Pract*. 2014;16:1–21.
2. Ramsey S, Palmer M. The management of female urinary retention. *Int Urol Nephrol*. 2006;38:533–535.
3. Thanagumtorn K. Accuracy of post-void residual urine volume measurement using an ultrasound bladder scanner among postoperative radical hysterectomy patients. *J Med Assoc Thai*. 2016;99:1061–1066.
4. Janardanan S, Moussa AEM, James P. False positive bladder scan in ascites with anuria. *Clin Case Rep*. 2019;7:1549–1550.
5. Bladderscan BVI 9400 operations & maintenance manual, April 2, 2019.
6. Verhamme KM, Sturkenboom MC, Stricker BH, et al. Drug-induced urinary retention: incidence, management and prevention. *Drug Saf*. 2008;31:373–388.
7. Billet M, Windsor TA. Urinary Retention. *Emerg Med Clin North Am*. 2019;37:649–660.
8. Wang X, Wang X, Li S, et al. Comparative effectiveness of oral drug therapies for lower urinary tract symptoms due to benign prostatic hyperplasia: a systematic review and meta-analysis. *PLoS ONE*. 2014;9:e107593.
9. Emberton M, Cornel EB, Bassi PF, et al. Benign prostatic hyperplasia as a progressive disease: A guide to the risk factors and options for medical management. *Int J Clin Pract*. 2008;62:1076–1086.
10. Li J, Shi Q, Bai Y, et al. Efficacy and safety of muscarinic antagonists as add-on therapy for male lower urinary tract symptoms. *Sci Rep*. 2014;4:3948.

CHAPTER 13

Bronchoscopy

Julie A. Murphy, PharmD ▪ Fadi Safi, MD

Background

Bronchoscopy is an endoscopic technique used to visualize the tracheobronchial tree for diagnostic and therapeutic purposes. The word "bronchoscopy" is derived from Greek words by combining the prefix "broncho" meaning "bronchus" and the verb "skopía" meaning "to view." Rigid bronchoscopy, which was first used in the 1920s, is less commonly used now, as it uses a more rigid piece of equipment that can only access the proximal airway. Flexible bronchoscopy is also known as standard white light bronchoscopy. Bronchoscopy is sometimes referred to as a "bronch."[1]

How to Use It

Bronchoscopy is used to examine a patient's airways and obtain samples of bronchoalveolar fluid or lung tissue using a cytology brush or transbronchial needle aspiration (TNA) from the upper and lower respiratory tract. Theses samples can diagnose respiratory tract infections, lung cancer or other cancer types that metastasize to the lungs, and diffuse parenchymal lung diseases. Diffuse parenchymal lung diseases can be idiopathic, secondary to occupational exposures, as part of a generalized autoimmune disease such as connective tissues diseases, or caused by medications. Examples of causative medications include chemotherapy agents (bleomycin, gemcitabine, epidermal growth factor receptor [EGFR]-targeted agents, mechanistic target of rapamycin protein [MTOR] inhibitors, immune checkpoint inhibitors), rheumatological therapies (methotrexate, leflunomide, biologic disease-modifying antirheumatic drugs), antibiotics (nitrofurantoin and daptomycin), and amiodarone. Bronchoscopy is used to remove foreign bodies or mucus plugs from the airways, evaluate and manage hemoptysis and airway bleeding, destroy large central airway tumors, apply tracheal stents, or facilitate endotracheal intubations and percutaneous tracheostomy procedures. Post lung transplant, bronchoscopy may help determine rejection and its severity and rule out opportunistic infection. Endobronchial ultrasound (EBUS) uses ultrasound waves along with bronchoscopy to examine and sample mediastinal lymph nodes and surrounding structures. It is used to diagnose conditions affecting lymph nodes such as sarcoidosis, lymphoma, or malignancy. It assists in the staging of lung cancer.[1–5]

How It Is Done

Pulmonologists, intensivists, anesthesiologists, and surgeons can perform bedside emergent bronchoscopy under conscious sedation or general anesthesia. Bedside procedures are performed in the emergency room, intensive care unit, or step-down unit, usually to obtain lower airway specimens, facilitate intubation, or remove foreign body or mucus plugs. A physician, a nurse, and a respiratory therapist are usually present. Specialized bronchoscopies with adjunct procedures such as TNA, lung biopsies, and EBUS are performed by pulmonologists in designated endoscopy areas or operating rooms. These procedures require the presence of well-trained staff and are performed under conscious sedation or general anesthesia. In nonemergent situations, patients should withhold food and liquids for the appropriate amount of time prior to the procedure to reduce the risk of aspiration. See

Chapter 6: Introduction to Anesthesia for details about withholding food and liquid. The test entails using a bronchoscope, video monitor, light source, and image processor. The bronchoscope consists of the control handle, a flexible shaft, and camera. The flexible shaft has the working channel in it. The cytology brush, biopsy forceps, and needles are usually inserted through the working channel. After sedating the patient using general anesthesia for rigid bronchoscopy or conscious sedation (benzodiazepines [e.g., midazolam] and analgesics [e.g., fentanyl]) for flexible bronchoscopy, the physician passes the scope through the nasal cavity or mouth, into the larynx, vocal cords, trachea, and right and left bronchial segments. Occasionally, bronchoscopy is performed under monitored anesthesia care in the presence of an anesthesiologist, so if necessary, the bronchoscopy may be converted to using general anesthesia with propofol without intubation. To anesthetize the airways and minimize cough, 1% lidocaine solution is used. A normal test shows a normal airway. Abnormal exams include findings such as excessive or discolored airway secretions, distorted anatomy of the bronchial tree, bronchial hemorrhage, foreign body, tracheomalacia, mucosal lesions, endobronchial lesions, or extrinsic compression. Procedure-related mortality is extremely rare (0.01%), and reported complication rates are 0.08%–6.8%. Most complications occur during or in the first few hours following the procedure. They are mostly related to sedation (transient hypotension or hypoxemia) or due to associated procedures such as TNA or transbronchial biopsies (bleeding and pneumothorax). Bleeding rate after a transbronchial lung biopsy is approximately 2.8%. Most bleeding is usually mild and resolves spontaneously. In those with continued bleeding, epinephrine can be sprayed onto the bleeding lesion to induce vasoconstriction. The pneumothorax rate following transbronchial biopsy is 2%–4%. Many cases are managed conservatively, while the remainder require chest tube placement. Minor complications include sore throat and minor hemoptysis in the first 1–2 days following the procedure. Other rare complications include bronchospasm, epistaxis, cardiac arrhythmias, laryngeal injury, and methemoglobinemia from excessive lidocaine use.[6-9]

Medication Implications

- Balancing bleeding and thrombosis risk[10-13]:
  - To minimize bleeding, correct platelet count <50,000/mm^3, international normalized ratio (INR) >1.5, or activated partial thromboplastin time (aPTT) >50 seconds prior to bronchoscopy if there is a possibility of biopsy.
  - Aspirin is safe and does not increase bleeding during bronchoscopy. It may be continued.
  - In addition to bleeding risk related to specific bronchoscopic procedures, risk of thrombotic events as defined by the American College of Chest Physicians (ACCP) must be considered. Patients are considered low risk (using antiplatelet therapy for primary prevention of myocardial infarction or stroke) or high risk (placement of coronary stent within previous 3–6 months or myocardial infarction within previous 3 months). ACCP further states that patients receiving dual antiplatelet therapy for coronary stents defer procedures like bronchoscopy for at least 6 weeks (bare metal stent [BMS]) and 6 months (drug-eluting stent [DES]).
    - For low-risk patients, P2Y$_{12}$ inhibitors (e.g., clopidogrel, ticlopidine, ticagrelor, prasugrel) should be stopped 7 days before the procedure. If not on aspirin, aspirin therapy can be considered while the P2Y$_{12}$ inhibitor is held. Resume P2Y$_{12}$ inhibitors 24 hours after the procedure.
    - For high-risk patients, consult cardiology. P2Y$_{12}$ inhibitors may be stopped if >6 weeks since BMS or >6 months since DES. The risks and benefits of the bronchoscopy should be considered for individual patients. Aspirin should be continued. Intravenous bridging using reversible glycoprotein inhibitors (e.g., eptifibatide or tirofiban) may be considered. Cangrelor, an intravenous P2Y$_{12}$ inhibitor, may also be used. Clopidogrel may be resumed 24 hours after the procedure. Ticagrelor and prasugrel have a rapid

onset of action, so caution should be used when resuming these agents. See Chapter 20: Coronary Artery Bypass Grafting for more details about $P2Y_{12}$ inhibitors.

■ In addition to bleeding risk related to specific bronchoscopic procedures, risk of thromboembolism must be considered. According to ACCP, annual thromboembolism risk determines overall risk (high [>10%], moderate [5%–10%], or low [<5%]).

■ For low- to moderate-risk patients, stop warfarin 5 days before bronchoscopy and check the INR the morning of bronchoscopy. If the INR is not <1.5, the bronchoscopy will be delayed if the indication were to obtain tissue biopsies. Warfarin may be restarted 12–24 hours after bronchoscopy. Evaluate INR in 1 week.

■ For moderate- to high-risk patients, stop warfarin 5 days before bronchoscopy and bridge with therapeutic doses of low-molecular-weight heparin (LMWH) or unfractionated heparin (UH) when the INR falls below the lower limit of therapeutic goal. Stop LMWH 24 hours prior to and UH 6 hours prior to procedure. Warfarin may be restarted 12–24 hours after bronchoscopy. Resume therapeutic doses of LMWH or UH 48–72 hours after the bronchoscopy if no bleeding has occurred. This may be resumed earlier if only bronchial alveolar lavage, EBUS, or TNA are performed. Bridging therapy can be stopped 5 days after resuming warfarin and when the INR is above the lower limit of the therapeutic range.

■ For patients taking a direct oral anticoagulant (DOAC), regardless of risk, stop DOAC 1–5 days before bronchoscopy depending on the agent used and the patient's creatinine clearance in mL/minute, as detailed in Table 13.1. Of note, these are general dosing recommendations for invasive procedures, not specific to bronchoscopy.

■ DOAC therapy can be resumed 48–72 hours after bronchoscopy. These agents may be resumed earlier if only bronchial alveolar lavage, EBUS, or TNA are performed.

TABLE 13.1 ■ Recommended intervals for stopping DOACs prior to invasive procedures

DOAC	Creatinine clearance (mL/minute)	Days to hold prior to procedure
Dabigatran*	<30	2–4
	30–50	≥2
	>50	1
Rivaroxaban*	15–29	4
	30–59	3
	60–90	2
	>90	≥1
Apixaban	<50	5
	50–59	3
	>60	1–2
Edoxaban	15–49	2–3
	50–80	1–2
	>80	1

*May be withheld longer before high-risk bleeding procedures

- For blood glucose control in patients with type 1 diabetes[14]
  - Continue basal rate insulin replacement (typically around 0.2–0.3 units/kg/day of a long-acting insulin)
- For blood glucose control in patients with type 2 diabetes[15,16]:
  - Metformin: avoid evening before and morning of bronchoscopy
  - Sulfonylureas, glinides, alpha-glucosidase inhibitors, dipeptidyl peptidase-4 (DPP-4) inhibitors, sodium-glucose cotransporter-2 (SGLT2) inhibitors: avoid morning of bronchoscopy
  - Thiazolidinediones: avoid several days before bronchoscopy
  - Glucagon-like peptide-1 (GLP-1) analogues: avoid injection morning of bronchoscopy
  - Long-acting insulin: stop or reduce (give 25% less) dose
  - Combination or premixed insulin: deliver 40%–50% of patient's usual total daily dose as long-acting insulin
  - While patient is taking nothing by mouth (NPO), fingerstick glucose monitoring may be done every 4–6 hours with short-acting (e.g., insulin aspart, insulin lispro) supplemental insulin used to correct hyperglycemia.
  - See Chapter 5: Glycemic Considerations for Tests and Procedures for more details about glycemic management.
- For blood pressure control[17]:
  - Angiotensin-converting enzyme inhibitors (ACEIs), angiotensin II receptor blockers (ARBs), and renin inhibitors: hold day of bronchoscopy due to risk of hypotension
  - Diuretics: hold day of bronchoscopy due to risk of hypokalemia and hypovolemia
  - Other antihypertensives may be taken at least 2 hours before bronchoscopy with a sip of water
- If bronchoscopy reveals infection (bacterial, fungal, or parasitic), treat according to current standards and considering patient-specific factors.
- If bronchoscopy reveals cancer (primary or metastatic), treat according to current standards and considering patient-specific factors and goals.
- If bronchoscopy reveals interstitial lung disease that is most likely due to a medication, avoid additional medication exposure and initiate systemic glucocorticoids.[18]
- If bronchoscopy reveals sarcoidosis, approximately one-third of patients will need treatment with glucocorticoids. Other cytotoxic agents like methotrexate, azathioprine, mycophenolate, or leflunomide may be necessary. If no response to these therapies, anti-tumor necrosis factor (TNF) therapy (e.g., infliximab or adalimumab) may be indicated.[19]

References

1. Paradis TJ, Dixon J, Tieu BH. The role of bronchoscopy in the diagnosis of airway disease. *J Thorac Dis.* 2016;8:3826–3837.
2. Feinsilver SH, Fein AM, Niederman MS, et al. Utility of fiberoptic bronchoscopy in nonresolving pneumonia. *Chest.* 1990;98:1322–1326.
3. Tan BB, Flaherty KR, Kazerooni EA, et al. The solitary pulmonary nodule. *Chest.* 2003;123:89S–96S.
4. Faro A, Visner G. The use of multiple transbronchial biopsies as the standard approach to evaluate lung allograft rejection. *Pediatr Transplant.* 2004;8:322–328.
5. Skeoch A, Weatherley N, Swift AJ, et al. *J Clin Med.* 2018;7:pii:E356.
6. Bolliger CT, Mathur PN, Beamis JF, et al. ERS/ATS statement on interventional pulmonology. European Respiratory Society/American Thoracic Society. *Eur Respir J.* 2002;19:356–373.
7. Facciolongo N, Patelli M, Gasparini S, et al. Incidence of complications in bronchoscopy. Multicentre prospective study of 20,986 bronchoscopies. *Monaldi Arch Chest Dis.* 2009;71:8–14.
8. Smith RS, Whisler DL, Safi F, et al. Dark chocolate arterial blood gas after bronchoscopy. *Am J Med Sci.* 2013;345:154.
9. Brady M, Kinn S, Stuart P. Preoperative fasting for adults to prevent perioperative complications. *Cochrane Database Syst Rev.* 2003:CD004423.
10. Herth FJ, Becker HD, Ernst A. Aspirin does not increase bleeding complications after transbronchial biopsy. *Chest.* 2002;122:1461–1464.

11. Youness HA, Keddissi J, Berim I, et al. Management of oral antiplatelet agents and anticoagulation therapy before bronchoscopy. *J Thorac Dis.* 2017;9:S1022–S1033.
12. Douketis JD, Spyropoulos AC, Spencer FA, et al. Perioperative management of antithrombotic therapy: Antithrombotic therapy and prevention of thrombosis, 9th ed: American College of Chest Physicians evidence-based clinical practice guidelines. *Chest.* 2012;141:e326S–e350S.
13. Baron TH, Kamath PS, McBane RD. Management of antithrombotic therapy in patients undergoing invasive procedures. *N Engl J Med.* 2013;368:2113–2124.
14. Meneghini LF. Perioperative management of diabetes: transitioning evidence into practice. *Cleve Clin J Med.* 2009;76:S53–S59.
15. Sudhakaran S, Surani SR. Guidelines for perioperative management of the diabetic patient. *Surg Res Pract.* 2015 2015:article ID 284063.
16. Cosson E, Catargi B, Cheisson G, et al. Practical management of diabetes patients before, during and after surgery: a joint French diabetology and anaesthesiology position statement. *Diabetes Metab.* 2018;44:200–216.
17. ACC/AHA Task Force on Practice Guidelines. Guideline on perioperative cardiovascular evaluation and management of patients undergoing noncardiac surgery. *JACC.* 2014;64:e77–e137.
18. Schwaiblmair M, Behr W, Haeckel T, et al. Drug induced interstitial lung disease. *Open Respir Med J.* 2012;6:63–74.
19. Ungprasert P, Ryu JH, Matteson EL. Clinical manifestations, diagnosis, and treatment of sarcoidosis. *Mayo Clin Innov Qual Outcomes.* 2019;3:358–375.

CHAPTER 14

Carotid Endarterectomy

Hira Shafeeq, PharmD

Background

Carotid endarterectomy (CEA) is a surgical procedure that involves the removal of plaque from the carotid arteries. Carotid arteries are the two major arteries located in the neck, which branch off from the aorta and supply blood to the brain. Plaque formation in the carotid arteries can result in stroke or transient ischemic attack (TIA). This extracranial atherosclerosis, or blockage in the arteries that supply blood to the brain, accounts for 15%–20% of all ischemic strokes. All patients presenting to the hospital with ischemic stroke or TIA should be worked up for carotid artery disease. Patients with carotid artery stenosis of ≥70% can be considered for CEA for prevention of future stroke.[1]

How to Use It

All patients admitted to the hospital for ischemic stroke or TIA workup should be screened for carotid artery stenosis via carotid duplex ultrasonography, a noninvasive and sensitive method for detecting the disease. Patients with carotid artery blockage of ≥70% can benefit from CEA for prevention of future strokes, especially patients presenting with TIA. Prior to CEA, carotid artery stenosis should be correlated by at least one additional imaging resource such as magnetic resonance angiography (MRA) or computed tomography (CT) angiography.[1] Asymptomatic patients can be screened for carotid artery stenosis by auscultating the carotid arteries. Presence of carotid bruits during physical examination should prompt further workup for carotid artery disease.

How It Is Done

CEA is usually performed by a vascular surgeon. The procedure can be performed under local or general anesthesia, although most physicians prefer performing the procedure under general anesthesia. Recommendations for fasting when using general anesthesia can be found in Chapter 6: Introduction to Anesthesia. The incision is made on the side of the neck along the blocked carotid artery. The surgeon makes an incision from behind the ear to above the collarbone. The blood supply to the carotid artery is clamped and a shunt is placed to enable cerebral blood circulation during the procedure. The carotid artery is incised, and the plaque is cut and removed from within the artery. There is a variation of surgical techniques that can be used to close the carotid artery incision. Many surgeons choose to close the artery using a patch to increase the diameter of the artery. This has implications for improving carotid artery blood flow for the affected artery, reducing residual or recurrent stenosis. Patch closure, however, also carries an increased risk of thrombosis due to additional time required to suture the patch. A specific surgical approach has not been proven to be beneficial. The preferred method depends on surgeon preference.[1,2] After the procedure, the patient may be transferred to an intensive care unit (ICU) or an inpatient service. Close neurologic monitoring may be required during the first 24 hours post-procedure. Most patients can be discharged 1–2 days after the procedure.

Medication Implications

BEFORE THE PROCEDURE

- Perioperative medical optimization of the patient includes the following:
  - Antithrombotic therapy: all patients should be initiated on aspirin 81–325 mg daily and continued before and after the surgical procedure. Patients allergic to aspirin can be initiated on clopidogrel 75 mg daily. The decision to discontinue clopidogrel prior to CEA should be made on a case-by-case basis[1,3]
  - Blood pressure goal is ≤140/80 mmHg
  - Beta blockade heart rate goal is 60–80 beats/minute
  - Statin therapy: patients should be initiated on a statin for plaque stabilization prior to the procedure. There is no optimal dose or agent recommended for initiation prior to CEA at this time. Intensive lipid-lowering therapy with a high-potency statin (e.g., atorvastatin 80 mg orally daily) may be recommended for most patients post-stroke or TIA for secondary prevention of stroke[1,4,5]
- CEA is often an elective procedure; therefore, oral anticoagulation should be discontinued prior to the procedure. For patients receiving warfarin, target international normalized ratio (INR) prior to surgery has not been defined and may be surgeon-dependent. Direct oral anticoagulation (e.g., dabigatran, apixaban, rivaroxaban, and edoxaban) are generally discontinued 1–3 days prior to the surgery but varies on a number of factors, namely renal function.[6] See Chapter 4: Anticoagulation Management in the Periprocedural Period for more details.
- Preoperative infectious prophylaxis should include administration of cefazolin 2 g (3 g for patients weighing ≥120 kg) or cefuroxime 1.5 g infused intravenously 1 hour prior to the surgical incision. Patients with a beta-lactam allergy can be administered vancomycin. Vancomycin 15 mg/kg (maximum of 2000 mg) should be administered intravenously 2 hours before surgical incision due to the longer time required to complete the infusion (maximum of 500 mg per 30 minutes). Infectious prophylaxis should be discontinued within 24 hours postoperatively.[7]

DURING THE PROCEDURE

- Surgeons may administer heparin 3000–5000 units intravenously prior to clamping the carotid artery during the procedure.
- There is debate whether protamine needs to be administered to reduce the risk of neck hematoma after the procedure. One concern is that the administration of protamine may lead to an increased risk of thrombosis after the procedure. Therefore, administration of protamine is based on patient risk factors and surgeon preference.[1,8]

AFTER THE PROCEDURE

- Postoperative hypertension can lead to increased risk of neck hematoma. It is recommended to maintain systolic blood pressure <170 mmHg in the postoperative period. Medications such as labetalol 10–20 mg or hydralazine 10 mg via intravenous push can be utilized to treat uncontrolled hypertension in the first 24 hours postoperatively.[4]
- Baroreceptor reflex responses such as bradycardia, hypotension, and vasovagal reactions occur in 5% to 10% of the cases. The response is usually self-limiting and often does not require an intervention postoperatively.[1]
- There is a small possibility (less than 1% of cases) that a clot can break off during surgery and cause a cerebrovascular event. Therefore, close neurologic evaluation postoperatively is recommended for all patients to monitor for signs and symptoms of stroke. Patients may be

transferred to an ICU during the first 24 hours postoperatively for close neurologic monitoring.[1]

- Medical therapy initiated for medical optimization prior to the surgical procedure, such as aspirin, beta blockade, and statin therapy, should be continued postoperatively once the patient is able to tolerate enteral medications (see details in "Before the procedure," above).

References

1. Brott TG, Halperin JL, Abbara S, et al. 2011 ASA/ACCF/AHA/AANN/AANS/ACR/ASNR/CNS/SAIP/SCAI/SIR/SNIS/SVM/SVS Guideline on the management of patients with extracranial carotid and vertebral artery disease. *J Am Coll Cardiol*. 2011;57:e16–e94.
2. Ooi YC, Gonzalez NR. Management of extracranial carotid artery disease. *Cardiol Clin*. 2015;33:1–35.
3. Alonso-Coello P, Bellmunt S, McGorrian C, et al. Antithrombotic therapy in peripheral artery disease. *Chest*. 2012;141:e669S–e690S.
4. Naylor AR. Medical treatment strategies to reduce perioperative morbidity and mortality after carotid surgery. *Semin Vasc Surg*. 2017;30:17–24.
5. Kernan WN, Ovbiagele B, Black HR, et al. Guidelines for the prevention of stroke in patients with stroke and transient ischemic attack: a guideline for healthcare professionals from the American Heart Association/American Stroke Association. *Stroke*. 2014;45:2160–2236.
6. Tomaselli GF, Mahaffey KW, Cuker A, et al. 2020 ACC Expert consensus decision pathway on management of bleeding in patients on oral anticoagulants. *J Am Coll Cardiol*. 2020;76:594–622.
7. Bratzler DW, Dellinger EP, Olsen KM, et al. Clinical practice guidelines for antimicrobial prophylaxis in surgery. *Am J Health-Syst Pharm*. 2013;70:195–283.
8. Ricotta JJ, AbuRahma A, Ascher E, et al. Updated Society for Vascular Surgery guidelines for management of extracranial carotid disease. *J Vasc Surg*. 2011;54:e1–e31.

Chest Tube

Julie A. Murphy, PharmD ■ Fadi Safi, MD

Background

A thoracostomy tube is a hollow plastic tube or catheter that is used to drain air, fluid, pus, or blood from the intrathoracic space (Fig. 15.1). The word "thoracostomy" combines the prefix "thoraco" meaning "chest wall" and the suffix "stomy" meaning "opening." Thoracostomy tube may sometimes be referred to as a chest tube (the term that will be used throughout this chapter), intrapleural drain, or pigtail (Fig. 15.2). The procedure to place the chest tube is called tube thoracostomy.

How to Use It

Indications for a chest tube include pneumothorax, hemothorax, and pleural effusions. Primary spontaneous pneumothorax occurs without predisposing factors or significant lung disease, and the male sex and smoking are risk factors. Iatrogenic pneumothorax occurs most commonly due to central line placement. Traumatic pneumothorax occurs with blunt or penetrating trauma to the chest. Pneumothorax after lung resection may develop from a persistent air leak or a bronchopleural fistula that does not resolve. Tension pneumothorax, the accumulation of air in the chest under positive pressure, is a life-threatening condition that leads to hemodynamic instability and requires immediate decompression by a needle or a chest tube. Hemothorax results from blunt or penetrating trauma to the chest wall or after a fall. It can also develop following cardiac events, thoracic surgery, or aortic conditions. Using Light's criteria, pleural effusions are defined as exudate or transudate according to pleural fluid protein and lactate dehydrogenase (LDH) values. If the pleural fluid/serum protein ratio is greater than 0.5, the pleural fluid/serum LDH ratio is greater than 0.6, or the pleural fluid LDH value is greater than two-thirds the upper limit of the normal serum LDH, the fluid is exudative indicating infection, inflammation, or malignancy. Some medications such as methotrexate, bromocriptine, nitrofurantoin, and amiodarone may lead to an exudative pleural effusion. The most common causes of transudative pleural effusion include congestive heart failure and cirrhosis with ascites. In the case of recurrent effusions, chest tubes may be used to instill sclerosing agents into the pleural space to induce pleurodesis. When adhesions are present in the pleural space, ultrasound guidance is the preferred method for tube insertion.[1–5]

How It Is Done

Pulmonologists, intensivists, emergency room physicians, interventional radiologists, or general, trauma, or thoracic surgeons can insert a chest tube. Most chest tube insertions are completed at bedside. The patient's arm should be placed behind the head to expose the axillary area. The area for insertion is determined by locating the fourth to fifth intercostal space in the anterior axillary line at the level of the nipple. This is referred to as the triangle of safety, which is the triangle between the apex of the axilla, the anterior margin of the latissimus dorsi, and lateral margin of the pectoralis major at the level of the nipple. The skin and the subcutaneous tissue at the insertion site should be anesthetized by locally injecting 10–20 mL of 1% lidocaine solution. An incision of 1.5 to 2.0 cm in length is made parallel to the rib, and a Kelly clamp is used to cut through the

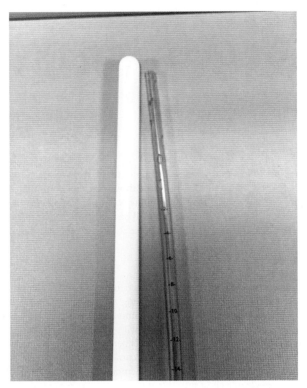

Fig. 15.1   Chest tube (24 French) with drainage holes.

intercostal muscles to the pleural space. The tube is then directed vertically in case for pneumothorax or basally for effusion. Conscious sedation (benzodiazepines [e.g., midazolam] and analgesics
[e.g., morphine or fentanyl]) can be used in nonemergent cases according to physician preference
or patient comfort level.

There are two methods to place chest tubes: the dissecting method places larger-bore
(20-French or larger) tubes and the Seldinger method uses smaller (14-French or smaller) tubes
and is done under ultrasound guidance. The dissecting method is usually performed at bedside
or in the operating room (OR), and the Seldinger method can be performed at bedside or in a
radiology suite. The size of the tube usually depends on the indication for the procedure (pneumothorax vs. effusion), the effusion characteristics (transudate vs. exudate), and patient condition.
Most hospitals have presterilized chest tube insertion trays. The trays contain a scalpel, dissecting
instruments, syringes, needles, sutures, and tubes of different sizes. Following lung resection or
other thoracic procedures, a chest tube that was placed in the OR may remain with the patient
when being transferred to the medical ward. For a pneumothorax, the tube can be removed once
bubbling (air leak) ceases and the lung is fully expanded on chest X-ray. A pleural drainage system
attaches to the tube once it is placed (Fig. 15.3). For pleural effusion, the drainage volume should
be less than 200 mL in 24 hours to consider removal of the tube. Relative contraindications
to chest tube placement include use of anticoagulant medications, coagulopathy, bleeding disorders, diaphragmatic hernia, or overlying infection. Complications of chest tube placement include
hemorrhage, infection, or inadvertent laceration of the liver or spleen. Long-term complications
include tube clogging or persistent air leak.[6,7]

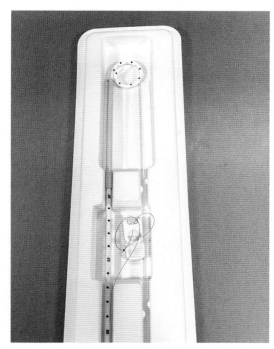

Fig. 15.2 Pigtail catheter (14 French).

Medication Implications

- Chest tube insertion is most commonly performed as an emergency procedure, so there is little time for preparation. As such, use of anticoagulant medications is a relative contraindication to chest tube placement. Continuation of clopidogrel may be safe in patients undergoing small-bore chest tube insertion.[8]
- Prophylactic intravenous antibiotics may reduce the risk of developing empyema and pneumonia in patients receiving a chest tube due to blunt and penetrating chest trauma. Patients receiving prophylactic intravenous antibiotics were found to have a shorter length of stay than those who received placebo. However, the optimal type, dose, and duration of antibiotic therapy has not been established.[9]
- In the case of recurrent effusions, chest tubes may be used to administer sclerosing agents into the pleural space for chemical pleurodesis. Bilateral simultaneous pleurodesis should not be attempted.[10–12]
    - Doxycycline: This is an inexpensive alternative to bleomycin and may have fewer adverse effects than talc. Prior to doxycycline administration, a negative history of allergy to tetracycline and its derivatives must be confirmed. Chest tube placement should be confirmed via chest X-ray, and there should be satisfactory drainage of the accumulated fluid (<50–100 mL in 24 hours). As above, an analgesic and anxiolytic should be administered. Approximately 3–4 mg/kg of lidocaine 1% solution should be instilled into the pleural space through the chest tube. The tube should be clamped and the patient rotated to spread the anesthetic over pleural membranes. Doxycycline 0.5–1 g for intravenous injection is reconstituted into 2 mL sterile water for injection and further diluted with sterile 0.9% NaCl to a final volume of 25–50 mL. The doxycycline solution is instilled into the pleural space

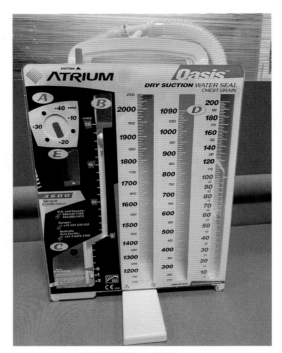

Fig. 15.3 Pleural drainage system.

through the tube and the tube is flushed with 10 mL of sterile 0.9% NaCl. The chest tube is clamped for 6–12 hours, and the patient is instructed to change positions every 15–30 minutes. After 6–12 hours, the chest tube is reconnected to water-seal drainage and suction. The patient is monitored for relief of symptoms, allergic reactions, pain, fever, and drainage volume. The procedure is repeated 48–72 hours later if 24-hour drainage is >150 mL. The chest tube is discontinued once drainage is 50–100 mL per 24 hours.

- Talc: This is an inexpensive and highly effective pleurodesis agent. Talc must be sterilized and asbestos-free with dosing not to exceed 5 g. The most common adverse effects are fever and pain. Fever usually occurs 4–12 hours after instillation and may last for up to 72 hours. All pleural fluid should be removed prior to talc instillation. Talc may be administered one of two ways:
  - Talc poudrage: Complete collapse of the lung is necessary to provide a good view of the pleural cavity, the opportunity to biopsy lesions, and for wide and even distribution of the talc. This method is generally performed in the OR under local anesthesia with conscious sedation or by video-assisted thoracic surgery.
  - Talc slurry: Talc is mixed with 50 mL of 0.9% NaCl and instilled through a chest tube. The tube is clamped for 1 hour, and patient rotation is recommended. Disadvantages include lack of uniform distribution, accumulation in dependent areas of the pleural space, and decreased direct contact time with the pleural surface.
- Bleomycin: Most studies have used a dose of 60 units of bleomycin mixed with 50–100 mL of sterile 0.9% NaCl. Direct studies comparing talc and bleomycin have demonstrated a superior pleurodesis success rate with talc.
- For complicated pleural effusions and early empyemas, the routine use of intrapleural fibrinolytic therapy with a combination of intrapleural tissue plasminogen activator and DNAse has been

increasingly utilized in hospital settings to drain the residual fluid in the thoracic cavity. While the Multicenter Intrapleural Sepsis Trial-2 (MIST2) found that such therapy had statistical and clinical improvement in pleural drainage and reduction in hospital stay, overall long-term outcomes including pulmonary reserve after treatment and time to return to full activity is lacking. More clinical trials will be needed in the future to assess the effectiveness of such therapy.[13,14]

■ If analysis of the pleural fluid from the chest tube reveals infection (bacterial, fungal, or parasitic), it should be treated according to current standards and considering patient-specific factors.

■ In the case of empyema specifically, thoracentesis with pleural drain placement is useful in the treatment of early-stage empyema. Intrapleural administration of antibiotics is not indicated. For community-acquired empyema, a parenteral second- or third-generation cephalosporin with metronidazole or parenteral aminopenicillin with β-lactamase inhibitor is recommended. For hospital-acquired or postprocedural empyema, parenteral antibiotics with activity against methicillin-resistant *Staphylococcus aureus* and *Pseudomonas aeruginosa* are indicated. Of note, aminoglycosides should be avoided. When possible, antibiotic therapy should be based on culture results and local resistance patterns. Duration of therapy is based on organism, adequacy of source control, and clinical response.[13]

■ If analysis of the pleural fluid from the chest tube reveals malignancy (primary or metastatic), it should be treated according to current standards and considering patient-specific factors and goals.

■ If analysis of the pleural fluid from the chest tube is indicative of congestive heart failure, subsequent tests, such as an echocardiogram, may be ordered. See Chapter 25: Echocardiography for details about this test.

■ If analysis of the pleural fluid from the chest tube is indicative of cirrhosis with ascites, the severity of the ascites will determine treatment. For mild to moderate ascites, spironolactone with or without a loop diuretic may be used. More severe cases may need paracentesis followed by albumin infusion and diuretic therapy.[15]

References

1. Sahn SA, Heffner JE. Spontaneous pneumothorax. *N Engl J Med*. 2000;342:868–874.
2. Kulshrestha P, Munshi I, Wait R. Profile of chest trauma in a level I trauma center. *J Trauma*. 2004;57:576–581.
3. Light RW, Macgregor MI, Luchsinger PC, et al. Pleural effusions: the diagnostic separation of transudates and exudates. *Ann Intern Med*. 1972;77:507–513.
4. Chetty KG. Transudative pleural effusions. *Clin Chest Med*. 1985;6:49–54.
5. Huggins JT, Sahn SA. Drug-induced pleural disease. *Clin Chest Med*. 2004;25:141–153.
6. Laws D, Neville E, Duffy J, et al. BTS guidelines for the insertion of a chest drain. *Thorax*. 2003;58:ii53–ii59.
7. Dev SP, Nascimiento B, Simone C, et al. Chest-tube insertion. *N Engl J Med*. 2007;357:e15.
8. Pathak V, Allender JE, Grant MW. Management of anticoagulant and antiplatelet therapy in patients undergoing interventional pulmonary procedures. *Eur Respir Rev*. 2017;26:170020.
9. Ayoub F, Quirke M, Frith D. Use of prophylactic antibiotic in preventing complications for blunt and penetrating chest trauma requiring chest drain insertion: a systematic review and meta-analysis. *Trauma Surg Acute Care Open*. 2019;4:e000246.
10. Andrews CO, Gora ML. Pleural effusions: pathophysiology and management. *Ann Pharmacother*. 1994;28:894–903.
11. Walker-Renard P, Vaughan LM, Sahn SA. Chemical pleurodesis for malignant pleural effusions. *Ann Intern Med*. 1994;120:56–64.
12. American Thoracic Society. Management of malignant pleural effusions. *Am J Respir Crit Care Med*. 2000;162:1987–2001.
13. Shen KR, Bribriesco A, Crabtree T, et al. The American Association for Thoracic Surgery consensus guidelines for the management of empyema. *J Thorac Cardiovasc Surg*. 2017;153:e129–e146.
14. Rahman NM, Maskell NA, West A, et al. Intrapleural use of tissue plasminogen activator and DNase in pleural infection. *N Engl J Med*. 2011;365:518–526.
15. Biecker E. Diagnosis and therapy of ascites in liver cirrhosis. *World J Gastroenterol*. 2011;17:1237–1248.

CHAPTER 16

Chest X-Ray

Samantha Moore, PharmD

Background

A chest X-ray (CXR) is a noninvasive imaging procedure that uses ionizing radiation to produce a shadow image of the anatomic structures in the thoracic cavity. The term "X-ray" refers to the type of high-energy electromagnetic radiation used in the imaging procedure, which was discovered by the German physicist, Dr. Wilhelm Roentgen.[1] A CXR is also known as a plain chest roentgenogram, a plain (chest) film, or a chest radiograph.

How to Use It

A CXR produces a two-dimensional image of the contents of the chest and nearby structures by beaming X-rays through the chest and onto a digital plate or film.[2] Different tissues attenuate (absorb) the X-rays to varying degrees, producing an image based on the amount of radiation that reaches the digital plate. The higher the attenuation, the more radiodense (or white) an object will appear in the image (Table 16.1).[3] A CXR enables the clinician to diagnose multiple cardiopulmonary conditions, including pneumothorax, pulmonary edema, pneumonia, cardiomegaly, metastatic disease, aortic dissection, pericardial effusion, drug-induced pulmonary toxicity, and rib fractures. CXRs also provide useful information about the upper gastrointestinal tract, such as the presence of intraperitoneal air.[3,4] The presence and location of invasive devices, including central venous catheters (CVCs), endotracheal tubes, feeding tubes (oro- and nasogastric), pulmonary artery catheters, and chest tubes, are also visible on CXR.[5] See Chapter: 37: Intravenous Access for details about CVCs. See Chapter 42: Nasogastric Tube for details. See Chapter 15: Chest Tube for details.

How It Is Done

CXRs are quick, noninvasive, painless, and relatively inexpensive. Patients do not need to fast before CXR, and procedural sedation is usually not indicated, as shooting an X-ray takes only a fraction of a second to obtain an image. A rare exception is an agitated and combative trauma patient, who may require sedation before a bedside CXR can be obtained by the radiology technician. During CXR, patients are exposed to a low dose of radiation, approximately 0.1 mSv or the equivalent of 10 days of normal background radiation.[6] CXRs can be taken from different views, which must be specified by the ordering clinician. For most indications, the posteroanterior (PA) view is preferred. The patient is asked to inhale deeply and stand with their chest against a film cassette, with an X-ray source located at the patient's back (Fig. 16.1). To better identify abnormalities obscured on the PA view, a left lateral view is also obtained (Fig. 16.2) by turning the patient a quarter-turn to the left. A PA and lateral CXR can be obtained in the outpatient or inpatient setting in a radiology suite as long as the patient is stable and able to cooperate. Portable X-ray machines can also be used to obtain an anteroposterior (AP) view at the bedside. A radiology technician will place a film cassette behind the patient's chest and a portable X-ray source in front of the patient's chest. Again, full inspiration is preferable to better visualize the patient's

TABLE 16.1 ■ **Radiographic Density Appearance on X-Ray**

Material	Radiographic Appearance	
Air	Black	
Fat	Dark-gray	
Water (Soft Tissue)	Light-gray	
Bone	Off-white	
Metal	White	

lungs. Compared with the PA view, the AP view increases cardiac magnification (artificially increasing heart size) and reduces anatomical resolution.[1,2,4] After taking the CXR, the technician will upload the image to a picture archiving and communication system. The CXR will be interpreted by a radiologist who will document their findings in a written report. Non-radiologist providers caring for the patient may also review the CXR while awaiting the report.

There are many described methods for interpreting CXRs. Regardless of the chosen method, the most important factor is to use a systematic approach, as this will minimize diagnostic errors.[3] Generally, the first step is to ensure the image is of the correct patient and of the correct date and time. Whenever possible, a previous CXR should be used as a comparator. Next, providers will assess the quality of the X-ray by noting the degree of inspiratory effort, the adequacy of X-ray penetration, and the positioning of the patient by checking that the trachea is midline and the clavicles appear straight. The reviewer should also inspect the lungs for signs of pulmonary

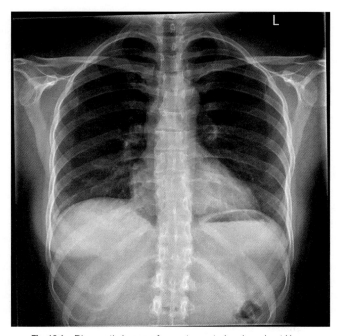

Fig. 16.1 Diagnostic image of a posteroanterior view chest X-ray.

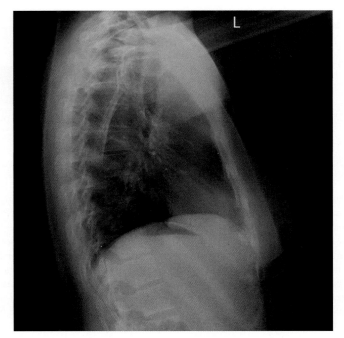

Fig. 16.2   Diagnostic image of a left lateral view chest X-ray.

infiltrates, assess the clarity of the costophrenic angles, evaluate for possible enlargement of the cardiac silhouette, and check for any rib fractures. The chest wall should be inspected for abnormalities, and the presence and location of any invasive medical devices should be noted.[4] Many clinicians use a mnemonic such as "ABCDE" as part of their systematic approach to interpreting CXRs. While there are several versions, one example is A: airway, B: bones or breathing (lungs/lung fields), C: cardiac/mediastinum, D: diaphragm, E: everything else. A normal CXR will show a nondeviated, midline trachea, seven to nine unfractured ribs above the diaphragm (this number generally demonstrates adequate inspiratory effort without hyperinflation), clear costophrenic angles and lung parenchyma, and a normal-sized cardiac silhouette (see Figs. 16.1 and 16.2).

Medication Implications

- Patients who are unable to swallow often have an orogastric or a nasogastric tube placed to allow for enteral feeding and medication administration. After placement of the tube, its location must be confirmed on CXR before it can be used to administer tube feeds or medications. The tip of the tube should be approximately 10 cm past the gastroesophageal junction.[5] See Chapter 42: Nasogastric Tube for details.
- There are several indications for CVC, including the administration of certain medications (e.g., hypertonic saline, total parenteral nutrition, vasopressors, chemotherapy). Except in emergency scenarios, the location of a subclavian or internal jugular placed CVC should be confirmed on CXR or ultrasound before it is used. The tip of the CVC should be in the superior vena cava, ideally just above the right atrium.[5] See Chapter 37: Intravenous Access for details about CVCs.

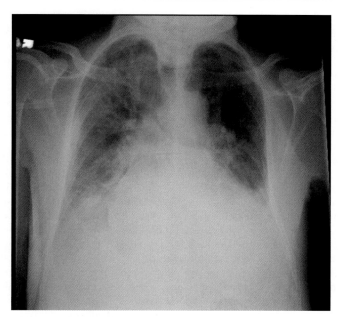

Fig. 16.3 Diagnostic image of an anteroposterior view chest X-ray in a patient with congestive heart failure and cardiogenic pulmonary edema who requires treatment with a loop diuretic. Note the enlarged cardiac silhouette, bilateral pleural effusions, and cephalization.

- A CXR may indicate the presence of pulmonary edema, which can be further classified as cardiogenic or noncardiogenic.
    - Cardiogenic pulmonary edema (CPE) is the result of elevated left-sided heart pressures (due to congestive heart failure, myocardial infarction, cardiomyopathy, arrhythmias, etc.) leading to increased pulmonary capillary pressure and fluid buildup in the lungs.[7] CXR findings consistent with CPE include cardiomegaly, cephalization, bilateral and symmetric interstitial and/or alveolar edema, Kerley B lines, and pleural effusion (Fig. 16.3).[4] After initial stabilization of the patient, the mainstay of therapy for CPE is to correct any reversible underlying cause and provide intravenous (IV) loop diuretics.[7] For patients who are using chronic diuretic therapy, the IV dose should be greater than or equal to their oral daily dose (e.g., if on furosemide 40 mg by mouth daily at home, administer furosemide ≥40 mg IV).[8] If a patient is loop diuretic–naive, an initial dose of furosemide 20–40 mg IV (or an equivalent dose of bumetanide [0.5–1 mg] or torsemide [10–20 mg]) is appropriate.[9] The diuretic can be given as intermittent boluses or a continuous infusion. Urine output and symptoms of fluid overload should be closely monitored with diuretic dose adjustments as necessary. If patients have an inadequate response to high-dose loop diuretics, a thiazide diuretic can be given 30 to 60 minutes before the loop diuretic to augment diuresis by preventing rebound sodium and fluid reabsorption in the distal tubule. Vasodilators and inotropes may also be indicated in select patients.[7,8]
    - Noncardiogenic pulmonary edema (NCPE) has several etiologies, including acute respiratory distress syndrome, neurogenic pulmonary edema, high-altitude pulmonary edema, opioid overdose, and transfusion-related acute lung injury. Compared with CPE, CXR findings consistent with NCPE include a peripheral distribution of bilateral infiltrates with no significant pulmonary vascular congestion or cardiomegaly.[5,10] However, it is often impossible to differentiate between CPE and NCPE on imaging alone, and patients

may also have overlapping etiologies.[5] The mainstay of treatment of NCPE is to correct the underlying cause. The use of loop diuretics to treat NCPE is not universally indicated but may be appropriate depending on the underlying cause and clinical scenario.[10]

- Patients with suspected pneumonia require a CXR as part of their standard workup. Pneumonia results in bacteria and neutrophils filling the alveoli, which can be observed on CXR as a pulmonary opacity.[11] An opacity is an area of increased radiodensity that may be surrounded by darker aerated lung or cause the loss of differential radiographic density between the lungs and adjacent organs (the silhouette sign). Air bronchograms may also be present. These CXR findings are not specific for pneumonia and must be assessed in the appropriate clinical context.[4,5]

  - Patients diagnosed with pneumonia require treatment with antibiotics. Whenever possible, respiratory and blood cultures should be obtained before antibiotic administration for patients diagnosed with hospital-acquired or ventilator-associated pneumonia.[12] Cultures should also be obtained for patients hospitalized with community-acquired pneumonia if it is severe or the patient has risk factors for methicillin-resistant *Staphylococcus aureus* or *Pseudomonas aeruginosa*.[13] The appropriate antibiotic regimen depends on many factors, including where the patient acquired pneumonia, risk factors for resistant organisms, and the severity of illness. Readers are encouraged to review the applicable guidelines for more information on antibiotic selection.[12,13] Repeat CXRs to monitor for pneumonia resolution are not required, as radiographic improvement usually lags days to weeks behind clinical improvement.[13] See Chapter 21: Culture – Blood for more details. See Chapter 22: Culture – Sputum for details about cultures and the use of antibiotics for pneumonia.

- Rib fractures are often identified on a CXR, although it is less sensitive than a computed tomography (CT) scan. However, if there is no other indication for a CT scan, many patients can have their fractures managed without further imaging.[14] The mainstay of treatment for rib fractures is analgesia, as inadequate pain control can result in poor respiratory effort and atelectasis.[15,16] Atelectasis refers to reduced lung inflation, which can lead to significant respiratory complications, including hypoxia and pneumonia.[4,17]

  - To prevent patients with rib fractures from developing atelectasis, patients should receive multimodal analgesia, which involves the use of multiple classes of medications to optimize pain control while also reducing opioid requirements. Multimodal analgesics include acetaminophen, nonsteroidal anti-inflammatory drugs (NSAIDs), lidocaine patches, gabapentin, and low-dose ketamine infusion.[15,16,18] In retrospective studies, IV NSAIDs have been shown to improve pain control, reduce opioid requirements, and reduce the risk of pneumonia in patients with rib fractures.[19,20] Regional analgesia including epidurals, paravertebral blocks, and intercostal blocks can also be used as part of multimodal analgesia. Epidural analgesia for rib fractures has been studied extensively and is considered by many providers to be the gold standard despite conflicting evidence regarding its superiority over nonregional analgesia regimens. Epidural analgesia may be most beneficial in patients who are older, have higher severity of injury, or have an inadequate response to other analgesic regimens.[15]

References

1. Raoof S, Feigin D, Sung A, et al. Interpretation of plain chest roentgenogram. *Chest*. 2012;141:545–558.
2. Zaer N, Amini B, Elsayes K. Overview of diagnostic modalities and contrast agents. In: Elsayes K, Oldham S, eds. *Introduction to Diagnostic Radiology*: McGraw-Hill; 2014.
3. Sachdeva A, Matuschak G. Interpreting chest x-rays, CT scans, and MRIs. In: Lechner A, Matuschak G, Brink D, eds. *Respiratory: An Integrated Approach to Disease*: McGraw-Hill; 2012. Accessed June 17, 2020. https://accessmedicine.mhmedical.com/content.aspx?bookid=1623&sectionid=105764262.

4. Barile M, Jacobson F. Basic chest radiography (CXR). In: McKean S, Ross J, Dressler D, Scheurer D, eds. *Principles and Practice of Hospital Medicine.* 2nd ed.: McGraw-Hill; 2017. Accessed June 17, 2020. https:// accessmedicine.mhmedical.com/content.aspx?bookid=1872&sectionid=146978418.

5. Qadir N, Matthew R. Imaging of the critically ill patient: radiology. In: Oropello J, Pastores S, Kvetan V, eds. *Critical Care*: McGraw-Hill; 2017. Accessed June 17, 2020. https://accessmedicine.mhmedical.com /content.aspx?bookid=1944&sectionid=143516056.

6. Radiation dose to adults from common imaging examinations. American College of Radiology. Accessed June 16, 2020. https://www.acr.org/-/media/ACR/Files/Radiology-Safety/Radiation-Safety/Dose -Reference-Card.pdf?la=en.

7. Iqbal M, Gupta M. Cardiogenic pulmonary edema In: *StatPearls [Internet]*. StatPearls Publishing; 2020. Accessed June 12, 2020. https://www.ncbi.nlm.nih.gov/books/NBK544260/.

8. Yancy CW, Jessup M, Bozkurt B, et al. 2013 ACCF/AHA guideline for the management of heart failure. *Circulation*. 2013;128:e147–e239.

9. Furosemide [package insert]. Shirley, NY: American Regent; 2011.

10. Clark S, Soos M. Noncardiogenic pulmonary edema In: *StatPearls [Internet]*. StatPearls Publishing; 2020. Accessed June 12, 2020. https://www.ncbi.nlm.nih.gov/books/NBK542230/.

11. ACR-SPR-STR practice parameter for the performance of chest radiography. American College of Radiology Practice Parameters. Published 2017. Accessed June 10, 2020. https://www.acr.org/-/media /ACR/Files/Practice-Parameters/ChestRad.pdf.

12. Kalil AC, Metersky ML, Klompas M, et al. Management of adults with hospital-acquired and ventilator-associated pneumonia: 2016 clinical practice guidelines by the Infectious Diseases Society of America and the American Thoracic Society. *Clin Infect Dis*. 2016;63:e61–111.

13. Metlay JP, Waterer GW, Long AC, et al. Diagnosis and treatment of adults with community-acquired pneumonia: an official clinical practice guideline of the American Thoracic Society and Infectious Diseases Society of America. *Am J Respir Crit Care Med*. 2019;200:E45–E67.

14. Chapman BC, Overbey DM, Tesfalidet F, et al. Clinical utility of chest computed tomography in patients with rib fractures CT chest and rib fractures. *Arch Trauma Res*. 2016;5:e37070.

15. Galvagno SM, Smith CE, Varon AJ, et al. Pain management for blunt thoracic trauma: A joint practice management guideline from the Eastern Association for the Surgery of Trauma and Trauma Anesthesiology Society. *J Trauma Acute Care Surg*. 2016;81:936–951.

16. Witt CE, Bulger EM. Comprehensive approach to the management of the patient with multiple rib fractures: a review and introduction of a bundled rib fracture management protocol. *Trauma Surg Acute Care Open*. 2017;2:1–7.

17. Hansell D, Bankier A, MacMahon H, et al. Fleischner Society: glossary of terms for thoracic imaging. *Radiology*. 2008;246:697–722.

18. Carver TW, Kugler NW, Juul J, et al. Ketamine infusion for pain control in adult patients with multiple rib fractures: results of a randomized control trial. *J Trauma Acute Care Surg*. 2019;86:181–188.

19. Yang Y, Young JB, Schermer CR, et al. Use of ketorolac is associated with decreased pneumonia following rib fractures. *Am J Surg*. 2014;207:566–572.

20. Bayouth L, Safcsak K, Cheatham ML, et al. Early intravenous ibuprofen decreases narcotic requirement and length of stay after traumatic rib fracture. *American Surg*. 2013;79:1207–1212.

CHAPTER 17

Computed Tomography Scan

Maria Sedky Saad, PharmD ■ Samantha Moore, PharmD

Background

A computed tomography (CT) scan is a noninvasive imaging modality that uses rotating X-ray beams and detectors to produce high-quality cross-sectional imaging of anatomic structures. The word "tomography" comes from the words "tomos" meaning "slice" and "graph" meaning "recording," referring to the cross-sectional image slices recorded with CT imaging. A CT scan may also be referred to as a computerized axial tomography (CAT) scan.

How to Use It

CT revolutionized the fields of radiology and medicine when it was introduced in the 1970s. Similar to a chest X-ray, CT scanning produces grayscale images of anatomic structures based on the different radiodensities of tissues. See Chapter 16: Chest X-Ray for more details. However, unlike conventional radiography (taken in the frontal/coronal or sagittal planes) in which body structures are superimposed on imaging, CT scans allow visualization of cross-sectional slices of the desired anatomy (in the axial/transverse plane). CT scans also provide significantly greater contrast resolution than conventional radiography, which allows for improved tissue differentiation and characterization.[1,2]

CT has numerous applications in patient care. For example, a noncontrast head CT is indicated in patients presenting with acute mental status changes, focal neurologic deficits, or head trauma. It can detect acute intracranial hemorrhage, intracerebral edema, hydrocephalous, and skull fractures. A chest CT can further characterize abnormalities detected on chest X-rays, including pleural abnormalities, chest masses/nodules, and pleural or pericardial fluid collections.[3] It is also used in the diagnostic evaluation of interstitial lung disease and is the best noninvasive method to assess for drug-induced lung disease.[4,5] CT pulmonary angiography is the preferred imaging modality to diagnose pulmonary embolism (PE).[6] CT is able to detect a wide range of intra-abdominal pathologies, including appendicitis, mesenteric ischemia, diverticulitis, pancreatitis, abdominal abscesses, and volvulus. Additionally, CT scans are often obtained to determine the location and severity of traumatic injuries and to help determine sources of bleeding.[3]

How It Is Done

CT scans are performed in both outpatient and inpatient settings and are often used in the diagnosis of medical emergencies. Unlike X-rays, which may be performed portably, CT scans cannot be performed at the bedside. Hospital emergency rooms may have adjacent radiology suites equipped with CT scanners to provide rapid diagnostic information; however, patients should be stabilized before they are transported to the radiology suite.

CT scans are noninvasive and painless and can often be completed within minutes. However, they are more expensive than plain radiographs and expose patients to much higher amounts of ionizing radiation. For example, patients undergoing an abdominal and pelvis CT are exposed to approximately 10 mSv or the equivalent of 3 years of background radiation.[7]

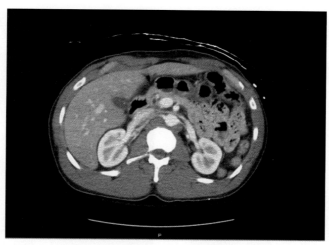

Fig. 17.1 Diagnostic image of an abdominal computed tomography scan with intravenous iodinated contrast media in the axial view.

The CT scanner consists of a sliding table where the patient is moved through a donut-shaped gantry that contains an X-ray source that rapidly rotates around the patient. The X-ray beam passes through the patient at multiple angles before reaching corresponding detectors. Similar to chest X-rays, the amount of X-ray attenuation depends on the radiodensity of the tissue the X-ray beam is passing through. See Chapter 16: Chest X-Ray for more details. The X-rays that pass though the patient to the detector are then transmitted to a computer that reconstructs cross-sectional images based on the degrees of attenuation at different points. While the axial/transverse view is standard (Fig. 17.1), modern CT technology allows for images to be reformatted and displayed in any anatomic plane, with sagittal (Fig. 17.2) and coronal/frontal (Fig. 17.3) reformations being the most common.[1]

Procedural sedation for a CT scan is generally not required for adult patients. One exception is an agitated or combative patient who may require sedation to remain still for the scan. Patients undergoing a CT scan with contrast are often required to fast for several hours before the scan. This is due to the risk of nausea, vomiting, and potential aspiration that can occur after administration of intravenous (IV) iodinated contrast. However, there is limited evidence to support fasting before IV contrast administration, and readers are encouraged to follow their local institutional policies.

Findings of a normal CT scan are specific to the region of the body being imaged. In general, a normal CT scan should show healthy tissues, organs, vasculature, lymph nodes, and bones without evidence of abscesses, masses, hematomas, hemorrhage, or free air. Findings should be interpreted in the context of the patient's history and current medical problems.

Medication Implications

- If a patient has an external portable infusion pump (e.g., insulin pump), it should not be directly exposed to the primary X-ray beam during the CT scan, as it may, albeit rarely, cause pump malfunction. If the pump will be exposed, options include temporary discontinuation (when safe) or moving the pump to another part of the body that will not be exposed. However, the risk of pump malfunction after direct X-ray exposure is extremely low (unlike magnetic resonance imaging [MRI] exposure) and should never preclude a CT scan that is medically indicated.[8] See Chapter 41: Magnetic Resonance Imaging for more details.

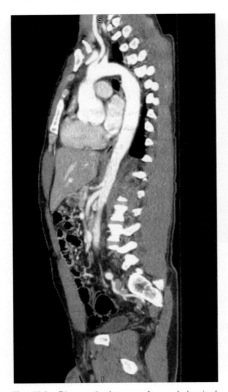

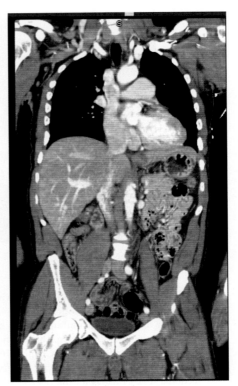

Fig. 17.2 Diagnostic image of an abdominal computed tomography scan with intravenous iodinated contrast media in the sagittal view.

Fig. 17.3 Diagnostic image of an abdominal computed tomography scan with intravenous iodinated contrast media in the coronal view.

- Patients with a PE detected on CT pulmonary angiography often require anticoagulation treatment. Initial anticoagulation options to treat a PE include unfractionated heparin, low-molecular-weight heparin, fondaparinux, or direct oral anticoagulants. Patients who have persistent arterial hypotension or obstructive shock as a result of a high-risk/massive PE should receive immediate reperfusion therapy with systemic fibrinolysis (alteplase 100 mg IV infused over 2 hours) if there are no contraindications.[6,9]

- A noncontrast head CT should be performed in patients with suspected stroke. Most ischemic strokes will not show immediately on head CT. However, a head CT is required to exclude the presence of hemorrhage prior to fibrinolytic administration (Figs. 17.4 and 17.5), which remains a mainstay of therapy for the treatment of ischemic stroke. The recommended dose of alteplase for ischemic stroke is a total of 0.9 mg/kg (maximum 90 mg) with 10% of the total dose given as an IV bolus over 1 minute and 90% of the total dose given as an infusion over 60 minutes.[10]

- Depending on the indication for CT, contrast agents may be administered to further enhance radiographic differentiation between tissues that normally have similar attenuation. Most contrast agents used for CT scans are "positive," meaning that they are radiodense with high attenuation properties and show up bright on imaging. IV iodinated contrast media (ICM) improves visualization of vascular structures, hypervascular tissues (e.g., tumors), and solid organ parenchyma.[1,2] Dilute ICM and barium contrast may be

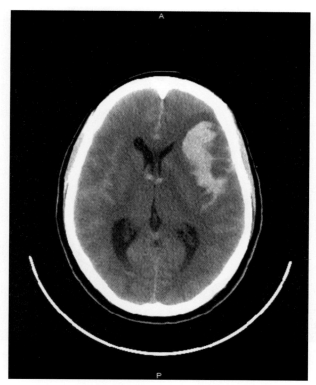

Fig. 17.4 Diagnostic image of a noncontrast head computed tomography scan in a patient presenting with stroke symptoms. This patient has an intracranial hemorrhage and is **not** a candidate for intravenous alteplase.

administered via the oral or rectal route prior to the CT scan to improve contrast between the bowel and adjacent structures.[2]

- One concern with the use of ICM, particularly IV ICM, is the risk of acute adverse reactions, which are classified as either allergic-like or physiologic. However, the risk of acute adverse reactions is relatively low (0.2%–0.7% of adult patients) with modern, nonionized, and low-osmolality ICM.[11,12]
- Most hypersensitivity reactions to ICM are not IgE-mediated and are referred to as "allergic-like." However, these reactions manifest similarly (with mild to life-threatening symptoms) and are treated as if they are a true allergic reaction.[12]
- Patients with a history of a prior allergic-like or unknown reaction to ICM are at the highest risk for a recurrent allergic-like reaction (incidence rate of 10%–35%) and should receive corticosteroid premedication (± an antihistamine) prior to future ICM administration (Table 17.1). However, the estimated number of patients that must be treated with premedication to prevent one reaction is high at 69.[13] Reactions can still occur despite premedication (a breakthrough reaction) and typically manifest with similar symptoms and severity as the patient's previous reaction. As a result, patients with a history of a severe life-threatening allergic-like reaction to ICM should not receive ICM in the future unless it is determined that the benefit of the imaging procedure outweighs the risk.[11,12]
- Risk factors that may increase the risk of an allergic-like reaction to ICM but do not require corticosteroid premedication include middle age, female sex, a history of asthma,

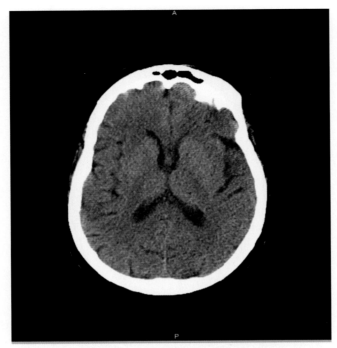

Fig. 17.5 Diagnostic image of a noncontrast head computed tomography scan in a patient presenting with stroke symptoms. This patient has no signs of intracranial hemorrhage and may be a candidate for treatment with intravenous alteplase for a suspected ischemic stroke.

TABLE 17.1 ■ Corticosteroid Premedication Regimens for Prophylaxis of Allergic-Like Reactions to Iodinated Contrast Media[11]

Premedication Indicated[a]	
Outpatient <u>or</u> emergency department patient/inpatient (in whom oral premedication will not adversely delay care) - use "Oral Regimen" below	Outpatient who arrives for CT scan without taking premedication <u>or</u> emergency department patient/inpatient in whom oral premedication would adversely delay care - use "Accelerated IV Regimen" below
Oral Regimen	**Accelerated IV Regimen**
Prednisone 50 mg[b] 13, 7, and 1 hour before contrast + diphenhydramine 50 mg PO/IV/IM 1 hour before contrast or Methylprednisolone 32 mg 12 and 2 hours before contrast ± diphenhydramine 50 mg PO 1 hour before contrast	Methylprednisolone succinate 40 mg <u>or</u> hydrocortisone 200 mg immediately and every 4 hours until contrast administration (usually 2 doses total) + diphenhydramine 50 mg IV 1 hour before contrast

[a]Corticosteroid premedication is indicated for patients who have had a previous allergic-like or unknown reaction to the same class of contrast media (e.g., iodinated contrast media).
[b]Patients unable to take oral medications may receive hydrocortisone 200 mg IV as an alternative for each dose.
CT, computed tomography; *IM,* intramuscularly; *IV,* intravenously; *PO,* orally.

atopy, and unrelated allergies. Patients with a history of shellfish or povidone-iodine allergy are not at any greater risk of an allergic-like reaction than patients with other medication or food allergies.[11]

- Physiologic adverse reactions to IV ICM are frequently dose- or concentration-dependent. Symptoms of physiologic reactions to IV ICM include nausea, vomiting, flushing, hypertension, vasovagal reactions, and rarely cardiac arrhythmias, cardiogenic pulmonary edema, and seizures. There is no role for corticosteroid premedication.[12]
- Contrast-induced nephropathy (CIN) is the acute deterioration in renal function (within 48 hours) directly caused by intravascular administration of IV ICM. CIN is a subset of postcontrast acute kidney injury (PC-AKI), which is the deterioration in renal function within 48 hours of IV ICM administration that *may or may not be directly related to the contrast*. Patients undergoing CT scans with IV ICM often have other coinciding nephrotoxic exposures that increase the risk of developing PC-AKI. True CIN is relatively rare and much less common than previously believed.[14]
  - The greatest risk factor for developing CIN is renal impairment prior to ICM administration, specifically AKI or chronic kidney disease (CKD) stage 4 or 5 (estimated glomerular filtration rate [eGFR] < 30 mL/minute/1.73 m²). These high-risk patients are considered to have a *relative but not absolute contraindication to IV ICM*, and whenever possible, other imaging modalities should be considered. However, some clinical scenarios will necessitate the use of IV ICM regardless of the risk of CIN. Patients with stage 5 CKD who are anuric on hemodialysis without a functioning transplant kidney are not at risk of CIN and may receive IV ICM.[14]
  - Isotonic IV fluids may reduce the risk of CIN and should be administered to high-risk inpatients (eGFR < 30 mL/minute/1.73m² or AKI). An example regimen is 0.9% sodium chloride at 100 mL/hour beginning 6 to 12 hours before and continuing 4 to 12 hours after IV ICM administration.[14]
  - There is insufficient evidence to support the use of sodium bicarbonate or N-acetylcysteine for CIN prophylaxis. Loop diuretics and mannitol may worsen renal function and should not be used for CIN prophylaxis.[14]
  - Patients at high risk of developing CIN should have **nonessential** nephrotoxic medications held for 24 to 48 hours before and 48 hours after IV ICM exposure, whenever possible. Commonly used nephrotoxic medications include nonsteroidal anti-inflammatory drugs, diuretics, renin-angiotensin-aldosterone system inhibitors, aminoglycosides, amphotericin, platins, zoledronate, and methotrexate. The necessity of a nephrotoxic medication should be determined on an individual patient basis.[15]
  - Metformin is a commonly prescribed oral antihyperglycemic that is renally eliminated. Metformin is not nephrotoxic and does not increase a patient's risk of developing CIN. However, patients with AKI (e.g., CIN) are at risk for metformin accumulation and metformin-induced metabolic acidosis.[15,16]
    - The American College of Radiology recommends that patients who are at high risk of CIN (AKI or an eGFR < 30 mL/minute/1.73 m²) or who are undergoing arterial catheter studies that may result in renal artery emboli should have their metformin held at the time of IV ICM administration and for at least 48 hours after. Additionally, they must have their renal function reassessed before resuming metformin. Patients who are not at an increased risk of CIN do not require interruption of their metformin therapy with IV ICM administration. Of note, this differs from the metformin package insert, which recommends withholding metformin after IV ICM administration in patients with an eGFR of 30–60 mL/minute/1.73 m².[15,16]

References

1. Zaer N, Amini B, Elsayes K. Overview of diagnostic modalities and contrast agents. In: Elsayes K, Oldham S, eds. *Introduction to Diagnostic Radiology*. New York, NY: McGraw-Hill; 2014. https://accessmedicine.mhmedical.com/content.aspx?bookid=1562&sectionid=95875179.

2. Ahern G, Brygel M, eds. Introduction. In: *Exploring Essential Radiology*, New York, NY: McGraw-Hill; 2014.

3. Jameson J, Fauci A, Kasper D, Hauser S, Longo D, Loscalzo J. Diagnostic imaging in internal medicine- *Harrison's Manual of Medicine*. 20th ed. New York, NY: McGraw-Hill; 2020.

4. Raghu G, Remy-Jardin M, Myers JL, et al. Diagnosis of idiopathic pulmonary fibrosis: an official ATS /ERS/JRS/ALAT clinical practice guideline. *Am J Respir Crit Care Med*. 2018;198:e44–e68.

5. Matsuno O. Drug-induced interstitial lung disease: mechanisms and best diagnostic approaches. *Respir Res*. 2012;13:39–48.

6. Konstantinides S, Meyer G, Bueno H, et al. 2019 ESC guidelines for the diagnosis and management of acute pulmonary embolism developed in collaboration with the European Respiratory Society (ERS). *Eur Heart J*. 2020;41:543–603.

7. Radiation dose to adults from common imaging examinations. American College of Radiology. Accessed June 16, 2020. https://www.acr.org/-/media/ACR/Files/Radiology-Safety/Radiation-Safety/Dose-Reference-Card.pdf?la=en.

8. US Food and Drug Administration. Interference between CT and electronic medical devices. Published 2018. Accessed June 17, 2020. https://www.fda.gov/radiation-emitting-products/electromagnetic-compatibility-emc/interference-between-ct-and-electronic-medical-devices.

9. Konstantinides S, Barco S, Lankeit M, et al. Management of pulmonary embolism: an update. *J Am Coll Cardiol*. 2016;67:976–990.

10. Activase (alteplase) [package insert]. South San Francisco, CA: Genentech; 2018.

11. ACR Committee on Drug and Contrast Media. Patient selection and preparation strategies before contrast medium administration. ACR Manual on Contrast Media. Published 2020. Accessed May 20, 2020. https://www.acr.org/-/media/ACR/files/clinical-resources/contrast_media.pdf.

12. ACR Committee on Drugs and Contrast Media. Allergic-like and physiologic reactions to intravascular iodinated contrast media. ACR Manual on Contrast Media. Published 2020. Accessed May 20, 2020. https://www.acr.org/-/media/ACR/files/clinical-resources/contrast_media.pdf.

13. Mervak BM, Davenport MS, Ellis JH, et al. Rates of breakthrough reactions in inpatients at high risk receiving premedication before contrast-enhanced CT. *AJR*. 2015;205:77–84.

14. ACR Committee on Drugs and Contrast Media. Post-contrast acute kidney injury and contrast-induced nephropathy in adults. ACR Manual on Contrast Media. Published 2020. Accessed May 20, 2020. https://www.acr.org/-/media/ACR/files/clinical-resources/contrast_media.pdf.

15. Davenport MS, Perazella M, Yee J, et al. Use of intravenous iodinated contrast media in patients with kidney disease: consensus statements from the American College of Radiology and the National Kidney Foundation. *Radiology*. 2020;294:660–668.

16. ACR Committee on Drugs and Contrast Media. Metformin. ACR Manual on Contrast Media. Published 2020. Accessed May 20, 2020. https://www.acr.org/-/media/ACR/files/clinical-resources/contrast_media.pdf.

CHAPTER 18

Continuous Glucose Monitoring

Joshua P. Rickard, PharmD

Background

Continuous glucose monitoring devices provide a way for patients to approximate their blood glucose by testing the interstitial fluid via the chemical reaction of fluorescence, every 1 to 5 minutes, with minimal "fingerstick" point-of-care glucose testing.[1-3] These devices are frequently referred to by the abbreviation "CGMs." There are two major types of CGMs called "real-time CGMs" or "intermittently scanning CGMs." The major difference between the two is related to how the data is transmitted between the sensor and receiver. The real-time CGMs automatically send glucose data to the receiver, allowing alerts to automatically be set for hyper- and hypoglycemia. Intermittently scanning CGMs require the patient to manually place the reading device near the sensor in order to receive glucose data, so no automatic alerts or alarms can be set.[4]

How to Use It

CGMs are useful for patients with type 1 and type 2 diabetes mellitus to reduce hypoglycemia and improve hemoglobin A1c.[4] They are especially helpful in patients who experience hypoglycemia unawareness.[4,5] The devices offer various ways in which data is presented for patients and healthcare providers. The devices display current glucose readings along with graphical presentation of the glucose trend throughout the day. They also have the ability to display to the user the future trend of their glucose, including the following: glucose remaining stable, slowly or rapidly rising, and slowly or rapidly decreasing.[6-11] The real-time CGMs can be programmed with alarms to alert the user of any of these trends along with hyper- and hypoglycemia self-set alert values.[6-10]

The American Diabetes Association (ADA) recommends considering CGMs in patients with type 1 diabetes who have not reached their blood glucose goals, have frequent episodes of hypoglycemia, or hypoglycemia unawareness. The ADA also recommends using CGMs in children and women who are pregnant with type 1 diabetes. In type 2 diabetes, the ADA states that CGMs can be helpful to reduce hemoglobin A1c or hypoglycemic events. All patients with diabetes should be counseled to use their CGMs daily to show benefit, and intermittently scanning CGMs should be scanned at least every 8 hours.[4]

How It Is Done

The CGM device system consists of three major components: sensor, transmitter, and receiver (which can also be patients' smart phones). The sensor is placed subcutaneously by either the patient or provider, and depending on the system and age of the patient, it will be placed in the abdomen, back of the arm, or top of the buttocks.[6-9,11] For example, the Senseonics Eversense® sensor needs to be implanted with an incision by the provider into the upper arm.[12] The reusable transmitter is then attached to the outside of the sensor by inserting it directly into a clip on the outside of the sensor or placed directly over it with adhesive.[6-10] In comparison, the Freestyle Libre® system has the transmitter built into the application of the sensor, so it is discarded along with the sensor each time it is changed.[11] The life of the sensor is different for each system.

Once the sensor and transmitter are in place, there is a "warm-up" period that ranges from 1 to 24 hours, depending on the system, which is followed by traditional fingerstick glucose calibrations.[6–11] After initial calibration, the Dexcom G4® and G5® and Medtronic Guardian® systems must be recalibrated every 12 hours via fingerstick testing.[6,7,9] The reader will prompt the patient when it is time to calibrate the device or change the sensor. Once the sensor has been calibrated, the sensor reads the interstitial glucose every 1 to 5 minutes, and the real-time CGMs' transmitter automatically sends glucose data every 5 to 15 minutes to the user's receiver. An intermittently scanning CGM only transmits on demand, like the Freestyle Libre ® receiver, which must be placed within 1.5 inches of the sensor to transmit the data.[6–10] One caveat of CGMs is that interstitial fluid glucose lags behind actual blood glucose concentrations by about 4 minutes and is further delayed when the glucose level is rapidly changing.[2] Continuous glucose monitors can be placed in clinic for professional use for the provider to assess trends from 10 to 14 days' worth of glucose data.[4]

Medication Implications

- The use of CGMs does not require any premedication.
- There are substances that interfere with the readings displayed by CGMs, and each system may have different interfering substances that will affect the reliability of the readings.[13] It is important to review each system individually, as each system may have different interfering substances.[6–11]
- Acetaminophen
  - When acetaminophen is oxidized at the sensor, it produces an electrochemical signal that may falsely elevate patients' glucose readings.[13,14] There is limited data regarding this effect.
  - One small pilot study enrolled 10 healthy patients who were each given 1 g of acetaminophen and measured their blood and interstitial glucose throughout the day, all fasting until the end of the study. Their blood glucose remained around 90 mg/dL throughout the day, while interstitial glucose readings averaged 30 mg/dL and 21 mg/dL higher in the Dexcom G4 Platinum® and Medtronic REAL-time Guardian® systems, respectively. The glucose levels on the CGM increased about 30 minutes after acetaminophen intake.[13]
  - Another study recorded data from 40 patients who were given 1 g of acetaminophen at breakfast. This study showed a statistically significant difference in glucose levels from the CGM compared with fingerstick glucose levels for 8 hours post-acetaminophen ingestion. The mean increase was 61 mg/dL in the CGM arm, and some patients who experienced hypoglycemia had CGM readings of 138 mg/dL and above.[14]
  - As of January 2020, the systems that are not affected by acetaminophen ingestion are the Dexcom G6®, Senseonics Eversense®, and Freestyle Libre®.[8,10,11,15,16]
- Albuterol
  - A small pilot study of 19 subjects saw some interference with a 4-mg oral dose of albuterol, but the response varied among subjects. Some readings were increased, decreased, or remained similar to blood glucose.
  - CGMs used in this study were Dexcom G4 Platinum® and Medtronic Guardian®.[17]
- Ascorbic acid
  - Ascorbic acid at doses 500 mg or higher have been shown to falsely increase glucose readings on Freestyle Libre® systems.[18,19]
- Aspirin
  - Aspirin at doses 650 mg or higher have been shown to falsely lower glucose readings on Freestyle Libre® systems.[18,19]

- Beta blockers
  - A small pilot study of 19 subjects saw some interference with a 100-mg dose of atenolol, but the response varied among subjects. Some readings were increased, decreased, or remained similar to blood glucose.
  - CGMs used in this study were Dexcom G4 Platinum® and Medtronic Guardian®. More variability was seen with the Medtronic Guardian.[17]
- Lisinopril
  - A small pilot study of 19 subjects saw some interference with a 20-mg dose of lisinopril, but the response varied among subjects. Some readings were increased, decreased, or remained similar to blood glucose.
  - In this study, five subjects had detectable interstitial fluid concentrations of lisinopril. The changes in glucose values on CGM seemed to align with the interstitial fluid concentrations of lisinopril.
  - CGMs used in this study were Dexcom G4 Platinum® and Medtronic Guardian®.[17]
- Mannitol and sorbitol
  - Mannitol has been shown to cause falsely elevated readings with the Senseonics Eversence® CGM system when used intravenously, as an irrigation solution, and in peritoneal dialysis.[12,16]
  - Sorbitol is frequently used in artificial sweeteners, and dietary consumption is not thought to affect sensor readings.[12]
- Tetracyclines
  - Tetracyclines have been shown to interfere with the Senseonics Eversence® CGM system by causing falsely low readings.[12,16]
- There may be times when patients suspect that their CGM glucose readings are inaccurate or that the patient feels symptoms of hypo- or hyperglycemia with a normal glucose reading on the CGM. If this occurs, the patient should test their fingerstick glucose with their home point-of-care device to compare against their GCM reading. If there is a discrepancy between testing methods, the patient should be instructed to treat based on their fingerstick blood glucose reading and recalibrate their CGM by following the instructions for their specific device, if applicable. The Freestyle Libre® device cannot be recalibrated, as this is done in the factory. The manufacturer recommends, if inconsistency occurs, to treat based on the fingerstick blood glucose.[20] Dexcom G6® is also factory calibrated; however, patients have the option to recalibrate if needed.[8] One study has shown that recalibrating Dexcom G6® may not improve its accuracy and may actually worsen its accuracy.[21]

References

1. Cappon G, Vettoretti M, Sparacino G, et al. Continuous glucose monitoring sensors for diabetes management: a review of technologies and applications. *Diabetes Metab J*. 2019;43:383–397.
2. Beck RW, Bergenstal RM, Laffel LM, et al. Advances in technology for management of type 1 diabetes. *Lancet*. 2019;394:1265–1273.
3. Funtanilla VD, Caliendo T, Hilas O. Continuous glucose monitoring: a review of available systems. *P T*. 2019;44:550–553.
4. American Diabetes Association. Diabetes technology: standards of medical care in diabetes–2020. *Diabetes Care*. 2020;43:S77–S88.
5. Garber AJ, Abrahamson MJ, Barzilay JI, et al. Consensus statement by the American Association of Clinical Endocrinologists and American College of Endocrinology on the comprehensive type 2 diabetes management algorithm—2019 executive summary. *Endocr Pract*. 2019;25:69–100.
6. Dexcom G4 Platinum: User's Guide. Dexcom. Accessed January 2020. Available at: https://s3-us -west-2.amazonaws.com/dexcompdf/LBL012590+Rev+003+User's+Guide%2C+G4+PLATINUM +(Pediatric)+with+Share+US+Web+with+cover.pdf.

7. Getting Started Guide for Dexcom G5® Mobile Continuous Glucose Monitoring (CGM) System. *Dexcom*. 2018. Accessed January 2020Available at. https://s3-us-west-2.amazonaws.com/dexcompdf/G5-Mobile-Getting-Started-Guide.pdf.

8. Dexcom G6: User Guide. Dexcom. 2019. Accessed January 2020. Available at: https://s3-us-west-2.amazonaws.com/dexcompdf/G6-CGM-Users-Guide.pdf.

9. Getting Started with Continuous Glucose Monitoring: My Guardian Connect System. *Medtronic*. 2018. Accessed January 2020. Available at: https://www.medtronicdiabetes.com/sites/default/files/library/download-library/references/getting-started.pdf.

10. Eversense® User Guide. Senseonics. March 2019. Accessed January 2020. Available at: https://resources.eversensediabetes.com/.

11. Freestyle Libre 14 Day Quick Start Guide. Abbott. 2018. Accessed January 2020. Available at: https://freestyleserver.com/Payloads/IFU/2018/ART39768-001_rev-A-Web.pdf.

12. Eversense CGM Sensor Insertion and Removal Instructions. Senseonics. Revised November 2017. Accessed January 2020. Available at: https://www.fda.gov/media/112159/download.

13. Basu A, Veettil S, Dyer R, et al. Direct evidence of acetaminophen interference with subcutaneous glucose sensing in humans: a pilot study. *Diabetes Technol Ther*. 2016;18:S2–43.

14. Maahs DM, DeSalvo D, Pyle L, et al. Effect of acetaminophen on CGM glucose in an outpatient setting. *Diabetes Care*. 2015;38:e158–e159.

15. Calhoun P, Johnson TK, Hughes J, et al. Resistance to acetaminophen interference in a novel continuous glucose monitoring system. *J Diabetes Sci Technol*. 2018;12:393–396.

16. Lorenz C, Sandoval W, Mortellaro M. Interference assessment of various endogenous and exogenous substances on the performance of the eversense long-term implantable continuous glucose monitoring system. *Diabetes Technol Ther*. 2018;20:344–352.

17. Basu A, Slama MQ, Nicholson WT, et al. Continuous glucose monitor interference with commonly prescribed medications: a pilot study. *J Diabetes Sci Technol*. 2017;1:936–941.

18. Kudva YC, Ahmann AJ, Bergenstal RM, et al. Approach to using trend arrows in the FreeStyle Libre flash glucose monitoring systems in adults. *J Endocr Soc*. 2018;2:1320–1337.

19. FDA: Summary of Safety and Effectiveness Data (SSED): Freestyle Libre 14 Day Indication and Important Safety Information. Abbott. Accessed May 2021. Available at: https://provider.myfreestyle.com/safety-information.html.

20. Freestyle Libre 14-Day Flash Glucose Monitoring System: User's Manual. Abbott. Accessed April 2020. Available at: https://freestyleserver.com/Payloads/IFU/2018/ART39764-001_rev-A-Web.pdf.

21. Wadwa RP, Laffel LM, Shah VN, et al. Accuracy of a factory-calibrated, real-time continuous glucose monitoring system during 10 days of use in youth and adults with diabetes. *Diabetes Technol Ther*. 2018;20:395–402.

CHAPTER 19

Continuous Renal Replacement Therapy

Yuriy Khanin, MD

Background

Continuous renal replacement therapy (CRRT) is commonly used in the intensive care unit (ICU) setting and can consist of continuous venovenous hemodialysis (CVVHD), continuous venovenous hemofiltration (CVVH), or continuous venovenous hemodiafiltration (CVVHDF). Each of these procedures involves the slow passage of blood, continuously (24 hours a day), through a filter to remove various waste products and/or fluid.[1]

How to Use It

CRRT is often referred to as a gentler form of hemodialysis (HD), as the infusion of the dialysate or replacement fluid is much slower. This is ideal for patients in the ICU who require dialysis but are hemodynamically unstable, on vasopressors, and cannot tolerate large fluid shifts over a short period of time. Generally speaking, a 24-hour session of CRRT is equivalent to a single 3-hour session of HD. Despite this advantage, no randomized trial has shown a mortality benefit for CRRT versus intermittent HD, though these trials excluded the treatment of the sickest patients with HD. Current Kidney Disease: Improving Global Outcomes guidelines recommend initiating CRRT for hemodynamically unstable patients.[2]

How It Is Done

CRRT is initiated via a double lumen catheter inserted into either the jugular or femoral vein, like some catheter placements for HD. See Chapter 34: Hemodialysis Access for more details. Unlike HD, arteriovenous access cannot be used in CRRT, as there is significant risk of damage to the artery during the continuous blood flow. Dialyzers for CRRT fall in the high-flux category. Dialysate and replacement fluid come premixed in 2.5–5 L bags; the most common suppliers are Baxter and Nxstage. One should refer to the package inserts for the exact chemical composition of the fluid. Replacement fluids are generally needed with convection to restore volume and maintain the body's physiological electrolyte composition. CVVHD refers to a continuous form of renal replacement that utilizes only dialysis solution (no replacement fluid is given), and the primary method of solute removal is diffusion. CVVH is a form of CRRT that utilizes only replacement fluid and relies on convection for solute clearance. A transmembrane gradient between the blood compartment and ultrafiltrate compartment causes water to be filtered across the membrane; as water crosses the membrane, it sweeps along with it (nonprotein-bound) small and large molecules (pore size permitting). CVVHDF is a combination of the two modalities listed above. The clearance of molecules is similar in the aforementioned modalities, and the modality utilized is at the discretion of the individual institution and nephrologist.[1,3]

Medication Implications

- Vascular access for CRRT is identical to some types of catheter access for HD. See Chapter 34: Hemodialysis Access for more details.
- Filter clotting is one of the most common complications associated with CRRT. This leads to extracorporeal blood loss (roughly 100–150 mL) and a reduction in dialysis efficiency, as a new circuit must be started.
  - Anticoagulation can be used to reduce filter clotting; however, as patients in the ICU are critically ill with significant comorbidities, such as gastrointestinal bleeding, coagulopathies, and thrombocytopenia, a risk/benefit discussion must occur with the ICU team prior to initiation. If anticoagulation is contraindicated, keeping blood flow at 200 mL/minute or greater can minimize clotting.[1]
  - Unfractionated heparin is the most common anticoagulant used in CRRT. Citrate, infused pre-filter, is an additional anticoagulation option, though it does hold some caveats. It works by chelating calcium and thereby inhibiting the coagulation cascade. This can lead to profound hypocalcemia, and therefore frequent monitoring of the ionized calcium concentration is warranted. An infusion of calcium chloride post-filter is generally required to maintain adequate calcium levels. The major contraindication to citrate therapy is liver dysfunction, as these patients are unable to metabolize the citrate into bicarbonate.[1,3]
- The main advantages of CRRT over HD is that it is better tolerated from a hemodynamic standpoint, is highly effective in volume removal, has less of an effect on intracranial pressure (important in cerebral edema), and results in better control of electrolyte and acid-base disturbances due to steady-state chemistries.
- Hypophosphatemia during CRRT is a common complication, as conventional CRRT fluids have no phosphorus. Therefore, frequent monitoring and supplementation with phosphorus is given when necessary. Phoxillum is the only commercially available solution that contains phosphorus; however, it is not available at all institutions.
- The ideal dose of CRRT is not known, as there are conflicting studies. One major study showed a 16% reduction in mortality in a prescribed effluent flow of 35–45 mL/kg/hour compared with 20 mL/kg/hour. However, a subsequent study comparing 40 mL/kg/hour with 20 mL/kg/hour failed to show any mortality benefit in the higher dose.[4,5]
- When aiming for a higher flow (and therefore clearance), one should also be cognizant that the higher clearance may lead to inadequate concentrations of important medications such as antibiotics. It is imperative to dose antibiotics to the prescribed effluent dose. This can be particularly difficult in a patient who experiences multiple episodes of clotting, because the prescribed effluent rate and the delivered effluent rate may differ significantly due to time off of the machine.
- Medication clearance in CRRT is complex, and due to the variability in techniques, it may be extremely challenging to predict. Molecular weight, extent of protein binding, and the volume of distribution of a medication will all factor into the clearance. In addition, the prescribed prescription of CRRT (i.e., dialysate/effluent rate) will influence the clearance of a medication. Higher flow rates will increase clearances, and higher doses of medications will be required.[1]
- An additional factor that is unique in CRRT is the variable residual renal function. Patients on CRRT are critically ill and can have highly fluctuating residual renal function within a given day; it is extremely important to account for this especially when dosing antibiotics.
- As there are so many variables for medication dosing in CRRT, it is always best to use a reference such as Drug Prescribing in Renal Failure: Dosing Guidelines for Adults and Children or The Renal Drug Handbook.[6,7]

References

1. Daugirdas JT, Blake PG, Ing TS. *Handbook of Dialysis*. 5th ed. Philadelphia, PA: Wolters Kluwer Health; 2015.
2. Kellum JA, Lameire N, Aspelin P, et al. Kidney Disease: Improving Global Outcomes (KDIGO) acute kidney injury work group. KDIGO clinical practice guideline for acute kidney injury. *Kidney Int Suppl*. 2012;2:1–38.
3. Gilbert S, Weiner D. *National Kidney Foundation Primer of Kidney Disease*. 7th ed. London: Elsevier Health Sciences; 2017.
4. Ronco C, Bellomo R, Homel P, et al. Effects of different doses in continuous veno-venous haemofiltration on outcomes of acute renal failure: a prospective randomized trial. *Lancet*. 2000;355:26–30.
5. Bellomo R, Cass A, Cole L, et al. Intensity of continuous renal-replacement therapy in critically ill patients. *N Engl J Med*. 2009;361:1627–1638.
6. Aronoff GR, et al. *Drug Prescribing in Renal Failure: Dosing Guidelines for Adults and Children*. 5th ed. Philadelphia, PA: American College of Physicians; 2007.
7. Dunleavy A, Ashley C. *The Renal Drug Handbook: The Ultimate Prescribing Guide for Renal Practitioners*. 5th ed.: CRC Press; 2018.

CHAPTER 20

Coronary Artery Bypass Grafting

Amit Alam, MD ▪ Ali Seyar Rahyab, MD

Background

Cardiovascular disease is the leading cause of death in the United States. An American suffers from a myocardial infarction approximately every 40 seconds. On average, men are 65 years old and women are 72 years old at the time of the first myocardial infarction. The death rate for coronary artery disease (CAD) has decreased by 31.8% over the 10-year period from 2006 to 2016. This has been attributed to effective treatment and prevention, which includes coronary artery bypass grafting (CABG).[1]

CABG is a surgical procedure to treat ischemic heart disease due to obstruction of the coronary arteries. The procedure involves redirecting blood flow around (or bypassing) an obstruction in a coronary artery using a vessel from an alternative location. Approximately 371,000 CABG procedures are performed annually in the United States.[1]

How to Use It

The diagnosis of CAD is made using coronary angiography when a patient has a myocardial infarction or angina symptoms. Subsequently, most medical centers will employ a "heart team" approach in which the results of the angiography are discussed among the cardiologists and cardiothoracic surgeons. If a patient is deemed to be a CABG candidate, the patient will undergo the operation. CABG is performed with the intention to treat CAD that has already been diagnosed, and typically no further diagnostic evaluation is undertaken during the CABG procedure itself.

The choice to proceed with CABG versus percutaneous coronary intervention (PCI) is a clinical decision taking into account baseline patient characteristics, such as functional status along with the coronary anatomy (including the location and severity of the obstructing lesions), and the patient's ability to tolerate and comply with the dual antiplatelet therapy required after PCI. In general, patients with diabetes mellitus and multivessel CAD undergo CABG.[2] For patients with triple-vessel or complex CAD, the preferred treatment is also CABG.[3] Patients who require dual antiplatelet agents for another indication or who are at high risk for surgery will typically undergo PCI. See Chapter 46: Percutaneous Coronary Intervention for more details about this procedure.

How It Is Done

CABG is performed by a cardiothoracic surgeon in the operating room. The main incision is the median sternotomy in which the anterior sternum is exposed. The surgeon will select a blood vessel to serve as the bypass blood vessel. The goal is to provide blood flow beyond the point of a blockage in a coronary artery. This is done by connecting a new blood vessel (the graft vessel), which comes with its own blood supply, to the distal part of the blocked coronary artery at a point past the blockage. In this manner, the blockage is bypassed and blood flow is restored to the coronary artery distal to the blockage.

The most common graft vessels are the left internal thoracic artery, the right internal thoracic artery, and the greater saphenous vein from the leg. The internal thoracic arteries typically remain connected to the subclavian artery proximally and are connected to the coronary artery distally. The greater saphenous vein is harvested from the leg and connected to the aorta proximally and to the diseased coronary artery distally. A radial artery may also be utilized, and it is harvested from the forearm and subsequently connected to the aorta proximally and the diseased coronary artery distally.[4]

In order to perform a CABG operation, the heart must remain still, and the body must remain oxygenated and perfused. This is achieved using a cardiopulmonary bypass device in which blood is routed away from the heart and lungs to an external oxygenator and is returned to the aorta distal to the clamped proximal aorta. The heart is purposely stopped during this time (known as cardioplegia) to reduce myocardial oxygen demand and prevent myocardial damage. This is typically achieved using cold fluids, chemicals, or via electrical stimulation. Once the appropriate graft vessels have been harvested and connected to the target coronary arteries, the heart is disconnected from the cardiopulmonary bypass and normal circulation is restored. The patient is monitored for appropriate blood flow in the operating room, and subsequently the sternum is closed using wires and sutures. With a successful CABG, patients will experience a resolution of angina symptoms, and the overall risk of death and myocardial infarction is significantly reduced.

Medication Implications
BEFORE THE PROCEDURE

- Antiplatelet agents:
  - Aspirin 100–325 mg daily should be continued before CABG.
  - Any other additional antiplatelet agent needs to be discontinued prior to the procedure due to concern for bleeding. The guidelines discussed below provide recommendations for discontinuing dual antiplatelet agents prior to CABG; however, emergent or urgent cases may proceed with a minimum of 24 hours off the second agent based on the surgeon's assessment of bleeding and the clinical urgency.[5] These agents include:
    - Clopidogrel: Prodrug that becomes an active metabolite that is an irreversible inhibitor of the P2Y12 ADP receptor on platelets.[6] The guidelines recommend discontinuing it 5 days prior to CABG.[5] There are significant drug interactions that need to be considered. These include:
      - Omeprazole/esomeprazole: These two proton pump inhibitors inhibit the activity of clopidogrel due to inhibited cytochrome P450 2C19 activation and other cytochrome P450 2C19-inhibiting medications will have the same effect. Pantoprazole, lansoprazole, and dexlansoprazole have less of an impact on clopidogrel activity. The clinical relevance of these interactions is a controversial issue.
      - Opioids reduce the absorption of clopidogrel.
      - Selective serotonin reuptake inhibitors (SSRIs), serotonin-norepinephrine reuptake inhibitors (SNRIs), and nonsteroidal anti-inflammatory drugs (NSAIDs) also inhibit platelet activity and may increase the risk of bleeding if used with clopidogrel.
      - Clopidogrel will increase the concentration of repaglinide and may lead to hypoglycemia if both medications are used in combination.
    - Prasugrel: Irreversible inhibitor of the P2Y12 ADP receptor on platelets.[7] The guidelines recommend discontinuing it 7 days prior to CABG.[5] A lower dose is indicated in individuals weighing less than 60 kg, and it is contraindicated in patients with a history of stroke or transient ischemic attack (TIA). It may be used with medications that inhibit or induce cytochrome P450. It can be used with glycoprotein IIb/IIIa inhibitors, statins, digoxin, proton pump inhibitors, and histamine-2 blockers and no significant drug interactions have been noted. Common nonbleeding-related adverse effects include hypertension, hyperlipidemia, shortness of breath, back pain, headache, nausea, dizziness, cough, hypotension, fatigue, and chest pain.

- Ticagrelor: Reversible inhibitor of the P2Y12 ADP receptor on platelets.[8] The guidelines recommend discontinuing it 5 days prior to CABG.[5] A history of intracerebral hemorrhage is a contraindication, and there is a warning against use in severe hepatic impairment. The most common nonbleeding side effect is dyspnea, thought to be due to an increase in adenosine. Bradycardia and ventricular pauses have also been noted. There are significant drug interactions that need to be considered. These include:
  - Cytochrome P450 3A inhibitors (such as ketoconazole, clarithromycin, ritonavir) will lead to an increased concentration of ticagrelor.
  - Cytochrome P450 3A inducers (such as rifampin, phenytoin, carbamazepine, phenobarbital) will lead to a reduced concentration of ticagrelor.
  - Ticagrelor will increase the concentration of simvastatin and lovastatin.
  - Digoxin concentration can become increased due to p-glycoprotein inhibition and may need to be monitored.
  - Aspirin at doses greater than 100 mg daily can reduce the effectiveness of ticagrelor.
- Oral anticoagulants should be discontinued prior to a CABG procedure. For warfarin, the international normalized ratio (INR) should be less than 2.0. Direct oral anticoagulants (such as dabigatran, apixaban, rivaroxaban, edoxaban) are generally discontinued 3 days prior to the surgery.[9] Patients who require urgent CABG and cannot wait this period of time may be treated with reversal agents. Intravenous heparin may be continued as it will also be used during the procedure intraoperatively.
- Beta blockers (such as metoprolol or carvedilol) should be started in all patients prior to CABG and continued afterward to reduce the risk of postoperative atrial fibrillation.

DURING THE PROCEDURE

- Anticoagulation: A continuous heparin infusion is maintained throughout the CABG procedure to prevent blood clotting within the cardiopulmonary bypass device.
- Anesthetic agents and neuromuscular agents are utilized for general anesthesia and paralysis.
- Cardioplegia solution is given to reduce myocardial oxygen demand. It is a mixture that includes calcium, magnesium, potassium, saline, and may be mixed with lidocaine or procainamide.
- Blood pressure management: If the patient becomes hypotensive, the most common agent that is utilized is intravenous phenylephrine (alpha adrenergic agonist), which causes systemic vasoconstriction leading to an increase in blood pressure.
- Cardiac arrhythmias may occur and a lidocaine bolus is typically given as prophylaxis during the procedure to prevent ventricular arrhythmias.[10]

AFTER THE PROCEDURE

- If aspirin 100–325 mg daily was not given preoperatively, it should be started within 6 hours postoperatively and continued indefinitely.
  - Clopidogrel 75 mg daily is a reasonable choice if the patient is intolerant to aspirin, despite not having evidence as strong as that for aspirin.
  - The current guidelines from 2011 do not recommend the routine use of dual antiplatelet agents post CABG; however, there are ongoing randomized controlled trials evaluating the use of a second agent either instead of aspirin or in addition to it.[11] The current level of evidence is insufficient and has not led to an update of the guidelines. Dual antiplatelet agents are not routinely prescribed in all patients post CABG at this time. The decision to start or continue a second antiplatelet agent in certain patients, including when it should be started postoperatively, is an individualized decision that takes into account patient factors such as bleeding risk based on the operation and risk of graft vessel or native coronary artery stenosis based on the patient's anatomy.

- The most common cardiac event post CABG is the development of atrial fibrillation.
  - Beta blockers are utilized preoperatively and postoperatively to reduce the incidence of atrial fibrillation.
  - Anticoagulation for postoperative atrial fibrillation is typically instituted on day 3 after CABG to reduce the risk of bleeding in the first few days post procedure.
  - Choices for anticoagulation for atrial fibrillation include warfarin, dabigatran, rivaroxaban, apixaban, or edoxaban.[5]
  - There are no randomized controlled trial data comparing direct oral anticoagulants with warfarin or head-to-head in the post-CABG patient. A retrospective study demonstrated an increased risk for pericardial or pleural effusions in patients who received a direct oral anticoagulant compared with warfarin.[12] However, this data is limited, and the overall sample size was small. The choice of anticoagulation is an area that requires further research and prospective randomized controlled studies.
- Beta blockers and statins should be prescribed to all patients upon discharge unless contraindicated. Angiotensin-converting enzyme inhibitors or angiotensin II receptor blockers should be prescribed to all patients with a compelling indication (i.e., diabetes mellitus, heart failure with reduced ejection fraction, hypertension, chronic kidney disease) unless contraindicated.
- Nonsteroidal anti-inflammatory cyclooxygenase-2 inhibitors should be avoided in the postoperative period, and they are specifically contraindicated in a "black box" warning due to increased risk of myocardial infarction and stroke.[5,13]

References

1. Benjamin EJ, Muntner P, Alonso A, et al. Heart disease and stroke statistics-2019 update: a report from the American Heart Association. *Circulation.* 2019;139:e56–e528.
2. Kappetein AP, Head SJ, Morice MC, et al. Treatment of complex coronary artery disease in patients with diabetes: 5-year results comparing outcomes of bypass surgery and percutaneous coronary intervention in the SYNTAX trial. *Eur J Cardiothorac Surg.* 2013;43:1006–1013.
3. Kappetein AP, Feldman TE, Mack MJ, et al. Comparison of coronary bypass surgery with drug-eluting stenting for the treatment of left main and/or three-vessel disease: 3-year follow-up of the SYNTAX trial. *Eur Heart J.* 2011;32:2125–2134.
4. Okada S, Robertson JO, Saint LL, et al. Acquired Heart Disease. In: Brunicardi F, Andersen DK, Billiar TR et al, eds. *Schwartz's Principles of Surgery.* 10th ed. New York, NY: McGraw-Hill; 2015. http://access-medicine.mhmedical.com/content.aspx?bookid=980&sectionid=59610863. Accessed April 02, 2020.
5. Hillis LD, Smith PK, Anderson JL, et al. 2011 ACCF/AHA guideline for coronary artery bypass graft surgery. a report of the American College of Cardiology Foundation/American Heart Association Task Force on practice guidelines. Developed in collaboration with the American Association for Thoracic Surgery, Society of Cardiovascular Anesthesiologists, and Society of Thoracic Surgeons. *J Am Coll Cardiol.* 2011;58:e123–e210.
6. Clopidogrel [package insert]. Quebec, Canada: Sanofi-Aventis; 2019.
7. Prasugrel [package insert]. Indianapolis, IN: Eli Lilly; 2019.
8. Ticagrelor [package insert]. Mississauga, Ontario: AzstraZeneca; 2019.
9. Godier A, Dincq AS, Martin AC, et al. Predictors of pre-procedural concentrations of direct oral anticoagulants: a prospective multicenter study. *Eur Heart J.* 2017;38:2431.
10. Dias RR, Stolf NA, Dalva M, et al. Inclusion of lidocaine in cardioplegic solutions provides additional myocardial protection. *J Cardiovasc Surg (Torino).* 2004;45:551–555.
11. Thuijs DJFM, Milojevic M, Head SJ. Doubling up on antiplatelet therapy after CABG: changing practice ASAP after DACAB? *J Thorac Dis.* 2018;10:S3095–S3099.
12. Yu PJ, Lin D, Catalano M, et al. Impact of novel oral anticoagulants vs warfarin on effusions after coronary artery bypass grafting. *J Card Surg.* 2019;34:419–423.
13. Celecoxib [package insert]. New York, NY: Pfizer; 2019.

CHAPTER 21

Culture - Blood

Nicholas W. Van Hise, PharmD, BCPS

Background

Blood culture is the most efficient way of identifying organisms in the blood. For someone who does not have an infection, blood should always be sterile.[1] The most common organisms identified in the blood are bacteria and fungi, and their presence is called bacteremia and fungemia, respectively.[1] Despite their possible presence in the blood, viruses are not typically identified through traditional blood culture technique because the isolation properties are targeted toward identifying bacteria or fungi.[1] This chapter will mainly discuss bacteremia, as bacteria are the most commonly identified microorganisms.

How to Use It

Identifying bacteria or fungi in the blood is important when treating infections. Following an initial positive result, the first step is to identify whether a culture is a true bacteremia or contamination. This determination can be quite difficult and should consider many factors, including the patient's clinical scenario, history, risk factors, surrogate markers of infection (e.g., white blood cell count, C-reactive protein, erythrocyte sedimentation rate [ESR], procalcitonin), estimated inoculum, and identity of the organism.[2-4] The most notable risk factors for blood stream infections include indwelling catheters, advanced age, immunosuppression, and loss of skin integrity. All other risk factors will stem from these.[2-4] For example, total parenteral nutrition (TPN) is a risk factor for both bacteremia and fungemia due to use of a chronic central line.

Various surrogate markers of infection have shown to be useful. Procalcitonin, the newest of these markers, is relatively specific to bacterial infections. The ESR, which is based on the turnover of red blood cells, can be an important determinant in someone with low-grade bacteremia from a deep-seeded source.[5] As mentioned earlier, the inoculum size is also an important factor. Inoculum size means the amount of bacteria in the blood at the given time of culture. In traditional culturing techniques, the amount of an organism needed to typically grow from a blood culture is 10^5 bacteria per bottle.[6] Currently, many facilities also use molecular diagnostics, which identify through polymerase chain reaction (PCR)-based techniques. These techniques can identify the presence of a single microorganism.[6] Traditional culturing versus PCR technology is an important factor to consider, as most adults who are presenting with an infection to a healthcare facility have low-grade bacteremia with less than 1 colony-forming unit (CFU) per mL, which PCR-based techniques can detect.[7] As discussed in the next section, the rate of positivity along with the identification of which draw site (i.e., bottle) tested positive can help identify whether a bacteremia is true or a contamination. For example, if there is a line infection from dialysis access, it is likely that the inoculum will be higher from that access site than a separate peripheral blood culture. If the dialysis access becomes positive first, this is called "first to positivity."[8] In the same sense, if the dialysis access culture tests positive and a separate peripheral intravenous access culture does not test positive, this may show potential contamination of the dialysis access sample.

When evaluating positive blood cultures, the organism that is identified is very important. *Staphylococcus epidermidis* (a coagulase-negative *staphylococcus*) is a common colonizer of skin flora and catheters, which in turn means that this is the most common contaminant of blood cultures.[4] If only one of two cultures returns positive with *S. epidermidis*, this is more likely to be a contaminant. In turn, a gram-negative bacteria or a different gram-positive bacteria such as *Staphylococcus aureus* are less likely to be contaminants. *S. aureus*, due to its virulence and ability to cause deep-seeded infections, is never considered a contaminant. This organism should always be evaluated to be a true infection and investigated for a potential source.[9,10] The two most common organisms to contaminate blood cultures are *S. epidermidis* and enterococci.

Repeating blood cultures can be essential in the setting of true infection and in contamination. If a patient is clinically stable, has no signs of infection, and blood cultures show one bottle being positive with a common skin contaminant, this is likely a contaminant. If the patient was not started on antibiotics, one consideration may be to repeat blood cultures to see if the blood is sterile while keeping in mind that the immune system may clear the blood without antibiotics. Alternatively, repeat cultures are typically necessary to document clearance if a patient has an organism that can lead to high rates of deep-seeded infection or those that cause high-grade bacteremia, such as *S. aureus*, group A *Streptococcus*, or *Enterococcus*. These cultures can be repeated daily depending on the clinical scenario to document clearance. If cultures remain positive for 48 hours despite antibiotics, this is classified as high-grade bacteremia and further sources need to be identified.[9,10]

It is important to identify in which patients blood cultures are necessary. This decision should take into account all of the above risk factors and include any patient suspected of a systemic infection. Systemic infection can be defined in various ways, some of which include specific criteria such as the sequential organ failure assessment (SOFA) scoring for sepsis.

How It Is Done

Antibiotic timing is one of the most important factors to consider when drawing blood cultures in a potentially infected patient. One dose of antibiotics can cause blood cultures to be falsely negative in a low-inoculum infection. Blood cultures should be drawn from two different sites with both times documented to assess time to positivity. Prior to drawing cultures, bottle tops should be disinfected to make sure that skin flora does not contaminate the culture. For an adult patient, 10–20 mL is sufficient for each bottle of a blood culture draw. Each site requires both an aerobic and an anaerobic bottle, for a total of four bottles.[1,3,4] A minimum of 10 mL per bottle is important as low-volume blood cultures are associated with higher rates of false-negative results.[7] If an intravenous catheter is the suspected source, one of the sets needs to be drawn from the catheter. It is not recommended to culture the catheter tip as this has shown to increase antimicrobial usage and leads to a high rate of contamination. If drawing blood cultures before treatment with antibiotics is not an option in the setting of a worsening infection, it is important to draw blood cultures prior to the change of antibiotics.

The rate of positivity can depend on many factors as mentioned above, including the inoculum size and how quickly the organism grows during incubation.[11,12] Many gram-negative organisms may result as positive within 12–24 hours, whereas some gram-positive organisms, HACEK organisms (*Haemophilus, Aggregatibacter, Cardiobacterium hominis, Eikenella corrodens, Kingella*), or fungi may require many days to grow.[11,12]

The steps of a blood culture include the blood draw, incubation of the blood culture bottle, and, in some scenarios, rapid detection techniques (i.e., PCR-based method). If rapid detection is utilized, depending on the instrument, a PCR result showing resistance mechanisms may be available within hours. Once a blood bottle tests positive for an organism, even if rapid detection methods are not used, that organism is then subcultured onto a plate and identified through Gram stain. The Gram stain results will initially show gram positive or gram negative. Then, the organism will be put on an instrument to identify the genus and species, along with the sensitivity to a panel of antibiotics.

Medication Implications

- In the majority of patients, the technique for drawing blood cultures is through a simple intravenous blood draw from a peripheral or central venous catheter. This does not require premedication for the draw. See Chapter 37: Intravenous Access for more details about phlebotomy and venous access sites.
- When possible, a blood culture should be collected prior to administration of empiric antibiotics. Administration of antibiotics prior to blood cultures can yield false-negative results.
- If there is a high suspicion for bacteremia despite negative blood cultures, antibiotics should not be discontinued and blood cultures should be redrawn. Antibiotic selection will be discussed below, but empiric selection should be based on the patient history and antimicrobial resistance trends in the hospital/community.
- Assessing the clinical significance of positive blood cultures can be difficult in some cases. Characteristics that should be taken into consideration are the number of positive blood culture bottles, the time to positivity, the site(s) that became positive, surrogate markers of infection, and the organism recovered.
- Empiric antibiotic recommendations for bacteremia should be based on the suspected source of infection, antimicrobial resistance trends in the hospital/community, previous organisms isolated from the patient, along with pharmacokinetics and pharmacodynamics of the antibiotic that is being considered. For example, if a patient has methicillin-resistant *S. aureus* (MRSA) bacteremia, doxycycline would be an incorrect choice for treatment. Although doxycycline covers MRSA empirically and may report sensitive on culture, the serum concentration for the drug would not be adequate to treat a bacteremic patient. Another example is daptomycin for an MRSA pneumonia. Since daptomycin is bound by lung surfactant, this would not clear the source of the MRSA bacteremia. Although it may clear the blood intermittently, by not clearing the source, the infection will ultimately not resolve.
- Antibiotic recommendations for gram-negative bacteremia should be divided into two categories[13–18]:
    - Without sepsis:
        - For those without risk factors for resistance: third- or fourth-generation cephalosporin (e.g., ceftriaxone or cefepime) or beta-lactam/beta-lactamase inhibitor (e.g., piperacillin/tazobactam) or cefazolin
        - For those with risk factors for resistance: fourth-generation cephalosporin or beta-lactam/beta-lactamase inhibitor or an antipseudomonal carbapenem
    - With sepsis:
        - Fourth-generation cephalosporin or beta-lactam/beta-lactamase inhibitor or an antipseudomonal carbapenem or aztreonam (for those with penicillin allergies)
    - Fluoroquinolones are not typically recommended empirically due to the high level of resistance within most communities.
    - Risk factors for gram-negative multidrug resistance[13–18]:
        - Presence of healthcare exposures including hospitalizations, hemodialysis, or admission into a long-term care facility
        - Recent intravenous antibiotics, chemotherapy, or immunosuppression
- Antibiotic recommendations for *S. aureus* bacteremia (prior to availability of sensitivity results)[19]
    - In the setting of a potentially high-grade bacteremia, cefazolin or nafcillin (to cover methicillin-sensitive *S. aureus*) in addition to vancomycin (to cover MRSA) may be prudent until susceptibilities result.
- Antibiotic recommendations for enterococci bacteremia (prior to availability of sensitivity results)[20]

- Empiric therapy includes ampicillin plus either vancomycin or daptomycin
- Daptomycin should be considered in patients with high rates of vancomycin-resistant enterococci (VRE) in their community or for those that have isolated VRE in the past.
- Treatment of bacteremic septic patients with unknown source:
  - Empiric therapy includes a fourth-generation cephalosporin or beta-lactam/beta-lactamase inhibitor or an antipseudomonal carbapenem.
  - Patients with penicillin allergy: aztreonam plus vancomycin
  - The addition of double coverage is dependent on the risk factors for multidrug resistance.
    - In septic patients, double coverage of potential gram-negative bacteremia can be considered an aminoglycoside with the highest susceptibility rates. Of note, this is purely dependent on community/facility resistance rates along with history of multidrug resistance within the patient.
- Following empiric treatment, definitive treatment of bacteremia will depend on the resistance pattern of the organism found on sensitivity report.
- As bacteremia can be caused by a variety of sources, treatment specifics such as duration of therapy and antibiotic choices have many nuances. For example, some infections require only a week of antibiotics whereas others require several months. When possible, professional guidelines such as those published by the Infectious Diseases Society of America and the American Thoracic Society should be consulted.

References

1. Weinstein MP. Current blood culture methods and systems: clinical concepts, technology, and interpretation of results. *Clin Infect Dis*. 1996;26:40–46.
2. Magadia RR, Weinstein MP. Laboratory diagnosis of bacteremia and fungemia. *Infect Dis Clin North Am*. 2001;15:1009–1024.
3. Mirrett S, Weinstein MP, Reimer LG, et al. Relevance of the number of positive bottles in determining clinical significance of coagulase-negative staphylococci in blood cultures. *J Clin Microbiol*. 2001;39:3279–3281.
4. Beekmann SE, Diekema DJ, Doern GV. Determining the clinical significance of coagulase-negative staphylococci isolated from blood cultures. *Infect Control Hosp Epidemiol*. 2005;26:559–566.
5. Fritz JM, McDonald JR. Osteomyelitis: approach to diagnosis and treatment. *Phys Sportsmed*. 2008;36:50–54.
6. Weinstein MP, Mirrett S, Wilson ML, et al. Controlled evaluation of 5 versus 10 milliliters of blood cultured in aerobic BacT/Alert blood culture bottles. *J Clin Microbiol*. 1994:2103–2106.
7. Mermel LA, Maki DG. Detection of bacteremia in adults: consequences of culturing an inadequate volume of blood. *Ann Internal Med*. 1993;119:270–272.
8. Lambregts MM, Bernards AT, van der Beek MT, et al. Time to positivity of blood cultures supports early re-evaluation of empiric broad-spectrum antimicrobial therapy. *PloS One*. 2019;14:e0208819.
9. Lowy FD. *Staphylococcus aureus* infections. *N Engl J Med*. 1998;339:520–532.
10. Fowler VG, Justice A, Moore C, et al. Risk factors for hematogenous complications of intravascular catheter-associated Staphylococcus aureus bacteremia. *Clin Infect Dis*. 2005;40:695–703.
11. Baron EJ, Scott JD, Tompkins LS. Prolonged incubation and extensive subculturing do not increase recovery of clinically significant microorganisms from standard automated blood cultures. *Clin Infect Dis*. 2005;41:1677–1680.
12. Marra AR, Edmond MB, Forbes BA, et al. Time to blood culture positivity as a predictor of clinical outcome of Staphylococcus aureus bloodstream infection. *J Clin Microbiol*. 2006;44:1342–1346.
13. Kang CI, Kim SH, Park WB, et al. Bloodstream infections caused by antibiotic-resistant gram-negative bacilli: risk factors for mortality and impact of inappropriate initial antimicrobial therapy on outcome. *Antimicrob Agents Chemother*. 2005;49:760–766.
14. Canzoneri CN, Akhavan BJ, Tosur Z, et al. Follow-up blood cultures in gram-negative bacteremia: are they needed? *Clin Infect Dis*. 2017;65:1776–1779.
15. Shorr AF, Tabak YP, Killian AD, et al. Healthcare-associated bloodstream infection: a distinct entity? Insights from a large U.S. database. *Crit Care Med*. 2006;34:2588–2595.
16. Lee CC, Wu CJ, Chi CH, et al. Prediction of community-onset bacteremia among febrile adults visiting an emergency department: rigor matters. *Diagn Microbiol Infect Dis*. 2012;73:168–173.

17. Graff LR, Franklin KK, Witt L, et al. Antimicrobial therapy of gram-negative bacteremia at two university-affiliated medical centers. *Am J Med.* 2002;112:204–211.
18. Vidal F, Mensa J, Almela M, et al. Bacteraemia in adults due to glucose non-fermentative Gram-negative bacilli other than P. aeruginosa. *QJM.* 2003;96:227–234.
19. Holland TL, Arnold C, Fowler VG. Clinical management of *Staphylococcus aureus* bacteremia: a review. *JAMA.* 2014;312:1330–1341.
20. Antalek MD, Mylotte JM, Lesse AJ, et al. Clinical and molecular epidemiology of *Enterococcus faecalis* bacteremia, with special reference to strains with high-level resistance to gentamicin. *Clin Infect Dis.* 1995;20:103–109.

CHAPTER 22

Culture - Sputum

Andrew J. Crannage, PharmD, FNKF, FCCP, BCPS

Background

A sputum culture is often a noninvasive and most useful test in the assessment of lower respiratory tract infections. Sputum samples can be useful in other disease states such as certain cancers; however, sampling is predominately useful for infectious diseases. Obtained sputum can be tested and evaluated via Gram stain, microbiologic culture, and sensitivity testing. These procedures are most frequently performed simultaneously and interpreted together in the evaluation of a sputum sample.[1]

How to Use It

Pneumonia, an infection of the lower respiratory tract, is a cause of significant morbidity and mortality. Sputum is a secretion of the respiratory tract and via collection can aid in the identification of etiologic microorganisms of infection. More specifically, sputum is primarily composed of secretions from the tracheobronchial tree. Minimal secretions from the upper airway contribute to the composition of sputum. Due to these details on sputum origin, certain characteristics must be considered and evaluated to determine the adequacy of sputum sampling. In order to be adequate for culture, the sample must contain less than 10 squamous epithelial cells and greater than 25 neutrophils when observed under low-power field. Both of these criteria allow for affirmation of a lower, rather than upper, respiratory tract collection. Performing Gram staining, microbiologic culture, and sensitivity testing on the sputum sample allows for identification of etiologic microorganisms and selection of appropriate antimicrobial therapy in infections of the lower respiratory tract. These results provide important details on the bacteria present in the respiratory tract. First, the culture identifies if a bacteria is located in the respiratory tract. If positive, Gram staining describes whether the organism is gram positive or gram negative and the shape and orientation to aid in identification. The culture later provides specific bacterial identification. A sensitivity report identifies minimum inhibitory concentrations of antibiotics that are used to label expected bacterial responses to specific antibiotics as sensitive, intermediate, or resistant. All of this information is used together to guide treatment of a specific patient. No one finding should be used solely, but rather as components integral to patient management.[1,2]

How It Is Done

Pre-treatment sputum samples should be collected from patients in the hospital setting with severe community-acquired pneumonia (CAP), patients with pneumonia being treated empirically for methicillin-resistant *Staphylococcus aureus* (MRSA) or *Pseudomonas aeruginosa*, or with hospital-acquired pneumonia (HAP).[3,4] The majority of patients will be able to provide sputum in a noninvasive manner via spontaneous expectoration into a collection container. A sputum sample from a patient without pneumonia should yield no bacterial growth. However, some patients without pneumonia will still have bacterial growth, indicating bacterial colonization. Similarly, not all patients with pneumonia will have bacterial growth, most commonly due to inadequate sampling. In order to ensure an adequate sputum sample via expectoration, rather than saliva and upper respiratory tract secretions, patients should attempt to generate the sample from a deep cough of the lungs. In some patients who are unable to produce an adequate sample via expectoration, more invasive methods and procedures are available. Examples of these include bronchoalveolar lavage or protected specimen brush, performed during a bronchoscopy. See Chapter 13: Bronchoscopy for details about this procedure. Assessment and evaluation methods of samples from invasive techniques often vary and can be specific to the institution.[2]

Medication Implications

- In the majority of patients, the technique to obtain sputum is spontaneous expectoration, which is noninvasive and does not require administration of medications prior to or during the process.
- As hypovolemia is common in patients with infectious diseases, one cause for the inability to produce spontaneously expectorated sputum is dehydration or hypovolemia. Sputum production may be increased with correction of dehydration. Administration of intravenous fluids, particularly isotonic fluids such as lactated Ringer's or normal saline, can correct hypovolemia and be beneficial in increasing sputum production.[5] Crystalloid therapy is especially beneficial for critically ill patients.[6] Additionally, as radiography of the chest is often done together with sputum evaluations, correction of hypovolemia can improve identification of infiltrates, which become more pronounced in radiologic images. See Chapter 16: Chest X-ray for more details.
- Sputum expectoration may also be induced in patients who are not able to spontaneously expectorate. Inhaled hypertonic saline, often 6%–7% sodium chloride, is moisturizing to the pulmonary system but also irritating after inhalation, which can induce sputum expectoration.[1,7] Other therapies such as bronchodilator therapy are often used with hypertonic saline to prevent excessive bronchoconstriction.
  - Sputum induction may help improve the adequacy of sputum sampling.[8] Sputum induction with hypertonic saline is the most studied, though less evidence exists for other therapies, such as guaifenesin.
  - Sputum induction is not only limited to medications, but devices using acoustic waves may also aid in sputum clearance.
- When possible, a sputum sample should be collected prior to administration of empiric antibiotics. Administration of antibiotics prior to sample collection can inhibit growth of bacteria on microbiologic media. Yield rates for positive culture results are generally low in sputum cultures (30–50% of patients with pneumonia have negative sputum cultures) and are further reduced with the administration of antibiotics prior to sample collection.[2,9]
- If the patient has signs and symptoms suggestive of pneumonia, empiric antibiotics should be initiated after attempting collection of the sputum sample, even before culture results are available. Empiric antibiotic selections should be based on the categorization of CAP versus HAP.
- Empiric antibiotic recommendations for CAP in the outpatient setting are dependent upon the presence of comorbidities or risk factors for resistant pathogens.[3]
  - Comorbidities include chronic heart, lung, liver, or renal disease; diabetes mellitus; alcoholism; malignancy; or asplenia.
  - Risk factors for resistant pathogens include prior respiratory isolation of MRSA or *P. aeruginosa* or recent hospitalization along with receipt of parenteral antibiotics within the previous 90 days.
- Antibiotic recommendations for CAP in the outpatient setting with no comorbidities or risk factors for MRSA or *P. aeruginosa* include: amoxicillin, doxycycline, or macrolide therapy.[3]

- Antibiotic recommendations for CAP in the outpatient setting with comorbidities include[3]:
  - Combination treatment with amoxicillin/clavulanate or cephalosporin therapy PLUS macrolide therapy or doxycycline
  - Monotherapy with a respiratory fluoroquinolone (e.g., levofloxacin 750 mg daily or moxifloxacin 400 mg daily)
- Empiric antibiotic recommendations for CAP in the inpatient setting are dependent upon the level of severity and drug resistance risk factors.[3] Severity is determined by a combination of signs, symptoms, and laboratory values as defined in the Infectious Diseases Society of America guidelines.[3]
- Antibiotic recommendations for nonsevere CAP without risk factors for MRSA or *P. aeruginosa* in the inpatient setting include:
  - Combination treatment with beta-lactam therapy plus macrolide therapy, or monotherapy with a respiratory fluoroquinolone.[3]
- Antibiotic recommendations for severe CAP without risk factors for MRSA or *P. aeruginosa* in the inpatient setting include:
  - Combination treatment with beta-lactam therapy plus macrolide therapy, or beta-lactam therapy plus respiratory fluoroquinolone therapy.[3]
- Empiric antibiotic recommendations for HAP are dependent upon the risk of patient mortality and risk factors for MRSA.[4]
  - Patients with HAP should receive an antibiotic that provides empiric activity against *P. aeruginosa*; however, aminoglycosides should be avoided as monotherapy.[4]
  - Patients with HAP who have received intravenous antibiotics in the previous 90 days or have a high risk of mortality should receive two antibiotics from different classes with activity against *P. aeruginosa*.[4]
  - Antibiotic recommendations for patients with HAP who are not at high risk of mortality and have no risk factors for MRSA include agents with activity against methicillin-susceptible *S. aureus* (MSSA). Recommended agents include: piperacillin-tazobactam, cefepime, imipenem, meropenem, or levofloxacin.[4]
  - Antibiotic recommendations for patients with HAP with risk factors for MRSA or at high risk of mortality include: vancomycin or linezolid.[4]
  - Daptomycin is an agent usually reserved for severe MRSA infections. Regardless of sensitivity results, its use for pneumonia is not recommended, as daptomycin activity is severely limited by pulmonary surfactant.[10]
- Gram staining and culture techniques performed on sputum samples should be used to refine antibiotic selections. While broad-spectrum antibiotics are often common in the empiric treatment of multiple pneumonia types, narrow-spectrum agents are advantageous as additional patient factors, such as response and laboratory data, are obtained. De-escalation should be considered whenever possible to prevent and reduce resistance and adverse effects. As with all medication therapy, patient-specific considerations such as allergies, contraindications, drug interactions, and renally adjusted dosing must be fully considered in choosing empiric therapy and adjusting therapy based upon sputum culture results.

References

1. Jameson JL, Kasper DL, Longo DL, et al. *Harrison's Principles of Internal Medicine*. 20th ed. New York, NY: McGraw-Hill; 2018.
2. Lee M. *Basic Skills in Interpreting Laboratory Data*. 6th ed. Bethesda, MD: American Society of Health-System Pharmacists; 2017.
3. Metlay JP, Waterer GW, Long AC, et al. Diagnosis and treatment of adults with community-acquired pneumonia: an official clinical practice guideline of the American Thoracic Society and Infectious Diseases Society of America. *Am J Respir Crit Care Med*. 2019;200:e45–e67.

4. Kalil AC, Metersky ML, Klompas M, et al. Management of adults with hospital-acquired and ventilator-associated pneumonia: 2016 clinical practice guidelines by the Infectious Diseases Society of America and the American Thoracic Society. *Clin Infect Dis*. 2016;63:e61–e111.
5. Dipiro JT, Talbert JT, Yee GC, et al. *Pharmacotherapy: A Pathophysiologic Approach*. 10th ed. New York, NY: McGraw-Hill; 2017.
6. Alderson P, Schierhout G, Roberts I, et al. Colloids versus crystalloids for fluid resuscitation in critical ill patients. *Cochrane Database Syst Rev*. 2000;2:CD000567.
7. Elkins MR, Bye PT. Mechanisms and applications of hypertonic saline. *J R Soc Med*. 2011;104:S2–S5.
8. Seong GM, Lee J, Lee JH, et al. Usefulness of sputum induction with hypertonic saline in a real clinical practice for bacteriological yields of active pulmonary tuberculosis. *Tuberc Respir Dis (Seoul)*. 2014;76:163–168.
9. Bartlett JG. Diagnostic tests for agents of community-acquired pneumonia. *Clin Infect Dis*. 2011;52:s296–s304.
10. Humphries RM, Pollett S, Sakoulas G. A current perspective on daptomycin for the clinical microbiologist. *Clin Microbiol Rev*. 2013;26:759–780.

CHAPTER 23

Culture - Urine

Michael Kaplan, MD ■ Bruce E. Hirsch, MD

Background

Urinary tract infections (UTIs) have been around for as long as humans have had urinary tracts. Hippocrates believed that symptoms were caused by an imbalance of four humors. Ancient treatment regimens in the pre-antibiotic era ranged from bed rest to narcotics, and also included various herbs, enemas, and, in the heroic era of medical treatments, "judicious bleeding."[1]

While medicine has advanced a great deal since then, the diagnosis and management of UTIs remain nuanced, challenging, and fraught with complications. The overuse of antibiotics has changed medicine's relationship with UTIs and disease altogether, though humanity now finds itself facing epic levels of antimicrobial resistance, teetering on the brink of a post-antibiotic civilization. Excessive antibiotic use is also driving a national epidemic of *Clostridioides difficile* infection, with alarming rates of morbidity and mortality. It is, therefore, incumbent upon clinicians to understand when to use and when not to use antibiotics. Incorrectly interpreted urinalysis and urine cultures are too frequently the cause of inappropriate antibiotic prescription.

What follows is a guide to understanding the urine culture: a remarkably helpful test to guide antibiotic use, when appropriate. This chapter focuses on bacterial UTIs and largely side-steps fungal and viral UTIs. It concludes with a basic overview of the antibiotics used to treat UTIs, as outlined by the Infectious Diseases Society of America (IDSA), as well as some practical pearls regarding treatment of UTIs.

How to Use It

Urine culture <u>does not</u> indicate the presence of a UTI.
Urine culture does indicate:

- If there are any microbes living in the urine at the time of collection
  - Humans have natural flora in the genitourinary system just as in the gastrointestinal system.
  - Therefore, it is important to consider the clinical status of the patient.
    - It is the presence of *symptoms* (think irritation of the bladder wall; i.e., dysuria, frequency, some women report vaginal irritation, bladder spasm, pelvic pain, back pain, and of course systemic signs like fevers, etc.) that determines if a UTI is present.
  - *Pyuria,* the presence of white cells in the urine, does not establish the presence of infection. Its absence, however, renders a UTI very unlikely.
  - It is also possible to have a contaminated and thus "false-positive" urine culture (more likely with epithelial cells in the urinalysis) or "false-negative" leukocyte esterase in the urinalysis. See Chapter 58: Urinalysis for details about this test.
- The identity of any bacteria living there (e.g., *Escherichia coli*)
- The quantity of bacteria expressed in colony-forming units (CFUs)
  - 100,000 CFU is not sensitive or specific for a UTI.
    - Patients must be symptomatic to warrant treatment, otherwise this is probably colonization.

Susceptibility is derived by exposing organisms to antibiotics and seeing which ones inhibit their growth most effectively. Susceptibility is either reported as raw data using the minimum inhibitory concentration (MIC) or is interpreted using Clinical and Laboratory Standards Institute (CLSI) criteria.[2]

The CLSI interpretations provide a clinical assessment for whether certain bacteria are "susceptible," "resistant," or "intermediate" to a certain antibiotic. These interpretations are derived from both the MIC and pharmacokinetic knowledge of the antibiotic in question; therefore, the significance of MIC depends on which bacteria and antibiotic duo are being tested.[3] This is why MIC numbers cannot be meaningfully compared among antibiotics when looking at a sensitivity report.

A final word of caution—the results of antimicrobial susceptibility testing assume that in vitro antibiotic activity parallels in vivo reality. This is not always the case. Multiple host, bacterial, and drug-dependent factors may complicate the picture (e.g., absorption, biofilms). These are not accounted for by in vitro analysis.[2] As such, susceptibility data is meant to inform, not dictate, clinical decision making.

How It Is Done

Several milliliters of urine are obtained in the manner outlined in Chapter 58: Urinalysis. Bacteria are then isolated, cultured, and incubated.

There are multiple commercial methods to assess susceptibility, and most are designed to determine the MIC. The MIC is the lowest concentration of antibiotic that prevents growth of a given bacteria.[3] This is derived using a variety of methods (e.g., broth dilution, impregnated antibiotic strips on agar), but the logic is the same: standard concentrations of bacteria are exposed to serial dilutions of a given antibiotic, thereby revealing the concentration of antibiotic necessary to stop bacterial growth.[3]

Alternatively, the disk diffusion susceptibility method is when an antibiotic disk is placed in the middle of a bacterial inoculum grown on an agar plate. The plate is then incubated, and one measures to the nearest millimeter the "zone of inhibition"—a circle devoid of growth around the disk, an indirect marker of antibiotic susceptibility. Again, these data are interpreted using CLSI criteria. Finally, there are a series of automated instruments approved by the Food and Drug Administration that allow for more rapid susceptibility testing. These machines use sensitive optical detection that allows for subtle detection of changes in bacterial growth.[3]

Medication Implications

Antibiotics taken prior to urine culture may render a "false negative."

- A few small studies have demonstrated noninferiority of a single dose of fosfomycin in clearing asymptomatic bacteriuria in pregnancy (though importantly, the IDSA still recommends a 4- to 7-day course of antibiotics for treatment of pregnant women with asymptomatic bacteriuria).[4,5]
- Single doses of antibiotics, then, can render the urine culture "negative," despite a patient having a UTI requiring a complete course of antibiotics as outlined below.

TREATMENT OF ACUTE UNCOMPLICATED CYSTITIS AND PYELONEPHRITIS[6]

UTI (acute cystitis)

- Trimethoprim/sulfamethoxazole (TMP/SMX): one double-strength (800 mg/160 mg) tablet by mouth twice daily for 3 days
- Nitrofurantoin 100 mg by mouth twice daily for 5 days

- Fosfomycin 3 g by mouth once
- Fluoroquinolones are not first line for cystitis given risks. If using, treat for 3 days.
  - Concern for side effects: seizures, tendon rupture, hypoglycemia, QTc prolongation, exacerbation of myasthenia gravis, peripheral neuropathy, aortic aneurysm
- Beta-lactams in 3- to 7-day regimens
- Avoid amoxicillin or ampicillin empirically

Pyelonephritis

- Fluoroquinolones are first line
  - Ciprofloxacin 500 mg twice daily for 7 days or levofloxacin 750 mg for 5 days
- Oral TMP/SMX is acceptable if the bacteria is susceptible.

PEARLS REGARDING URINARY TRACT INFECTION MANAGEMENT

- Avoid ordering a urine culture in the elderly without specific urinary symptoms. Asymptomatic pyuria as well as asymptomatic bacteriuria are not uncommon in this population.
- Avoid nitrofurantoin in patients over 65 years old with creatinine clearance less than 30 mL/minute; it may predispose to pulmonary toxicity, hepatotoxicity, and neuropathy, especially with longer courses.[7]
- TMP/SMX is associated with disease flares and high rates of adverse drug reactions in patients with systemic lupus erythematosus (SLE).[8,9]
- Emerging data suggests that UTI-relevant antibiotics may actually predispose to the development of and flaring of rheumatoid arthritis.[10]
  - Sulfonamides and TMP antibiotics are associated with a 70% increased risk of rheumatoid arthritis flare at 1–3 months and an elevated risk persists at 1 year.
- TMP/SMX and nitrofurantoin are relatively contraindicated in glucose-6-phosphate dehydrogenase (G6PD) deficiency.
- Fosfomycin, given in two or three sequential oral doses, is an option for outpatient treatment of extended-spectrum beta-lactamase (ESBL) cystitis.
  - There is currently no other oral treatment available for infections caused by ESBL-producing organisms.
  - Consult with an infectious disease physician prior to using fosfomycin for this indication.
- The antibiotic history of the patient helps determine initial empiric antibiotic choice. An antibiotic given within the previous 3 months is more likely to fail due to acquired resistance.
- The urine of patients with chronic indwelling urethral catheters are <u>always</u> positive on culture.
  - Urine cultures from catheterized patients should not be done unless the clinical symptoms of the patient suggests infection.
- Asymptomatic bacteriuria should not be treated, with the following exceptions: upcoming urologic surgery and pregnancy.

PEARLS REGARDING ANTIBIOTIC STEWARDSHIP IN URINARY TRACT INFECTIONS

- The ultimate question, even if a patient has a UTI: Is it better for this patient to get antibiotics, or not? Many patients who are otherwise healthy can recover from UTIs with hydration and nonsteroidal anti-inflammatory drugs alone. If they are not manifesting systemic symptoms or are not predisposed to systemic illness, thinking in this way may help curb unnecessary antibiotic prescribing.
- It is the author's opinion that antibiotics should not be used to treat bacteriuria when the suspected symptom is delirium in noncatheterized elderly persons. These patients are very frequently admitted for "altered mental status" secondary to a UTI.

- There is no high-quality data to suggest that patients with delirium and asymptomatic bacteriuria do better with antibiotics.[11]
- Acute uncomplicated cystitis is benign: up to 42% of untreated women in studies reported early resolution of symptoms.[12] As such, given that most UTIs throughout history have been self-limited, a course of watchful waiting may be in these patients' best interests.
  - Exceptions to watchful waiting include: if the patient is significantly ill (e.g., meets systemic inflammatory response syndrome [SIRS] criteria), immunocompromised, pregnant, or has an upcoming urologic instrumentation.

References

1. Nickel JC. Management of urinary tract infections: historical perspective and current strategies: part 1—before antibiotics. *J Urol*. 2005;173:21–26.
2. Antimicrobial Susceptibility Testing: What does it mean? University of Pennsylvania Medical Center Guidelines for Antibiotic Use. Available at: http://www.uphs.upenn.edu/bugdrug/antibiotic_manual/amt.html. Accessed 1/17/2020.
3. Reller LB, Weinstein M, Jorgensen JH, et al. Antimicrobial susceptibility testing: a review of general principles and contemporary practices. *Clin Infect Dis*. 2009;49:1749–1755.
4. Guinto VT, De Guia B, Festin MR, et al. Different antibiotic regimens for treating asymptomatic bacteriuria in pregnancy. *Cochrane Database Syst Review*. 2010;9. Available at: https://www.ncbi.nlm.nih.gov/pubmed/20824868.
5. Infectious Disease Society of America guidelines: Management of Asymptomatic Bacteriuria: 2019 Update by the Infectious Disease Society of America. Available at: https://www.idsociety.org/practice-guideline/asymptomatic-bacteriuria/. Accessed 1/17/2020.
6. International Clinical Practice Guidelines for the Treatment of Acute Uncomplicated Cystitis and Pyelonephritis in Women: A 2010 Update by the Infectious Disease Society of America and the European Society for Microbiology and Infectious Diseases. Available at: https://academic.oup.com/cid/article/52/5/e103/388285. Accessed 1/17/2020.
7. American Geriatrics Society 2019 Updated AGS Beers criteria for potentially inappropriate medication use in older adults. *J Am Geriatr Soc*. 2019;00:1–21.
8. Suyama Y, Okada M, Rokutanda R, et al. Safety and efficacy of upfront graded administration of trimethoprim-sulfamethoxazole in systemic lupus erythematosus: a retrospective cohort study. *Modern Rheumatology*. 2016;26:557–561.
9. Johns Hopkins Lupus Center. 5 things to avoid if you have lupus. 2020. Available at: https://www.hopkinslupus.org/lupus-info/lifestyle-additional-information/avoid/. Accessed 1/17/2020.
10. Nagra NS, Robinson DE, Douglas I, et al. Antibiotic treatment and flares of rheumatoid arthritis: a self-controlled case series study analysis using CPRD GOLD. *Sci Rep*. 2019;9:8941.
11. McKenzie R, Stewart MT, Bellantoni MF, et al. Bacteriuria in individuals who become delirious. *Am J Med*. 2013;127:255–257.
12. Hooton TM. Uncomplicated urinary tract infection. *N Engl J Med*. 2012;366:1028–1037.

CHAPTER 24

Dexamethasone Suppression Test

Jamie M. Pitlick, PharmD, BCPS, BC-ADM

Background

The dexamethasone suppression test (DST), low-dose DST, overnight DST, or 1-mg DST is a dynamic endocrine test in which hormone levels are evaluated based on the principles of bio-feedback regulation.[1,2] A suppression test, in general, involves giving the patient a substance that would normally cause the inhibition of the release of the hormone.[1] However, due to the excessive amounts of hormone or hyperfunction of the endocrine organ, a patient with the disease state would fail to have the hormone levels suppressed.[1] A 48-hour, 2-mg DST can be used in certain populations that may have overactivation of the hypothalamic-pituitary-adrenal axis but without true Cushing's syndrome.[2,3]

How to Use It

DST is used for evaluation of Cushing's syndrome, a group of clinical signs and symptoms that result from chronic exposure to excess glucocorticoids, whatever the etiology.[2,4] In Cushing's syndrome, the normal circadian rhythm of cortisol is disrupted. Serum cortisol concentration normally peaks around 8:00 am and reaches its nadir around 1:00 am to 3:00 am.[3] Dexamethasone is used, as it does not cross-react in the cortisol assay and will not interfere with the measurement of serum cortisol.[5]

The test should be performed when there is clinical suspicion of Cushing's syndrome and is used in combination with other tests (midnight plasma cortisol, late-night salivary cortisol, and/or 24-hour urinary free cortisol) to confirm the diagnosis.[2–4] The initial evaluation and testing may be performed by a non-endocrinologist, but if the initial test is abnormal, the patient should be referred to an endocrinologist for further evaluation.[2]

Some of the more common signs and symptoms that may prompt testing include central adiposity, facial rounding, proximal myopathy, striae, amenorrhea, hirsutism, impaired glucose tolerance, diastolic hypertension, and osteoporosis.[2–4] Iatrogenic Cushing's syndrome is the most common etiology, caused by administration of exogenous glucocorticoids (oral, rectal, inhaled, injectable, or topical administration).[3] Therefore, a thorough medication history should be completed prior to biochemical testing to avoid unnecessary testing.[2]

How It Is Done

As mentioned above, there are multiple types of DSTs. The most common approach is for a supraphysiologic dose of dexamethasone (1 mg) to be administered orally at 11:00 pm, followed by a fasting plasma cortisol level drawn at 8:00 am.[3] This generally is an outpatient test.[2] In a healthy individual, this dose of dexamethasone would suppress adrenocorticotropic hormone (ACTH), a pituitary hormone in the negative feedback loop of cortisol regulation, and subsequently suppress additional release of cortisol resulting in a fasting plasma cortisol level <1.8 mcg/dL.[3] In a patient with Cushing's syndrome, the negative feedback loop is ineffective. This results in the lack of suppression of cortisol release, and thus elevated fasting plasma cortisol levels.[3]

While a fasting plasma cortisol level greater than 5 mcg/dL is consistent with Cushing's syndrome, lower levels (>1.8 mcg/dL) may not fully rule out Cushing's syndrome, as some patients may be able to slightly suppress cortisol.[2] This lower level may increase the sensitivity but at the expense of the specificity. The Endocrine Society recommends use of 1.8 mcg/dL as the threshold to rule out Cushing's syndrome.[2] Unlike antibody-based immunoassays (e.g., enzyme-linked immunosorbent assay [ELISA]), the more commonly used structurally based assays (e.g., HPLC and tandem mass spectrometry) are not affected by cross-reactivity with cortisol metabolites and synthetic glucocorticoids.[2]

Medication Implications

- Anything that decreases the amount of dexamethasone in the patient may result in less of a suppression of endogenous cortisol, increasing the risk for a false positive. Conversely, anything that increases the amount of dexamethasone in a patient may result in more than expected suppression of endogenous cortisol, increasing the risk for a false negative.
- Drugs that increase the metabolism of dexamethasone by induction of cytochrome P450 (CYP) 3A4 may increase the possibility of a false positive, as these medications essentially reduce the body's exposure to dexamethasone.[2–4] Examples include: phenobarbital, phenytoin, carbamazepine, primidone, rifampin, rifapentine, ethosuximide. A more complete and up-to-date list of CYP 3A4 inducers can be found at https://drug-interactions.medicine.iu.edu/MainTable.aspx.[6]
- Drugs that decrease the metabolism of dexamethasone by inhibition of CYP 3A4 may increase the possibility of a false negative.[2–4] Examples include: aprepitant/fosaprepitant, itraconazole, ritonavir, fluoxetine, diltiazem, cimetidine. A more complete and up-to-date list of CYP 3A4 inhibitors can be found at https://drug-interactions.medicine.iu.edu/MainTable.aspx.[6]
- Conditions that may reduce the clearance of dexamethasone and increase the possibility of a false negative include liver and renal failure.[2,3]
- Drugs and conditions that increase cortisol-binding globulin (CBG) concentration (e.g., estrogens, mitotane, and pregnancy) increase the false-positive rates for DST.[2,3] Patients taking estrogen should be off the drug for 4 to 6 weeks before testing.[2,4]
- Conditions that decrease CBG or albumin (e.g., critically ill or nephrotic patients) may increase the rate of false-negative results.[2]
- Synthetic glucocorticoids (e.g., hydrocortisone) will only interfere with immunoassays (i.e., ELISA) for serum cortisol resulting in a high cortisol level (false positive).[2]

TREATMENT FOR A POSITIVE DEXAMETHASONE SUPPRESSION TEST

- If DST is positive, the next step is to determine the cause of the excess glucocorticoids (e.g., exogenous steroid use, adrenal tumor, Cushing disease, or ectopic ACTH syndrome) with additional testing/imaging.[2]
- Once the etiology is known, the treatment is very specific to the etiology.[3,4] For example, if the cause is excess exogenous steroid exposure, the goal would be to decrease the amount of steroid the patient is exposed to, if possible. For most other etiologies (e.g., adrenal tumor, Cushing disease, ectopic ACTH syndrome), the cause for the hypercortisolism is a tumor, in which the treatment of choice would be surgery to remove the tumor. Medications may be used if the patient is not a surgical candidate or as adjunctive therapy before or after the surgery.[3]
- The choice of drug that is chosen is dependent on the site of the tumor.[3]
    - Ectopic ACTH syndrome: metyrapone, ketoconazole

- Pituitary-dependent: mitotane, metyrapone, mifepristone, cabergoline, pasireotide
- Adrenal adenoma: ketoconazole
- Adrenal carcinoma: mitotane
- Steroidogenesis inhibitors (e.g., metyrapone and ketoconazole) block the production of cortisol and other steroids, depending on the specific agent.[3]
  - Metyrapone causes a sudden decrease in cortisol within hours; however, there is a compensatory increase in ACTH.[7] This increase in ACTH causes increased production of other steroids (androgens) in the adrenal glands, which can lead to adverse reactions of hirsutism and acne.[3,7] Currently, metyrapone is only available from the manufacturer for compassionate use.
  - Ketoconazole inhibits steroidogenesis when used in large doses over several weeks of therapy.[3] In contrast to metyrapone, ketoconazole has antiandrogenic activity that leads to gynecomastia and hypogonadism in men.[3,7] Risk of severe hepatotoxicity limits the use of ketoconazole. If used, liver functions tests including aspartate aminotransferase (AST), alanine aminotransferase (ALT), total bilirubin, alkaline phosphatase (ALP), prothrombin time, and international normalized ratio (INR) should be monitored at baseline, with continued monitoring of ALT weekly. In addition, there are many drug-drug interactions that need to be monitored for (as ketoconazole is a potent inhibitor of CYP 3A4), and ketoconazole requires an acidic environment in order to be absorbed.[3,7]
  - Etomidate may be used at low doses in patients with acute hypercortisolemia requiring emergency treatment or in preparation of surgery, as it is only available in a parenteral formulation.[3] Because of risk of excess sedation, this drug requires monitoring in an intensive care unit.[3,7]
- Adrenolytic agents inhibit cortisol and corticosterone synthesis in the adrenal cortex.[3]
  - Mitotane, when dosed for weeks to months, can cause sustained cortisol suppression for 80% of patients and may last upon discontinuation in up to one-third of the patients.[3] If used for too long, mitotane, a cytotoxic drug, will result in atrophy of the adrenal cortex and may ultimately necessitate steroid replacement therapy if too much tissue is damaged.[7] Neurologic (lethargy and somnolence) and gastrointestinal (nausea and vomiting) adverse effects limit the use of this medication.[3,7]
- Neuromodulatory agents target neurotransmitters (i.e., serotonin, gamma-aminobutyric acid [GABA], acetylcholine, and catecholamines) that normally mediate pituitary secretion of ACTH.[3]
  - Cabergoline, a dopamine D_2-receptor agonist, initially reduces ACTH secretion in approximately 50% of patients; however, the reduction is only sustainable in about 30%–40% of patients.[3,7]
  - Pasireotide, a somatostatin analog, inhibits the release of corticotrophin-releasing hormone from the hypothalamus and thus decreases the production of ACTH in the pituitary.[3] Patients need to be monitored for hyperglycemia because of impaired insulin secretion with long-term therapy.[3,7]
- Glucocorticoid receptor-blocking agents antagonize progesterone and glucocorticoid receptors.[3]
  - Mifepristone has the ability to block activation of glucocorticoid receptors and decrease the symptoms of hypercortisolism (e.g., hyperglycemia, hypertension, and weight gain).[3] These are particularly beneficial in patients with history of diabetes mellitus or glucose intolerance.[7] With antagonism of the receptors, the endogenous levels of ACTH and cortisol do increase, so cortisol levels cannot be used to monitor efficacy of this drug therapy.[3,7] Adverse effects include fatigue, nausea, arthralgia, peripheral edema, and hypokalemia.

References

1. Jameson J. Approach to the patient with endocrine disorders. In: Jameson J, Fauci AS, Kasper DL, et al, eds. *Harrison's Principles of Internal Medicine*. 20th ed. New York, NY: McGraw-Hill; http://accesspharmacy.mhmedical.com/content.aspx?bookid=2129&sectionid=179924007. Accessed January 09, 2020.
2. Nieman LK, Biller BMK, Findling JW, et al. The diagnosis of Cushing's syndrome: an Endocrine Society Clinical Practice Guideline. *JCEM*. 2008;93:1526–1540. doi:10.1210/jc.2008-0125.
3. Smith SM, Garland SG, Gums JG. Adrenal gland disorders. In: DiPiro JT, Yee GC, Posey L, et al., eds. *Pharmacotherapy: A Pathophysiologic Approach*. 11th ed. New York, NY: McGraw-Hill; http://accesspharmacy.mhmedical.com/content.aspx?bookid=2577&sectionid=221104771. Accessed January 17, 2020.
4. Arlt W. Disorders of the adrenal cortex. In: Jameson J, Fauci AS, Kasper DL, et al., eds. *Harrison's Principles of Internal Medicine*. 20th ed. New York, NY: McGraw-Hill; http://accesspharmacy.mhmedical.com/content.aspx?bookid=2129&sectionid=192287137. Accessed January 09, 2020.
5. Schimmer BP, Funder W. Adrenocorticotropic hormone, adrenal steroids, and the adrenal cortex. In: Brunton LL, Hilal-Dandan R, Knollmann BC, eds. *Goodman & Gilman's: The Pharmacological Basis of Therapeutics*. 13th ed. New York, NY: McGraw-Hill; http://accesspharmacy.mhmedical.com/content.aspx?bookid=2189&sectionid=172482605. Accessed January 17, 2020.
6. Flockhart DA. Drug Interactions: Cytochrome P450 Drug Interaction Table. Indiana University School of Medicine (2007). https://drug-interactions.medicine.iu.edu. Accessed January 23, 2020.
7. Nieman LK, Biller BMK, Findling JW, et al. Treatment of Cushing's syndrome: an Endocrine Society Clinical Practice Guideline. *J Clin Endocrinol Metab*. 2015;100:1807–1831.

CHAPTER 25

Echocardiography

Amit Alam, MD ▦ Ali Seyar Rahyab, MD

Background

Echocardiography uses ultrasound imaging to visualize the structures of the heart. An ultrasound machine uses an electrical pulse that causes a sound wave that courses through tissue and results in an image based on the variable conductance through different parts of the body. There are two ways to obtain images in echocardiography, noninvasively and invasively. For the noninvasive approach, an ultrasound is placed externally on the chest, and this is referred to as a transthoracic echocardiogram (TTE). Alternatively, an ultrasound probe can be passed down the esophagus, and this invasive approach is referred to as a transesophageal echocardiogram (TEE). A TEE provides better resolution and improved image quality because the probe is in closer proximity to the heart; however, it carries the risk of being an invasive procedure. A TTE is noninvasive, easier to perform, carries little to no risk to the patient, and provides a great deal of useful information.[1]

How to Use It

Transthoracic echocardiography is the initial imaging test of choice to evaluate a patient's cardiac structure and function. The images obtained allow the cardiologist to evaluate[1]:
1. Left ventricular systolic function and diastolic function.
2. Left ventricular structure.
3. Right ventricular structure and function.
4. Aortic, pulmonic, mitral, and tricuspid valves for evidence of valvular pathology including stenosis, regurgitation, or structural deformities.
5. Prosthetic valves.
6. Diseases of the pericardium and proximal aorta.
7. Pulmonary hypertension.
8. Structure of the atria and congenital defects of the heart.

Transesophageal echocardiography is performed if the TTE is either nondiagnostic or if it identified an abnormality that requires further evaluation. In addition, a TEE may be performed during surgery, both in cardiac and noncardiac cases, and during percutaneous transcatheter procedures to guide the placement of the intervention device (such as in transcatheter aortic valve replacement [TAVR]). The most common indications for a TEE are:[1]
1. Evaluation of the left atrial appendage for the presence of a blood clot (such as prior to cardioversion or atrial fibrillation ablation).
2. Further evaluation of prosthetic valves including assessments for valve endocarditis or paravalvular abscess.
3. For patients with low-quality or nondiagnostic TTE images including patients who are intubated and on mechanical ventilation.
4. During surgical procedures to evaluate cardiac structure/function.

Given that a TEE is an invasive procedure, it must not be performed if there is significant esophageal pathology such as esophageal trauma, perforation, tumor, prior esophageal surgery, or active or recent bleeding. Consultation by a gastroenterologist may be necessary for evaluation of the esophagus via esophagogastroduodenoscopy (EGD) prior to a TEE in some cases. See Chapter 32: Gastrointestinal Endoscopy - Upper for more details.

A stress TTE is performed to evaluate a patient's left ventricular systolic function in order to deduce if exercise or a pharmacologic agent can lead to inducible ischemia from underlying coronary artery disease. This is particularly useful for patients with symptoms that are concerning for coronary artery disease. These may include exertional chest discomfort or shortness of breath. The cardiologist will consider the patient's history, physical examination, and baseline electrocardiogram (EKG) to determine if a stress TTE is appropriate. See Chapter 53: Stress Tests for more details.

How It Is Done
TRANSTHORACIC ECHOCARDIOGRAPHY

The images are obtained by a sonography technician or a cardiologist. Images can be obtained in the inpatient or outpatient settings, and a portable machine may be utilized for patients that cannot be moved. The technician places the patient in the appropriate position and obtains images by placing the ultrasound probe on the patient's chest. The images are uploaded to specialized cardiac imaging software that is used by the cardiologist to review the images and generate a report with the findings. There are even smaller handheld devices available that can be employed to conduct limited studies in certain situations, such as with a critically ill patient; however, these devices do not contain all of the functionality and thus do not replace the complete echocardiography study that is typically performed.

TRANSESOPHAGEAL ECHOCARDIOGRAPHY

The patient must be in an inpatient setting, either in an intensive care unit, in the transesophageal echocardiography procedure room, or in the operating room/cardiac catheterization laboratory. After an appropriate period of fasting, the patient is placed under sedation or general anesthesia for the duration of the procedure. The cardiologist passes the specialized transesophageal echocardiography probe (which is smaller than a transthoracic echocardiography probe) into the esophagus and, for certain views, into the stomach. The cardiologist externally manipulates the probe to obtain the images. A sonography technician assists by managing the ultrasound machine. Once image acquisition is complete, the probe is removed and the patient is monitored to ensure appropriate recovery after the sedation or general anesthesia.

STRESS TRANSTHORACIC ECHOCARDIOGRAPHY

This is typically performed in an outpatient stress laboratory. Upon arrival for a stress TTE, a patient first undergoes a TTE at rest to establish baseline left ventricular function. Subsequently, the patient either performs exercise or a pharmacologic agent is used to raise the heart rate and increase oxygen demand. Typical options for the exercise portion include either a standard treadmill or a recumbent exercise bike. The exercise bike is considered the better option, since it allows the sonography technician to obtain images while the patient is undergoing exercise. For patients who cannot exercise, usually due to musculoskeletal concerns, dobutamine is given, which causes an increase in cardiac contractility and heart rate. Once the patient is adequately "stressed" (i.e., reaches his/her goal heart rate), the sonography technician obtains a second set of TTE images to evaluate the left ventricular systolic function again. If a recumbent exercise bike is being used, images may be obtained without moving the patient off the bike. For treadmill tests, the patient is quickly laid down for image acquisition. A positive test would demonstrate inducible reduced function in one or more segments of the left ventricle under stress. See Chapter 53: Stress Tests for more details.

Medication Implications

BEFORE THE PROCEDURE

- There are no medication adjustments that need to be undertaken for a patient to undergo either a routine TTE or TEE.
- For patients who are on anticoagulation, the risks/benefits should be considered prior to performing a TEE. In general, anticoagulation is continued uninterrupted, unless there is a compelling clinical reason to withhold anticoagulation.
- For patients undergoing a stress TTE with dobutamine, they will need to discontinue any beta blocker prior to the test. A once-daily beta blocker should be held for 1 day prior to the test and a twice-daily beta blocker should be held 12 hours prior to the test.

DURING THE PROCEDURE

- Sedation or general anesthesia is used for a TEE. The choice of agent is institution-specific and may vary based on whether an anesthesiologist is involved. Typical agents most commonly used include:
  - Propofol is a lipophilic sedative that causes global central nervous system depression likely through activity via GABA receptors. The steady-state blood concentration is proportional to the infusion rate. It can cause cardiac and respiratory depression, which are more likely at higher infusion rates or with bolus dosing. Cardiac output and respiratory drive decrease and hypotension occurs with sometimes greater than 30% reduction in blood pressure. Contraindications are allergies to eggs, egg products, soybeans, and soy products.[2]
  - Combination of an intravenous benzodiazepine with an intravenous opioid such as midazolam with fentanyl are also commonly used.[3]
- Dobutamine for a stress TTE[4]
  - Dobutamine causes beta1 stimulation, which leads to increased cardiac output, heart rate, and blood pressure.
  - Adverse events are related to increases in heart rate and blood pressure, and dobutamine may predispose to ventricular arrhythmias. EKG and blood pressure monitoring should be done during dobutamine infusion.
  - Dosing during a stress TTE:
    - The initial dose is 10 mcg/kg/minute and is increased every 3–5 minutes by 10 mcg/kg/minute to achieve a goal heart rate of 85% of the maximum predicted heart rate (220 beats/minute – the patient's age = maximum predicted heart rate) up to a total dose of 40 mcg/kg/minute.
    - The dose is not escalated if the patient has symptoms, severe hypertension, or achieves 85% of the maximum predicted heart rate.
- Agitated saline (for a "bubble study" during the TTE or TEE): Normal saline (sodium chloride 0.9%) is vigorously mixed with room air, causing bubbles, which are then injected intravenously while imaging the four-chamber view of the heart (right atrium, left atrium, right ventricle, left ventricle) to evaluate for an inter-atrial communication that would be visualized as bubbles crossing from the right atrium into the left atrium.
- Ultrasound enhancing agents: These agents are composed of microbubbles that opacify the left ventricular cavity to provide a better estimate of the left ventricular systolic function. The enhancing agent is injected intravenously at the time of the TTE and is eliminated through the lungs as a gas. See Chapter 7: Abdominal Ultrasound for more details about these agents. Common agents include:

- Lumason[5]: Most common adverse reactions are headache and nausea. Mechanism: Sulfur hexafluoride lipid-type A microspheres make up Lumason and the microspheres reflect ultrasound beams creating an image that provides better contrast within the left ventricle.
- Optison[6]: Most common adverse reactions are headache, nausea, vomiting, dizziness, or flushing. Mechanism: Optison is a suspension of microspheres of human serum albumin with perflutren which creates a contrast effect in the blood. The albumin portion is metabolized in the body.
- Definity[7]: Most common adverse reactions include headache, nausea, back pain, flushing, chest pain, dizziness, and injection-site reactions. Mechanism: Definity is perflutren lipid microspheres, which enhance the intrinsic backscatter of blood under ultrasound imaging. The fatty acid portion is metabolized in the body.

AFTER THE PROCEDURE

- The patient's typical cardiac and noncardiac medications are resumed, and there are no additional specific medication recommendations for patients who underwent a TTE or TEE.
- If a new diagnosis was made as a result of echocardiography, the condition should be managed accordingly. See Chapter 36: Implantable Electronic Cardiac Devices for details about medications used in heart failure with reduced ejection fraction.

References

1. Solomon S, Wu J, Gillam L. *Essential Echocardiography*. Elsevier; 2017.
2. Propofol [package insert]. Lake Zurich, IL: Fresenius Kabi; 2017.
3. Hahn RT, Abraham T, Adams MS, et al. Guidelines for performing a comprehensive transesophageal echocardiographic examination: recommendations from the American Society of Echocardiography and the Society of Cardiovascular Anesthesiologists. *J Am Soc Echocardiogr*. 2013;26:921–964.
4. Dobutamine [package insert]. Bedford, OH: Bedford Laboratories; 2013.
5. Lumason [package insert]. Monroe Township, NJ: Bracco Diagnostics Inc; 2019.
6. Optison [package insert]. Marlborough, MA: GE Healthcare Inc; 2016.
7. Definity [package insert]. N. Billerica, MA: Lantheus Medical Imaging; 2018.

CHAPTER 26

Electrocardiography

Gregory J. Hughes, PharmD, BCPS, BCGP

Background

An electrocardiogram (EKG) is a noninvasive test that provides a visual representation of the electrical conduction of the heart. It is called EKG because the test produces a "-gram" (something written or drawn—e.g., telegram, diagram—the "G") of the electrical (the "E") conduction through the heart (cardio—the "K" or "C"). The abbreviation ECG can be used interchangeably with the more common EKG, a reflection of the original Dutch spelling of "electrokardiogram." There are different types of EKGs, but one of the most common is the 12-lead EKG, named so because the conduction is visualized in 12 directions, or vectors, in space.[1] The 12-lead EKG is the primary focus of this chapter.

How to Use It

The EKG is a useful tool in getting information about conduction through the myocardium. By providing a visual representation of conduction in 12 spatial planes, clinicians are able to envision a three-dimensional model of the heart. This information is used in diagnosing both cardiac and non-cardiac conditions, as well as for cardiovascular disease risk assessment. Abnormalities ranging from minor to severe can be identified. The EKG detects a variety of arrhythmias when they are suspected or need to be ruled out (i.e., tachycardia, bradycardia, atrial fibrillation, atrial flutter, supraventricular tachycardia, ventricular tachycardia, torsade de pointes, ventricular fibrillation, and conduction blocks). It can also detect ischemia or infarction (i.e., non-ST-segment elevation myocardial infarction [NSTEMI] or ST-segment elevation MI [STEMI]), hypertrophy, pulmonary emboli, pericarditis, electrolyte abnormalities (i.e., hyper- and hypokalemia or calcemia), and certain drug toxicities (e.g., digoxin).[1] Prior to administering a potentially pro-arrhythmic medication, the EKG identifies the baseline rhythm and may detect risk factors for a future arrhythmia (e.g., an already prolonged QTc interval). The EKG is also used to monitor for efficacy of antiarrhythmic therapy.

In addition to screening, diagnosing, and ruling out conditions, the EKG can be used in combination with traditional screening tools to assess cardiovascular disease risk. Examples of these tools include the American College of Cardiology/American Heart Association atherosclerotic cardiovascular disease pooled cohort equation (ASCVD risk estimator or PCE) and the Framingham Risk Score.[2] These tools include risk factors such as age, smoking status, cholesterol concentrations, and blood pressure. The EKG may add to the cardiovascular disease risk assessment for patients who have symptoms of ischemic heart disease or are at intermediate or high risk for cardiovascular disease. However, multiple organizations including the United States Preventive Services Task Force, the American Academy of Family Physicians, and the American College of Physicians recommend against resting- or exercise-EKG screening in asymptomatic patients at low risk of cardiovascular disease events.[3-5]

How It Is Done

The EKG can be performed by physicians or allied health professionals in the inpatient or outpatient setting and is not restricted to those specialized in cardiology. Often, a nurse will perform the test independently and the results will be transferred to the medical record. The EKG is

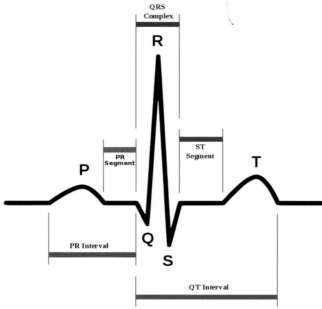

Fig. 26.1 Illustration of a normal electrocardiogram with labeled segments. (From https://en.wikipedia.org/wiki/File:SinusRhythmLabels.png.)

noninvasive, inexpensive, can be quickly arranged, and is brief (the actual rhythm observed and recorded is only a few seconds duration). The 12-lead EKG involves placing adhesive pads on 10 points on the body, 6 across the trunk in front of the heart and 4 on the limbs. Then an electrode (i.e., a wire with a clip on the end) is attached to each pad and the wires converge at a computer. The computer prints out one sheet of paper that contains the 12 planes of conduction. In each plane, the rhythm is represented by a line that deflects upward and downward with the conduction of the heart. A normal sinus rhythm (NSR) features a P wave (atrial depolarization), a QRS complex (ventricular depolarization), and a T wave (ventricular repolarization). See Fig. 26.1 for an illustration identifying the EKG segments. A normal heart rate is 60–100 beats/minute, PR interval is <200 ms, QRS duration is <120 ms, and QTc is <450–460 ms.[1]

Medication Implications

- The EKG is noninvasive and no medications are administered prior to or during the test. Neither sedation nor pain control is needed, and there is no recovery period. The patient does not need to be awake or able to follow directions besides briefly lying motionless. Tremors or seizures can produce artifacts, interfering with interpretation of the EKG. No medications need to be held prior to the test.
- If the EKG reveals heart block, certain medications may need to be avoided and a pacemaker may need to be implanted. Beta blockers and non-dihydropyridine calcium channel blockers may be used only in first-degree heart block (PR interval >200 ms). In second- and third-degree heart block, the progressive failure of the atrioventricular (AV) node to conduct to the ventricles, they are contraindicated (unless the patient also has a permanent pacemaker).[6,7] See Chapter 36: Implantable Cardiac Devices for details about these devices. Examples of beta blockers include carvedilol, metoprolol, and others (generic names all

ending in -lol). The two non-dihydropyridine calcium channel blockers are diltiazem and verapamil.

- If ischemia or infarction is detected, medications for acute coronary syndrome (ACS) may need to be initiated. Many patients will require antiplatelet therapy (possibly dual anti-platelet therapy [DAPT], which usually includes aspirin plus a P2Y12 antagonist), a beta blocker, an HMG-CoA reductase inhibitor ("statin"), renin-angiotensin-aldosterone system inhibitors, anticoagulation, and antianginal therapy. Patients who will undergo cardiac catheterization should generally have nephrotoxic agents held as the radiocontrast dye can cause nephropathy in the days following the procedure.[8,9] See Chapter 17: Computed Tomography Scan for details about contrast-induced nephropathy. If the 12-lead EKG does not confirm coronary injury, yet clinical suspicion remains high, alternative types of EKGs may be performed.
- If the EKG reveals left ventricular hypertrophy, subsequent tests, such as an echocardiogram, may be ordered. See Chapter 25: Echocardiography for details about this test.
- If the EKG reveals electrolyte abnormalities, the electrolyte abnormality needs to be corrected. Hypokalemia or hypocalcemia require intravenous and/or oral replacement, but hyperkalemia and hypercalcemia require other medications to correct them.
  - Treatment of hyperkalemia-induced EKG changes (often "peaked T waves") involves measures that:
    - Reduce myocardial excitability and risk for arrhythmias (e.g., intravenous calcium gluconate or calcium chloride).
    - Shift the potassium into the cells such as beta agonists (e.g., albuterol), insulin (e.g., insulin regular given intravenously), and alkalinizing medications (e.g., sodium bicarbonate) to correct acidemia.
    - Facilitate removal of potassium such as loop diuretics (e.g., furosemide), exchange resins (e.g., sodium polystyrene sulfonate), or dialysis.[10]
  - Hypercalcemia treatment may involve administration of fluids, loop diuretics, calcitonin, corticosteroids, and/or bisphosphonates depending on the presentation.[1]
- The EKG is a useful tool in identifying some drug toxicities. A prolonged QTc interval is worrisome because it can lead to a life-threatening arrhythmia (torsade de pointes). An antecedent QTc interval > 500 ms was present in 92% of torsade de pointes cases, so this duration is frequently used as a cutoff for initiation or dose escalation of many medications.[11,12]
  - Some of the medications more commonly associated with a prolonged QTc interval are antipsychotics, antiarrhythmics, macrolides (reported with azithromycin, erythromycin, and clarithromycin), fluoroquinolones, ondansetron, and methadone. There is no specific dose or combination of medications that creates a prolonged QTc interval or its conversion to torsade de pointes, so care should be taken to monitor for and correct risk factors. Follow-up EKGs should be performed to monitor the QTc interval as clinically warranted.[13]
  - Risk factors for torsade de pointes include hypokalemia, hypomagnesemia, bradycardia, bundle branch block, certain ion channel polymorphisms, female sex, cardiovascular disease (e.g., chronic heart failure, previous myocardial infarction), conversion from atrial fibrillation to NSR, rapid infusion or overdose of QTc interval-prolonging drugs, prolonged QTc interval at baseline, and family history of prolonged QTc interval.[13]
  - In 2013, the Food and Drug Administration (FDA) warned the public about the increased risk of fatal heart rhythms caused by azithromycin. While there is evidence that azithromycin does increase the QTc interval, this warning was based on retrospective data that compared cardiovascular event risk among azithromycin and other antimicrobial regimens in the outpatient setting. The risk of cardiovascular death was increased when using azithromycin compared to amoxicillin with risk varying drastically depending

on the patients' baseline cardiovascular risk (as there are numerous risk factors for torsade de pointes, mentioned previously). In patients at highest cardiovascular risk, relative to amoxicillin, azithromycin was associated with an increased risk of one cardiovascular death per roughly 4100 prescriptions. The risk was much less in lower-risk patients.[14] It is important to note that the increased risk of cardiovascular death occurred in patients taking azithromycin when compared with amoxicillin or ciprofloxacin but not when compared with those taking levofloxacin, in which the risk was equal. Azithromycin-prescribing information has been updated to warn prescribers of the risk of QTc prolongation in patients with a known prolonged QTc interval; a history of torsade de pointes, bradyarrhythmias, uncompensated heart failure; use of other drugs that prolong the QTc interval; or ongoing pro-arrhythmic conditions (such as hypokalemia or hypomagnesemia).[15]

- Fluoroquinolones as a class have been found to prolong the QTc interval. The risk of prolongation is thought to be higher with moxifloxacin as it has been shown to inhibit conduction channels at doses used therapeutically. By contrast, ciprofloxacin and levofloxacin require much higher doses to block the same channels. The risk of prolonged QTc interval and torsade de pointes is lowest with ciprofloxacin when used at therapeutic doses.[16]

- In 2011, the FDA warned about the risk of ondansetron causing QTc interval prolongation. This warning was specifically for the intravenous dose of 32 mg, but the effects of lower doses and the oral route have also come into question.[17] Two small prospective studies further explored the effect of lower doses using 4 mg administered intravenously in the emergency department. The QTc interval was prolonged by a mean of 20 ms in one study and by 16.2 ms in the other. No patients had ondansetron-related cardiac events. It should be noted that although these studies confirm an effect of a 4-mg intravenous dose on the QTc interval, they contained fewer than 50 patients and the clinical impact of 20-ms prolongation is unknown.[18,19] Also, little is known about the effects of oral ondansetron on QTc prolongation and the FDA warning does not apply to this formulation.

- Digoxin toxicity can result in several arrhythmias, namely premature ventricular contractions, bradycardia, atrial tachyarrhythmia with AV block, AV blockade, and others. Ventricular tachycardia with a fascicular block is a characteristic rhythm of digoxin toxicity. Treatment is situation specific but can include digoxin-specific antibody fragments (brand names Digibind and DigiFab), repletion of potassium, and correcting kidney failure. Of note, calcium administration for concomitant hyperkalemia is not recommended because digoxin toxicity involves excessive intracellular calcium.[20]

- The digoxin-specific antibody fragment is indicated in life-threatening or potentially life-threatening toxicity from digoxin. Other factors that influence whether to administer the antibody include acute versus chronic ingestion, known versus suspected overdose, serum digoxin concentration, serum potassium concentration, and the development and progression of cardiac and gastrointestinal toxicity. An important limitation of monitoring digoxin serum concentrations following acute ingestion is that it takes 4 to 6 hours to reach equilibrium with the myocardium.[20]

References

1. Electrocardiography. *Harrison's Principles of Internal Medicine.* 20th ed. AccessPharmacy: McGraw-Hill Medical. https://accesspharmacy.mhmedical.com/content.aspx?bookid=2129&sectionid=186950143&jumpsectionid=186950200. Accessed October 31, 2019.
2. Arnett DK, Blumenthal RS, Albert MA, et al. 2019 ACC/AHA guideline on the primary prevention of cardiovascular disease: a report of the American College of Cardiology/American Heart Association Task Force on Clinical Practice Guidelines. *Circulation.* 2019;140:e596–e646.
3. US Preventive Services Task Force. Screening for cardiovascular disease risk with electrocardiography: US Preventive Services Task Force Recommendation Statement. *JAMA.* 2018;319:2308–2314.

4. Clinical Preventive Services Recommendation. American Academy of Family Physicians. Available at: https://www.aafp.org/patient-care/clinical-recommendations/all/coronary-heart-disease.html. Accessed June 26, 2020.

5. Chou R. Cardiac Screening with electrocardiography, stress echocardiography, or myocardial perfusion imaging: advice for high-value care from the American College of Physicians. *Ann Intern Med.* 2015;162:438–447.

6. Coreg [package insert]. Research Triangle Park, NC: GlaxoSmithKline; 2005.

7. Cardizem CD [package insert]. Kansas City, MO: Sanofi-Aventis; 2009.

8. 2014 AHA/ACC Guideline for the management of patients with non–ST-elevation acute coronary syndromes. *Circulation.* 2014;130:e344–e426.

9. Ibanez B, James S, Agewall S, et al. 2017 ESC Guidelines for the management of acute myocardial infarction in patients presenting with ST-segment elevation. *Eur Heart J.* 2018;39:119–177.

10. Mount DB. Fluid and electrolyte disturbances. In: Jameson J, Fauci AS, Kasper DL, Hauser SL, Longo DL, Loscalzo J. eds. *Harrison's Principles of Internal Medicine.* 20th ed. McGraw-Hill; Accessed June 26, 2020. https://accesspharmacy.mhmedical.com/content.aspx?bookid=2129&sectionid=192013179.

11. Moss AJ, Schwartz PJ, Crampton RS, et al. The long QT syndrome. Prospective longitudinal study of 328 families. *Circulation.* 1991;84:1136–1144.

12. Bednar MM, Harrigan EP, Anziano RJ, et al. The QT interval. *Prog Cardiovasc Dis.* 2001;43:1–45.

13. Li EC, Esterly JS, Pohl S, et al. Drug-induced QT-interval prolongation: considerations for clinicians. *Pharmacotherapy.* 2010;30:684–701.

14. Ray WA, Murray KT, Hall K, et al. Azithromycin and the risk of cardiovascular death. *N Engl J Med.* 2012;366:1881–1890.

15. Zithromax [package insert]. New York, NY: Pfizer; 2017.

16. Briasoulis A, Agarwal V, Pierce WJ. QT Prolongation and torsade de pointes induced by fluoroquinolones: infrequent side effects from commonly used medications. *Cardiology.* 2011;120:103–110.

17. FDA Drug Safety Communication: New information regarding QTc prolongation with ondansetron (Zofran). Available at: https://www.fda.gov/drugs/drug-safety-and-availability/fda-drug-safety-com-munication-new-information-regarding-qt-prolongation-ondansetron-zofran. Accessed January 1, 2020.

18. Moffett PM, Cartwright L, Grossart EA, et al. Intravenous ondansetron and the QT interval in adult emergency department patients: An observational study. *Acad Emerg Med.* 2016;23:102–105.

19. Li K, Vo K, Lee BK, et al. Effect of a single dose if i.v. ondansetron and QTc interval in emergency department patients. *Am J Health Syst Pharm.* 2018;75:276–282.

20. Antidotes in Depth. *Goldfrank's Toxicologic Emergencies.* 10th ed. AccessPharmacy. McGraw-Hill Medical. https://accesspharmacy.mhmedical.com/content.aspx?bookid=1163&sectionid=65087766. Accessed October 31, 2019.

CHAPTER 27

Electroencephalography

Ebtesam Ahmed, PharmD, MS

Background

An electroencephalography is a test to measure the electrical activities of the brain, allowing for the detection of abnormal brain activity.[1] It is often abbreviated as EEG. The suffix "-graphy" ("G") refers to the presentation of the results found from the electrical ("E") impulses measured in the brain (encephalo - "E").[1]

How to Use It

The EEG is useful for the diagnosis/monitoring of conditions that affect the brain, such as epilepsy, stroke, and Alzheimer's disease. It detects voltage differences between two electrodes (points in the brain). The differences in the electric potentials leads to a series of upward and downward waves, which can convey information depending on differences with the reference points.[1] These waves are distinguished into four primary types: delta (frequency <3 Hz), theta (slow frequency, 3.5–7.5 Hz), alpha (7.5–13 Hz), and beta (fast activity, >13 Hz).[1]

The EEG records spontaneous electrical activity in the cortical neurons, which is "highly influenced and synchronized by subcortical structures."[2] It is assumed that these efferent impulses are responsible for "entraining cortical neurons to produce characteristic rhythmic brain-wave patterns, such as alpha rhythm and sleep spindles."[2]

How It Is Done

The EEG is noninvasive, and no medications, sedation, or pain control is necessary before or during the procedure. The patient must have a clean head without any hair products. Prior to the EEG, patients must discontinue interfering medications, avoid consuming any food or drinks containing caffeine for 8 to 12 hours, and refrain from fasting the night before or the day of the procedure.[2] Environmental factors such as caffeine and low blood sugar must be excluded, as they influence the results of the recording.[3] There may also be EEG abnormalities if the patient is unresponsive due to catatonia, structural brain disease, or drug overdose (e.g., a drug overdose shows diffuse beta activity, which is called a beta coma).[4]

Patients will have their heads measured to designate the electrode placement. Silver-silver chloride or gold disk electrodes held on by collodion are recommended, as they are free of inherent noise and drift.[5] Twenty-one electrodes are applied following the 10-20 system by placing the electrodes at estimated intervals of 10% to 20% of the hemi-circumference of the head.[2,5] It is essential to have an adequate number of electrodes to "ensure that EEG activity having a small area of representation on the scalp is recorded and to analyze the distribution of more diffuse activity."[5] A square wave calibration of at least 10 seconds should be done at the beginning of every EEG recording. The EEG recording should include periods of when the eyes are open and when they are closed, hyperventilation, photic stimulation in a room with a dimmed light placed 30 cm away from the patient's face, or period of sleep.[2,5] Photic stimulation should be performed after all hyperventilation-related EEG changes have been resolved. Photic stimulation and hyperventilation can potentially cause seizures in susceptible patients, as it is "intended to elicit epileptiform discharges."[5] These tasks are done to monitor if any changes are seen in the EEG and will help arrive at a more complete diagnosis.[6]

The recording should contain at least 20 minutes of technically satisfactory recording, although a longer recording may be more informative.[5] It is often common practice to use video telemetry when recording an EEG in a hospital inpatient setting. While it is not a requirement, it is useful in "interpreting clinical events as well as identifying artifacts" when analyzing the EEG.[5]

Medication Implications

- If the EEG reveals that the patient suffers from epilepsy, caution should be used with drugs that lower the seizure threshold. Examples of such drugs include antidepressants (e.g., tricyclic antidepressants [TCAs], serotonin-specific agents [e.g., sertraline]), antipsychotics (e.g., clozapine), narcotics (e.g., opioid analgesics, psychostimulants), and antibiotics (e.g., isoniazid, carbapenems, cefepime). There are multiple classes of drugs that can treat epilepsy, such as levetiracetam, gabapentin, valproic acid, and phenobarbital.[7]
- Long-term video-EEG monitoring (LTM) is a tool used to evaluate patients with epilepsy to determine seizure type, for localization of epileptogenic foci, or understand the nature of episodic events, such as psychogenic nonepileptic seizures.[8] LTM needs to be able to record a sufficient number of seizures. Occurrence of seizures is unpredictable, so prior to the LTM, sleep deprivation, hyperventilation, or withdrawal of antiepileptic drugs (AEDs) is done in order to reduce LTM duration.[8] These interventions reduce the monitoring duration necessary by allowing seizures to occur earlier.
    - In an open-label randomized controlled trial, patients were randomly separated into one of two groups: rapid AED taper or slow AED taper. The primary endpoint is the mean difference in LTM duration in days between a rapid and slow taper of AEDs.[8]
    - Results of the primary outcome were found to be statistically significant. The mean difference in LTM duration between the two groups was -1.8 days (95% confidence interval: -2.9 to -0.8, $P = .0006$). The study concluded the advantage of rapid AED tapering in reducing LTM duration over slow tapering, without major adverse events.[8]
- Patients who suffer from schizophrenia will often show two changes on their EEG test: the mismatch negativity and P3a (one of the electrical waves of an EEG).[9] These differences were shown to be reduced in schizophrenic patients, leading to their social cognitive deficits. These patients should be treated with antipsychotic drugs such as risperidone, olanzapine, or haloperidol.[10]
- A study on bipolar disorder demonstrated that there is reduced brain synchronization and alterations of network topologies, primarily in the alpha bands.[11] These changes were specifically shown in the fronto-central and central-parietal lobes of the brain.[11] These changes can be treated with lithium, anticonvulsants (e.g., valproic acid, lamotrigine), antipsychotics, or a combination of these.[11]
- Early manifestations of Parkinson's disease can also be detected by an EEG. The beta-band and wavelet entropy was shown to be shorter in patients with early manifestations of Parkinson's disease than in those without early manifestations of the disease.[12] Patients with Parkinson's disease should be treated primarily by a combination of carbidopa and levodopa, but can also use other therapies, such as dopamine agonists (e.g., ropinirole, pramipexole) and monoamine oxidase-B inhibitors (e.g., selegiline, rasagiline, safinamide).[12] These patients should also try to avoid drugs that inhibit dopamine, such as metoclopramide and haloperidol, as they can result in parkinsonism or substantially worsen motor symptoms in patients with Parkinson's disease and may lead to neuroleptic malignant syndrome.[13]

- Patients who have generalized anxiety disorder (GAD) demonstrated higher levels of gamma activity when using an EEG in times of stress/worry.[14] Gamma brain waves are found throughout the central nervous system, but are notably seen in areas related to processing emotions.[14]
  - A study that evaluated EEG results for patients with GAD used worry as a negative experience to monitor EEG changes. The study included 30 participants, 15 of whom had GAD, according to the Diagnostic and Statistical Manual of Mental Disorders, fourth edition (DSM-IV) criteria, and 15 control patients.[14] EEG was done for baseline, relaxation, and worry tasks. During worry tasks, higher levels of gamma activity were seen in the GAD group than in the control group.[14] After 14 weeks of psychotherapy, gamma activity in the GAD group decreased compared with the initial worry tasks EEG performed at the beginning of the study.[14]
  - Treatment options for GAD include cognitive behavioral therapy and relaxation as first-line agents. If ineffective, pharmacotherapy options include certain Food and Drug Administration (FDA)-approved serotonin-norepinephrine reuptake inhibitors (SNRIs) (e.g., venlafaxine, duloxetine), selective serotonin reuptake inhibitors (SSRIs) (e.g., paroxetine), benzodiazepines, and buspirone.[15] There are also many other medications that can be used off-label for treatment of GAD.[15]
- In Alzheimer's disease, well-known EEG abnormalities include slowing of the dominant posterior alpha rhythm, appearance of theta and delta activity, and generalized bursts of slow activity that are usually maximal in frontal and temporal leads.[16] Cholinesterase inhibitors such as galantamine, rivastigmine, and donepezil are used in the treatment of mild to moderate Alzheimer's disease, while donepezil and N-methyl D-aspartate (NMDA) antagonists such as memantine are used in the treatment of moderate to severe Alzheimer's disease.[17] The FDA has also approved a combination product including memantine and donepezil for the treatment of moderate to severe Alzheimer's disease.[17]
- In patients with delirium, EEG shows unreactive alpha with dropout, generalized slowing, and occipital slowing.[16] However, persistent and prolonged slowing indicate that the patient has delirium complicating dementia.[16] Patients with delirium can be treated with antipsychotics such as haloperidol and atypical antipsychotics such as risperidone, olanzapine, or quetiapine.[17]
- In patients with attention-deficit hyperactivity disorder (ADHD), the EEG displays changes in the theta/beta ratio, although these changes are not to be relied on as a sole diagnostic tool. Typically, what is observed on the EEG is elevated power of slow/theta waves and/or beta waves with decreased power.[18]
  - In July 2013, the FDA had approved the neuropsychiatric EEG-Based Assessment Aid (NEBA) to help clinicians to diagnose more accurately children/adolescents (6–17 years). By using NEBA, clinicians can further determine if a patient's symptoms are due to ADHD or another undiagnosed medical condition.[19]
  - Upon diagnosis with ADHD with or without the EEG, FDA-approved medications that can be initiated are stimulants such as amphetamine and methylphenidate, or non-stimulants such as atomoxetine, guanfacine, and clonidine.[20]
- The EEG can also be used in psychiatric medicine to monitor for psychotropic drug toxicity (e.g., closely monitoring clozapine for epileptic discharge) and to predict the response to psychiatric therapy.[4]
- The EEG can also act as a "pharmaco-sparing agent" where it can act as a natural antiepileptic by rewarding the brain for holding particular frequencies.[4] The patient eventually learns to produce the "desirable brain wave pattern" to continue the neurofeedback loop to continue being rewarded which can improve different mental states depending on the frequency (e.g., beta state improves arousal and depression, while sensory motor rhythm produces calmness and relaxation).[4,17]

References

1. Electroencephalogram (EEG). Electroencephalogram (EEG) | Johns Hopkins Medicine. https://www.hopkinsmedicine.org/health/treatment-tests-and-therapies/electroencephalogram-eeg. Accessed July 3, 2020.
2. Diagnostic Testing in Neurologic Disease. In: Ropper AH, Samuels MA, Klein JP, Prasad S. eds. *Adams and Victor's Principles of Neurology, 11e*. McGraw-Hill; Accessed September 14, 2020. https://accessmedicine.mhmedical.com/content.aspx?bookid=1477&sectionid=855363.
3. Siepmann M, Kirch W. Effects of caffeine on topographic quantitative EEG. *Neuropsychobiology*. 2002;45(3):161–166.
4. Chandra SR, Asheeb A, Dash S, et al. Role of electroencephalography in the diagnosis and treatment of neuropsychiatric border zone syndromes. *Indian J Psychol Med*. 2017;39(3):243–249.
5. Sinha SR, Sullivan L, Sabau D, et al. American Clinical Neurophysiology Society Guideline 1: minimum technical requirements for performing clinical electroencephalography. *J Clin Neurophysiol*. 2016;33(4):303–307.
6. Britton JW, Frey LC, Hopp JL, et al. *Electroencephalography (EEG): An Introductory Text and Atlas of Normal and Abnormal Findings in Adults, Children, and Infants*. Chicago: American Epilepsy Society; 2016. https://www.ncbi.nlm.nih.gov/books/NBK390346/.
7. Chen HY, Albertson TE, Olson KR. Treatment of drug-induced seizures. *Br J Clin Pharmacol*. 2016;81(3):412–419.
8. Kumar S, Ramanujam B, Chandra PS, et al. Randomized controlled study comparing the efficacy of rapid and slow withdrawal of antiepileptic drugs during long-term video-EEG monitoring. *Epilepsia*. 2018;59(2):460–467.
9. Garrido MI, Kilner JM, Stephan KE, et al. The mismatch negativity: a review of underlying mechanisms. *Clin Neurophysiol*. 2009;120(3):453–463.
10. Ibáñez-Molina AJ, Lozano V, Soriano MF, et al. EEG multiscale complexity in schizophrenia during picture naming. *Front Physiol*. 2018;9:1213.
11. Kim DJ, Bolbecker AR, Howell J, et al. Disturbed resting state EEG synchronization in bipolar disorder: A graph-theoretic analysis. *Neuroimage Clin*. 2013;2:414–423.
12. Han CX, Wang J, Yi GS, et al. Investigation of EEG Abnormalities in the early stage of Parkinson's disease. *Cogn Neurodyn*. 2013;7(4):351–359.
13. Burkhard PR. Acute and subacute drug-induced movement disorders. *Parkinsonism Relat Disord*. 2014;20:S108–S112.
14. Oathes DJ, Ray WJ, Yamasaki AS, et al. Worry, generalized anxiety disorder, and emotion: evidence from the EEG gamma band. *Biol Psychol*. 2008;79(2):165–170. doi:10.1016/j.biopsycho.2008.04.005.
15. National Institute for Health and Care Excellence (NICE). Generalised anxiety disorder and panic disorder in adults: management. https://www.nice.org.uk/guidance/cg113. Published January 2011.
16. Winslow BT, Onysko MK, Stob CM, et al. Treatment of Alzheimer disease [published correction appears in Am Fam Physician. 2014 Aug 15;90(4):209]. *Am Fam Physician*. 2011;83(12):1403–1412.
17. Fong TG, Tulebaev SR, Inouye SK. Delirium in elderly adults: diagnosis, prevention and treatment. *Nat Rev Neurol*. 2009;5(4):210–220.
18. Lenartowicz A, Loo SK. Use of EEG to diagnose ADHD. *Curr Psychiatry Rep*. 2014;16(11):498.
19. Food and Drug Administration. De novo classification request for neuropsychiatric EEG-based assessment aid for ADHD (NEBA) system regulatory information. Published December 8, 2011. https://www.accessdata.fda.gov/cdrh_docs/reviews/K112711.pdf. Accessed September 9, 2020.
20. National Institute for Health and Care Excellence (NICE). Attention deficit hyperactivity disorder: diagnosis and management. NICE clinical guideline NG87. London, UK: National Institute for Health and Care Excellence. https://www.nice.org.uk/guidance/ng87/chapter/recommendations. Published March 2018.

CHAPTER 28

Endoscopic Retrograde Cholangiopancreatography

Julie A. Murphy, PharmD, FASHP, FCCP, BCPS ■
Basil E. Akpunonu, MD, MSC, FACP ■ Shahab Ud Din, MD ■
Jeannine Hummell, CNP

Background

Endoscopic retrograde cholangiopancreatography (ERCP) is an invasive test used to visualize the common bile duct (CBD) and pancreatic duct for diagnostic and therapeutic purposes in a variety of biliary and pancreatic disorders. The term *endoscopic* is derived from Greek by combining the prefix "endo" (within) and "scope" (to view). The term *cholangiopancreatography* is also derived from Greek by combining "chole" (bile), "angio" (vessel), "pancreato" (pancreas), and "graphy" (write). ERCP was developed in 1968 by Drs. McCune, Shorb, and Moscovitz as a diagnostic tool. Until this time, endoscopy had never been used to visualize the pancreatic duct or CBD.[1,2]

How to Use It

ERCP has evolved from a diagnostic procedure to an almost exclusively therapeutic procedure for abnormalities of the CBD, pancreatic duct, and ampulla. The diagnostic component has been replaced by noninvasive techniques such as computed tomography (CT) scan, endoscopic ultrasound (EUS), and magnetic resonance imaging (MRI). Once choledocholithiasis (gallstones in the CBD) is identified, ERCP may be performed to clear stones and allow for biliary drainage. This may be especially useful for patients who are not candidates for cholecystectomy. ERCP is the gold standard for the diagnosis (malignant or benign) and treatment (benign) of biliary strictures. The stricture is visualized, and brushings are obtained via ERCP to allow for tissue diagnosis. Treatment for benign strictures involves stenting, with stent replacements to prevent cholangitis, and eventual stent removal. Primary sclerosing cholangitis may occur in patients with dominant strictures (stenosis of <1.5 mm in the CBD or <1 mm in the hepatic duct). Dilation with or without stenting is the preferred treatment for patients with dominant strictures. Since these patients are at an increased risk of developing cholangiocarcinoma, additional evaluation including MRI or CT scan, CA 19-9 levels, and repeated ERCP with brushings and biopsies should be conducted. For patients with cholangiocarcinoma distal to the hepatic duct bifurcation, a stent is recommended to relieve obstructive jaundice. ERCP assists in the diagnosis and staging of ampullary tumors through tissue biopsies. If ampullectomy is done, a pancreatic duct stent is placed via ERCP to minimize pancreatitis. Patients with acute gallstone pancreatitis with synchronous cholangitis require urgent ERCP and sphincterectomy to reduce morbidity and mortality. In cases of chronic pancreatitis, ERCP is used not only to identify the presence of pancreatic duct strictures and stones but also to place stents or remove stones as needed. Malignancy must be excluded if pancreatic duct strictures are identified. For pancreatic duct leaks from surgical or procedural complications, stenting of the pancreatic duct across the area of the leak may be performed using ERCP. ERCP also allows for pseudocysts to be drained if they are symptomatic, infected, or progressively enlarging. The most common indication for ERCP during pregnancy is choledocholithiasis.[1,3–10]

How It Is Done

ERCP is a technically demanding procedure that should be performed by a specially trained gastroenterologist. The procedure may be performed in the inpatient or outpatient setting. A plastic mouth guard is placed in the patient's mouth to prevent damage to the teeth and the scope. After sedating the patient using general anesthesia for high-risk cardiopulmonary patients or conscious sedation (benzodiazepines [e.g., midazolam] and analgesics [e.g., fentanyl]), the physician passes the endoscope through the mouth, throat, esophagus, stomach, and into the duodenum where the papilla is located. Once the papilla is identified, a catheter is passed through the working channel of the endoscope and contrast dye is injected to allow for adequate visualization on X-ray of the biliary and pancreatic ducts. With a cutting wire, an incision is made at the papilla (sphincterectomy) to allow for a wider opening for bile drainage, passage and removal of stones, or stent placement. In addition to the cutting wire, the endoscope has tools that allow for flushing, suctioning, brushing for tissue biopsy, and aspiration of fluid for analysis. In the case of choledocholithiasis in pregnancy, the procedure can be modified to reduce radiation exposure. When sphincterectomy or biopsies are anticipated, a complete blood count and prothrombin time/international normalized ratio (PT/INR) should be obtained. Mortality rates are low after diagnostic and therapeutic ERCPs, 0.2% and 0.4%–0.5%, respectively. The most common serious adverse event after ERCP is pancreatitis, occurring in 3%–10% of patients. Bleeding after sphincterectomy during ERCP occurs in 0.3%–2% of patients. Infections such as cholangitis (0.5%–3%) or cholecystitis (0.5%) may occur. Risk of perforation during ERCP is approximately 0.08%–0.6%. Minor complications associated with anesthesia (e.g., nausea, vomiting, aspiration pneumonitis, hypoxemia, and cardiac arrhythmias) occur in 5%–7% of patients. The patient is not allowed to eat or drink for 6–8 hours before the test. Some patients may continue to fast, slowly advancing the diet to clear liquids with resumption of a normal diet over 24 hours. Others, at low risk of complications, may safely advance the diet over 4–6 hours after the procedure.[1,4,11,12]

Medication Implications

- Holding antiplatelets and anticoagulants prior to ERCP is based on procedure bleeding risk (e.g., biliary or pancreatic sphincterectomy [high risk], stent placement without sphincterectomy [low risk]). In case of a planned high-risk procedure[13]:
  - Low-dose aspirin and nonsteroidal anti-inflammatory drugs (NSAIDs) may be continued.
  - Clopidogrel and prasugrel should be held for 5–7 days and ticagrelor should be held for 3–5 days prior to ERCP.
  - Stop warfarin 5 days prior to ERCP. For patients at high risk of thromboembolism, bridge with therapeutic doses of low-molecular-weight heparin (LMWH) or unfractionated heparin (UH) when the INR falls below the lower limit of therapeutic goal. Stop LMWH 24 hours prior to procedure, and stop UH 6 hours prior to procedure. Warfarin may be restarted on the same day as the procedure assuming there is no ongoing bleeding. Resume therapeutic doses of LMWH or UH 48–72 hours after the ERCP if no bleeding has occurred. Bridging therapy can be stopped 5 days after resuming warfarin and when the INR is above the lower limit of the therapeutic range.
  - For patients taking a direct oral anticoagulant (DOAC), stop the DOAC 1–5 days before ERCP depending on agent used and creatinine clearance in mL/minute (Table 28.1).
  - Re-initiation of DOACs should be delayed until adequate hemostasis is ensured. If the DOAC cannot be restarted within 12–24 hours for a patient at high risk of thromboembolism, bridging with therapeutic doses of LMWH or UH should be considered.
- For blood glucose control in patients with type 1 diabetes:
  - See Chapter 30: Gastrointestinal Endoscopy - Capsule

TABLE 28.1 ■ **Recommended intervals for stopping D. .Cs prior to ERCP**

DOAC	Creatinine clearance (mL/minute)	Days to hold prior to procedure
Dabigatran	<30	4–6
	30–50	3–4
	>50	2–3
Rivaroxaban	15–29	4
	30–59	3
	60–90	2
	>90	≥1
Apixaban	15–29	4
	30–59	3
	>60	1–2
Edoxaban	≤15	No data
	>15	≥1

- For blood glucose control in patients with type 2 diabetes [14,15]:
  - See Chapter 30: Gastrointestinal Endoscopy - Capsule; a few differences are noted here.
  - Sodium-glucose cotransporter-2 (SGLT2) inhibitors (including combination products that include an SGLT2 inhibitor): avoid the morning of ERCP.
  - Thiazolidinediones: avoid several days before ERCP.
  - See Chapter 5: Glycemic Considerations for Tests and Procedures for more details about glycemic management.
- In the absence of cholangitis, periprocedural prophylactic antibiotic use is only recommended for patients with a history of liver transplant, patients with known or suspected biliary obstruction that may be incompletely drained, and in cases of infected pseudocyst or ductal leaks. Routine antibiotic prophylaxis is not recommended when complete drainage is anticipated.[16]
- In the presence of cholangitis, the American Heart Association suggests the inclusion of an agent active against enterococci within the antibiotic regimen.[17]
- Prevention of post-ERCP pancreatitis:
  - Rectal administration of indomethacin or diclofenac 50 mg or 100 mg immediately before or after the ERCP is recommended.[18–20]
  - Aggressive hydration with lactated Ringer's solution (e.g., 3 mL/kg/hour during the procedure, 20 mL/kg bolus after the procedure, and 3 mL/kg/hour for 8 hours after the procedure) reduced the incidence of post-ERCP pancreatitis and was not associated with fluid overload.[21,22]
- Treatment of post-ERCP pancreatitis:
  - The use of antibacterial agents with good penetration of pancreatic tissue (e.g., meropenem, imipenem, ciprofloxacin) may be indicated only in patients with severe disease to reduce the risk of pancreatic abscess and decrease mortality.[18]
- If gallstones or biliary sludge is identified, potential medication causes should be considered. Estrogens used for contraception, hormone replacement therapy, or for treatment of prostate cancer may increase risk. The glucagon-like peptide (GLP-1) analogs (e.g., liraglutide and exenatide) are associated with an increased risk of bile duct and gallbladder disease.

Fibrate derivatives have been found to increase the risk of gallstone formation. The overall incidence of gallstones and/or gallbladder sludge in patients receiving long-term octreotide is >50%; however, patients are usually asymptomatic. Symptomatic biliary sludge with ceftriaxone has been reported in rare instances. Most reports are in children.[23–27]

- If pancreatitis is identified, potential medication causes should be considered when other causes have been excluded. Some medication classes with the most evidence to support association include angiotensin-converting enzyme inhibitors, HMG-CoA reductase inhibitors (less likely with pravastatin), oral contraceptives/hormone replacement therapy, diuretics (e.g., furosemide and hydrochlorothiazide), valproic acid, and GLP-1 analogs (e.g., exenatide).[28]
- If gallstones are small (≤5 mm) or if a patient is not a candidate for surgery, ursodiol 8–10 mg/kg/day in two to three divided doses may be used to promote dissolution of the stones. Use beyond 24 months is not established.[29]
- If ERCP reveals biliary tract or ampullary carcinomas, treat according to current standards and considering patient-specific factors and goals. Chemotherapy may be indicated for those with unresectable, locally advanced disease or distant metastasis, or for those with recurrence after resection.[30]

References

1. Wanis KN, Haimanot S, Kantahn R. Endoscopic retrograde cholangiopancreatography: a review of technique and clinical indications. *J Gastroint Dig Syst.* 2014;4(4):1000208.
2. Kozarek RA. The past, present, and future of endoscopic retrograde cholangiopancreatography. *Gastroenterol Hepatol.* 2017;13(10):620–622.
3. Cohen S, Bacon BR, Berlin JA, et al. National Institutes of Health State-of-the-Science Conference Statement: ERCP for diagnosis and therapy, January 14-16, 2002. *Gastrointest Endosc.* 2002;56(6):803–809.
4. Adler DG, Baron TH, Davila RE, et al. ASGE guideline: the role of ERCP in diseases of the biliary tract and the pancreas. *Gastrointest Endosc.* 2005;62(1):1–8.
5. Clark CJ, Fino NF, Clark N, et al. Trends in the use of endoscopic retrograde cholangiopancreatography for the management of chronic pancreatitis in the United States. *J Clin Gastroenterol.* 2016;50(5):417–422.
6. Jeurnink SM, Poley JW, Steyerberg EW, et al. ERCP as an outpatient treatment: a review. *Gastrointest Endosc.* 2008;68(1):118–123.
7. Chapman R, Fevery J, Kalloo A, et al. Diagnosis and management of primary sclerosing cholangitis. *Hepatology.* 2010;51(2):660–678.
8. Coelho-Prabhu N, Baron TH. Endoscopic retrograde cholangiopancreatography in the diagnosis and management of cholangiocarcinoma. *Clin Liver Dis.* 2010;14(2):333–348.
9. Sharma VK, Howden CW. Metaanalysis of randomized controlled trials of endoscopic retrograde cholangiography and endoscopic sphincterotomy for the treatment of acute biliary pancreatitis. *Am J Gastroenterol.* 1999;94(11):3211–3214.
10. Christodoulou DK, Tsianos EV. Role of endoscopic retrograde cholangiopancreatography in pancreatic diseases. *World J Gastroenterol.* 2010;16(38):4755–4761.
11. Chandrasekhara V, Khashab MA, Muthusamy R, et al. Adverse events associated with ERCP. *Gastrointest Endosc.* 2017;85(1):32–47.
12. Park CH, Jung JH, Hyun B, et al. Safety and efficacy of early feeding based on clinical assessment at 4 hours after ERCP: a prospective randomized controlled trial. *Gastrointest Endosc.* 2018;87(4):1040–1049.
13. Acosta RD, Abraham NS, Chandrasekhara V, et al. The management of antithrombotic agents for patients undergoing GI endoscopy. *Gastrointest Endosc.* 2016;83(1):3–16.
14. Sudhakaran S, Surani SR. Guidelines for perioperative management of the diabetic patient. *Surg Res Pract.* 2015;2015:article ID 284063.
15. Cosson E, Catargi B, Cheisson G, et al. Practical management of diabetes patients before, during and after surgery: a joint French diabetology and anaesthesiology position statement. *Diabetes Metab.* 2018;44(3):200–216.
16. Khashab MA, Chithadi KV, Acosta RD, et al. Antibiotic prophylaxis for GI endoscopy. *Gastrointest Endosc.* 2015;81(1):81–89.
17. Wilson W, Taubert KA, Gewitz M, et al. Prevention of infective endocarditis: guidelines from the American Heart Association: a guideline from the American Heart Association Rheumatic Fever,

Endocarditis, and Kawasaki Disease Committee, Council on Cardiovascular Disease in the Young, and the Council on Clinical Cardiology, Council on Cardiovascular Surgery and Anesthesia, and the Quality of Care and Outcomes Research Interdisciplinary Working Group. *Circulation.* 2007;116(15):1736–1754.

18. Mine T, Morizane T, Kawaguchi Y, et al. Clinical practice guideline for post-ERCP pancreatitis. *J Gastroenterol.* 2017;52(9):1013–1022.

19. Elmunzer BJ, Scheiman JM, Lehman GA, et al. A randomized trial of rectal indomethacin to prevent post-ERCP pancreatitis. *N Engl J Med.* 2012;366(15):1414–1422.

20. Kochar B, Akshintala VS, Afghani E, et al. Incidence, severity, and mortality of post-ERCP pancreatitis: a systematic review by using randomized, controlled trials. *Gastrointest Endosc.* 2015;81(1):143–149.

21. Buxbaum J, Yan A, Yeh K, et al. Aggressive hydration with lactated Ringer's solution reduces pancreatitis after endoscopic retrograde cholangiopancreatography. *Clin Gastroenterol Hepatol.* 2014;12(2):303–307.

22. Zhang ZF, Duan ZJ, Wang LX, et al. Aggressive hydration with lactated ringer solution in prevention of postendoscopic retrograde cholangiopancreatography pancreatitis: a meta-analysis of randomized controlled trials. *J Clin Gastroenterol.* 2017;51(3):e17–e26.

23. Gurusamy KS, Davidson BR. Gallstones. *BMJ.* 2014;348:g2669.

24. Faillie J, Yu OH, Yin H, et al. Association of bile duct and gallbladder diseases with the use of incretin-based drugs in patients with type 2 diabetes mellitus. *JAMA Intern Med.* 2016;176(10):1474–1481.

25. Caroli-Bosc FX, Le Gall P, Pugliese P, et al. Role of fibrates and HMG-CoA reductase inhibitors in gallstone formation. *Dig Dis Sci.* 2001;46:540–544.

26. Trendle MC, Moertel CG, Kvols LK. Incidence and morbidity of cholelithiasis in patients receiving chronic octreotide for metastatic carcinoid and malignant islet cell tumors. *Cancer.* 1997;79(4):830–834.

27. Bickford CL, Spencer AP. Biliary sludge and hyperbilirubinemia associated with ceftriaxone in an adult: case report and review of the literature. *Pharmacotherapy.* 2005;25(10):1389–1395.

28. Jones MR, Hall OM, Kaye AM, et al. Drug-induced acute pancreatitis: a review. *Ochsner J.* 2015;15(1):45–51.

29. Abraham S, Rivero HG, Erlikh IV, et al. Surgical and nonsurgical management of gallstones. *Am Fam Physician.* 2014;89(10):795–802.

30. Furuse J, Takada T, Miyazaki M, et al. Guidelines for chemotherapy of biliary tract and ampullary carcinomas. *J Hepatobiliary Pancreat Surg.* 2008;15(1):55–62.

CHAPTER 29

Gastric Emptying Study

Julie A. Murphy, PharmD, FASHP, FCCP, BCPS ▦ Shuhao Qiu, MD, PhD
▦ Shahab Ud Din, MD

Background

Gastric emptying study (GES) is a noninvasive nuclear medicine test used to evaluate patients with suspected gastric motility disorders. As its name suggests, it is used to determine the amount of time required for the stomach to empty after a meal. The first GES to evaluate gastric motility was described in 1966 by Dr. G.H. Griffith and colleagues and consisted of "a standard breakfast of ordinary food" labeled with chromium-51. In 2008, an expert panel of gastroenterologists and nuclear medicine physicians developed consensus guidelines for GES, which is also referred to as gastric emptying scintigraphy.[1-3]

How to Use It

Located in the left upper quadrant of the abdomen, the stomach has four functional components: the fundus, body, antrum, and pylorus. These components work together. The fundus relaxes when solid and liquid food enters the body of the stomach, and then it provides a pressure gradient to move the meal distally by contraction. The stomach body then mixes the ingested meal, and subsequently, the antrum grounds the food into smaller particles (1–2 mm) through repetitive contractions. Once the particles are small enough, the pylorus will then pass the meals into the duodenum. GES correlates with the function of the stomach and determines the presence of normal, delayed, or accelerated emptying of the stomach. Indications for GES include unexplained nausea, vomiting, and dyspepsia, assessment of acid reflux symptoms unresponsive to therapy, assessment of gastric motility prior to fundoplication for gastroesophageal reflux disease, assessment of gastric motility prior to small bowel transplantation or colectomy for colonic inertia, and to screen for gastroparesis in patients with diabetes or rapid gastric emptying as in dumping syndrome.[4-8]

How It Is Done

GES is usually performed by a nuclear medicine technologist under the supervision of an imaging physician in a nuclear medicine department. The test may be performed in an outpatient or inpatient setting. It is best to perform the study in the morning when the rate of gastric emptying is increased. Patients should not eat or drink after midnight on the day of the test. At a minimum, patients should fast for at least 6 hours prior to the test. Medications that are allowed before the test, including serotonin receptor antagonists for severe nausea and vomiting, may be taken with some water when the patient awakens. Patients should not smoke the morning of or during the test, as smoking can slow gastric emptying. A focused medical history should be obtained prior to the GES. Diseases such as esophageal motility disorders, hiatal hernias, gastroesophageal reflux, and previous stomach or abdominal surgeries should be recorded. A standardized gastric emptying meal is prepared. The meal consists of liquid egg whites (120 g or 4 oz) mixed with 0.5 to 1 mCi technetium-99m sulfur colloid marker that is scrambled on a hot skillet or in a microwave.

The mixture should be stirred once or twice during cooking to the consistency of an omelet. Also included as a part of the gastric emptying meal are two slices of toasted white bread with 30 g of strawberry jam. The patient must ingest all the egg mixture and toast/jelly with water (120 mL or 4 oz) within 10 minutes. If the patient cannot eat the entire meal, they must eat at least 50% of each component. The technologist should record how much of the meal the patient consumes, how long it takes to consume the meal, and if the patient vomits at any time during the test. With the patient standing upright, images of the distal esophagus, stomach, and proximal small intestine are taken by scintigraphy (gamma camera) immediately upon ingestion of the meal and 1, 2, and 4 hours after ingestion. The percent of the meal remaining in the stomach at each time point is recorded. Normal values are 30%–90% (1 hour), 30%–60% (2 hours), and 0%–10% (4 hours). Alternative meals that include oatmeal or liquid nutrient supplements may be used for patients with egg allergies or intolerance to eggs; however, normal values are not available for these alternative meals. Some research indicates that even combining liquid and solid gastric emptying studies may add diagnostic benefit as some patients may have normal solid and liquid, abnormal liquid and normal solid, normal liquid and abnormal solid, or abnormal liquid and abnormal solid results. Between images, patients are advised to rest in the sitting position and minimize activity. Patients can resume normal activities after the procedure. The total length of the exam is approximately 4 hours. Allergic reactions to the meal or radiopharmaceuticals are rare and are treated as needed. For premenopausal women, it is best to schedule the study during the first 10 days of the menstrual cycle to avoid radiopharmaceutical exposure for a potentially pregnant woman and to avoid hormonal effects on gastrointestinal motility. GES is not recommended in pregnant patients. Since GES is performed for non-life-threatening conditions, the test should be delayed until breast feeding has finished.[2,3,8–14]

Medication Implications

- Many medications are known to alter gastric emptying and should therefore be avoided prior to the study, except when the purpose of the study is to evaluate a patient's response to therapy.
- Prokinetic agents stimulate smooth muscle contraction to enhance gastric emptying, so they should be stopped 2 days prior to GES. Examples include metoclopramide, tegaserod, erythromycin, and domperidone (not available in the United States).[2,3]
- Since opioid analgesic medications delay gastric emptying, their use could result in a false diagnosis of delayed gastric emptying, so they should be stopped 2 days prior to the study. Examples include morphine, oxycodone, codeine, hydrocodone, meperidine, fentanyl, and methadone.[2,3]
- Anticholinergic antispasmodic agents should be stopped 2 days prior to GES. Examples include atropine, dicyclomine, hyoscyamine, glycopyrrolate, methscopolamine, and hyoscyamine/atropine/scopolamine/phenobarbital.[2,3]
- Antidepressants, dihydropyridine calcium channel blockers, octreotide, theophylline, benzodiazepines, phentolamine, gastric acid suppressants, and aluminum-containing antacids should be discontinued 48 to 72 hours prior to GES.[2,3]
- Laxatives should be avoided the day before the test.[2,3]
- For patients with diabetes, blood glucose levels should be reasonably controlled, as hyperglycemia delays gastric emptying. Hypoglycemia may also influence gastric emptying. Ideally, the blood glucose concentration should be < 200 mg/dL. If the blood glucose concentration is > 275 mg/dL at the time of the test, either the GES should not be performed or the blood glucose concentration can be lowered to < 275 mg/dL with insulin. The blood glucose concentration prior to meal ingestion should be recorded.[2,3]
    - Patients with insulin-dependent diabetes should bring their insulin and glucose monitor with them to GES. They should monitor and adjust their insulin dose accordingly.

Usually, one-half of the usual morning insulin dose is administered with the standardized gastric emptying meal.

- There is no consensus on how to manage oral hypoglycemic agents on the day of GES.
- If GES reveals gastroparesis in a patient with diabetes, glycemic control is the goal, as hyperglycemia is associated with delayed gastric emptying. Pramlintide and glucagon-like peptide-1 analogs should be avoided, as they may delay gastric emptying. In addition, prokinetic therapy should be considered[15]:
  - Metoclopramide at the lowest effective dose should be administered in its liquid formulation to improve absorption. Because of its risk of side effects, including tardive dyskinesia, the Food and Drug Administration placed a black box warning on metoclopramide. Therapy should be discontinued if adverse effects, such as involuntary movements, occur. Metoclopramide may also be associated with QTc prolongation. Drug-drug interactions with agents that alter cytochrome P450 (CYP450) 2D6 function may occur.
  - Erythromycin administered intravenously (IV) may be considered when IV prokinetic therapy is needed in hospitalized patients. Long-term effectiveness of oral therapy is limited by tachyphylaxis due to downregulation of the motilin receptor. The decline in clinical response is usually seen at 4 weeks. Erythromycin may also be associated with QTc prolongation. Drug-drug interactions with agents that alter CYP450 3A4 function may occur.
- If GES reveals dumping syndrome, which may occur after gastric bypass surgery, dietary modifications, including increased protein and fiber intake and eating five to six small meals per day, are indicated. If patients do not respond to these dietary modifications, pharmacologic intervention may be needed[16]:
  - Octreotide has been used with short-term success in patients with both early and late dumping syndrome. Octreotide works by delaying gastric emptying, delaying transit through the small intestine, inhibiting the release of gastrointestinal hormones, inhibiting insulin secretion, increasing splanchnic vasoconstriction, and inhibiting postprandial vasodilation. The short-acting formulation is administered subcutaneously three times daily, and the long-acting formulation is administered intramuscularly every 2–4 weeks. The most common adverse effects are diarrhea, nausea, steatorrhea, gallstones, and injection site pain.
  - Acarbose slows carbohydrate digestion, so it may slow late dumping syndrome. Its use is limited by its adverse effects, including bloating, flatulence, and diarrhea.

References

1. Griffith GH, Owen GM, Kirkman S, et al. Measurement of rate of gastric emptying using chromium-51. *Lancet.* 1966;1(7449):1244–1245.
2. Abell TL, Camilleri M, Donohoe K, et al. Consensus recommendations for gastric emptying scintigraphy: a joint report of the American Neurogastroenterology and Motility Society and the Society of Nuclear Medicine. *Am J Gastroenterol.* 2008;103(3):753–763.
3. Farrell MB. Gastric emptying scintigraphy. *J Nucl Med Technol.* 2019;47(2):111–119.
4. Parkman HP, Jones MP. Tests of gastric neuromuscular function. *Gastroenterology.* 2009;136(5):1526–1543.
5. Harmon RC, Peura DA. Evaluation and management of dyspepsia. *Therap Adv Gastroenterol.* 2010;3(2):87–98.
6. Bielefeldt K. Gastroparesis: concepts, controversies, and challenges. *Scientifica (Cairo).* 2012;2012:424802.
7. Verne GN, Hocking MP, Davis RH, et al. Long-term response to subtotal colectomy in colonic inertia. *J Gastrointest Surg.* 2002;6(5):738–744.
8. Szarka LA, Camilleri M. Gastric emptying. *Clin Gastroenterol Hepatol.* 2009;7(8):823–827.
9. Gill RC, Murphy PD, Hooper HR, et al. Effect of the menstrual cycle on gastric emptying. *Digestion.* 1987;36(3):168–174.

10. Tougas G, Chen Y, Coates G, et al. Standardization of a simplified scintigraphic methodology for the assessment of gastric emptying in a multicenter setting. *Am J Gastroenterol.* 2000;95(1):78–86.
11. Miller G, Palmer KR, Smith B, et al. Smoking delays gastric emptying of solids. *Gut.* 1989;30(1):50–53.
12. Klingensmith WC 3rd, Rhea KL, Wainwright EA, et al. The gastric emptying study with oatmeal: reference range and reproducibility as a function of age and sex. *J Nucl Med Technol.* 2010;38(4):186–190.
13. Ziessman HA, Chander A, Clarke JO, et al. The added diagnostic value of liquid gastric emptying compared with solid emptying alone. *J Nucl Med.* 2009;50(5):726–731.
14. Ziessman HA, Okolo PI, Mullin GE, et al. Liquid gastric emptying is often abnormal when solid emptying is normal. *J Clin Gastroenterol.* 2009;43(7):639–643.
15. Camilleri M, Parkman HP, Shafi MA, et al. American College of Gastroenterology. Clinical guideline: management of gastroparesis. *Am J Gastroenterol.* 2013;108(1):18–37.
16. van Beek AP, Emous M, Laville M, et al. Dumping syndrome after esophageal, gastric or bariatric surgery: pathophysiology, diagnosis, and management. *Obes Rev.* 2017;18(1):68–85.

CHAPTER 30

Gastrointestinal Endoscopy - Capsule

Julie A. Murphy, PharmD, FASHP, FCCP, BCPS ▪ Basil E. Akpunonu, MD, MSC
▪ Shahab Ud Din, MD ▪ Jeannine Hummell, CNP

Background

Capsule endoscopy (CE) is a noninvasive test that was originally developed to visualize abnormalities of the small intestine but may now be used to diagnose and monitor various disease processes throughout the entire gastrointestinal (GI) tract. The word "endoscopy" is derived from the Greek by combining the prefix "endo" meaning "within" and the verb "skopía" meaning "to view." The discovery of CE technology dates to 1981 through the collaboration of Gavriel Iddan, Eitan Scapa, and Paul Swain. Application of Shuji Nakamura's invention of light-emitting diodes (LED) as a light source for optical devices led to further refinement of CE. CE is also referred to as video capsule endoscopy (VCE) and wireless capsule endoscopy (WCE).[1]

How to Use It

CE aids in the diagnosis of various diseases such as obscure GI bleeding, chronic iron deficiency anemia from GI loss, celiac disease, Crohn's disease, nonsteroidal anti-inflammatory drug (NSAID)-induced enteropathy, esophageal disease, and large colon disease. Some limitations of CE include the inability to obtain tissue biopsies, the lack of suctioning or flushing properties, and the possibility of overinterpretation of findings (e.g., reddened areas confused for vascular changes, lymphoid structures as inflammation, and intestinal folds as masses). Obscure GI bleeding is considered when the source of bleeding is not identified within the reach of lower and upper endoscopies. See Chapter 31: Gastrointestinal Endoscopy - Lower and Chapter 32: Gastrointestinal Endoscopy - Upper for more details about these procedures. Bleeding from lesions within the small intestine is responsible for the majority (80%) of obscure GI bleeding events and can manifest as iron deficiency anemia. Most of these lesions are angiodysplastic, which are characteristically small, bleed intermittently, and share similarities to ones that never bleed. In patients with suspicious obscure GI bleeding and unexplained chronic iron deficiency anemia, CE is recommended. CE should not be used to screen or diagnose colon cancer in the general population and especially in those with positive family history of colon cancer or with alarm symptoms of anemia, bleeding, or weight loss. Colon CE is approved by the Food and Drug Administration for use following an incomplete colonoscopy. It can be helpful in patients who do not wish to undergo colonoscopy or when sedation poses a major risk to the patient. CE is now used for screening for Barrett's esophagus, but it is not cost-effective in diagnosis and treatment compared with routine fiber-optic endoscopy. In patients with celiac disease, CE can aid in assessing inadvertent gluten use (gluten contamination). If patients experience unexplained symptoms despite appropriate treatment with a gluten-free diet, CE is recommended to identify complications such as ulcerative jejunoileitis, lymphoma, enteropathy-associated T-cell lymphoma, fibroepithelial polyps, and adenocarcinoma. In patients with Crohn's disease, CE has a sensitivity for detecting jejunal lesions (which are associated with high risk of relapse) reaching 100% when compared with computed tomography enterography and magnetic resonance imaging. CE is not recommended in patients with chronic abdominal pain or diarrhea with no evidence of positive biomarkers such as C-reactive protein. CE is less sensitive in detecting small bowel tumors because lesions in the duodenum and proximal jejunum are easily missed due to rapid transit of capsule and normal bulges are mistaken for masses. The use of CE has expanded our knowledge about the extent of NSAID-induced enteropathy to the small and large bowels.[2–14]

How It Is Done

The procedure should be performed by an endoscopist who is usually a gastroenterologist with documented competency in cognitive, technical, reporting, and interpretation of the capsule examinations. Routine laboratory tests are not required. CE functions are not affected in patients with pacemakers or automatic implantable cardioverter defibrillators (AICDs). However, images can be compromised in patients with left ventricular assist devices (LVAD). CE does not require sedation. For patients who can swallow, the vitamin-size capsule is swallowed orally with water. For patients who cannot swallow, the capsule is deployed by endoscopy. The patient is fitted with a belt containing antennae sensor array that can track the capsule and provide real-time viewing as in cases of GI bleeding or to be viewed later in those with nonacute indications. Activities of daily living should proceed with limitation of strenuous activities. The day before the CE, the patient should be instructed to have only a light breakfast and clear liquids the rest of the day. The patient should not eat or drink for 12 hours before the procedure. Clear liquids can be ingested 2 hours after capsule administration, and a light meal and/or medication(s) can be ingested at 4 hours. Informed consent detailing the benefits and potential complications of CE should be discussed. Complications of CE may include battery failure, missed lesions, and capsule retention in the stomach or areas of obstruction that might require endoscopic or surgical retrieval.[2,15]

Medication Implications

- Bowel preparation improves visualization; no specific type of preparation is recommended.[2,16,17]
  - Polyethylene glycol (PEG) 1, 2, or 4 L demonstrated better visualization and diagnostic yield than clear liquid diet with no other preparation.
  - Combination of PEG (1, 2, or 4 L) and simethicone versus simethicone alone improves visualization with no improvement in diagnostic yield or CE completion rates.
  - Low- versus high-volume PEG cleansing strategies before CE found no differences in visualization, transit times, cleansing scores, or completion rates.
  - European Society of Gastrointestinal Endoscopy recommends administration of simethicone 80–120 mg (optimal dose is not defined) before capsule ingestion.
  - Sodium phosphate improves diagnostic yield without affecting visualization quality.
  - Prokinetic agents do not improve completion rate.
  - PEG is well tolerated; patients may experience minor electrolyte changes, nausea, and bloating.
  - Sodium phosphate is well tolerated; patients may experience minor electrolyte changes, dizziness, and anal irritation.
- The colonic cleansing preparation for a colon CE must be close to perfect to provide excellent pictures. Typically, 3 L of PEG is ingested the evening prior to the procedure with the remaining 1 L administered the morning of the procedure. Use of low-volume oral sodium phosphate and water approximately 2 hours after capsule ingestion, only if the capsule has exited the stomach, may help stimulate the progression of the capsule through the GI tract.[18,19]
- Retrospective cohort studies did not show increased risk of incomplete CE or CE retention related to narcotic use.[20]

- The following medications should be stopped 5–7 days prior to the procedure[21]:
    - All iron supplements (including multivitamins)
    - Antidiarrheal medications (loperamide, bismuth subsalicylate)
    - Fiber supplements (psyllium, methylcellulose)
- For blood glucose control in patients with type 1 diabetes[22]:
    - Continue basal rate insulin replacement (typically around 0.2–0.3 units/kg/day of a long-acting insulin)
- For blood glucose control in patients with type 2 diabetes[23–25]:
    - Thiazolidinediones and sodium-glucose cotransporter-2 (SGLT2) inhibitors (including combination products that include an SGLT2 inhibitor): avoid day before and morning of CE
    - Metformin: avoid evening before and morning of CE
    - Sulfonylureas, glinides, alpha-glucosidase inhibitors, dipeptidyl peptidase-4 (DDP-4) inhibitors, glucagon-like peptide-1 (GLP-1) analogs: avoid morning of CE
    - Long-acting insulin: stop or reduce (give 25% less) dose
    - Combination or premixed insulin: deliver 40%–50% of patient's usual total daily dose as long-acting insulin
    - While patient is taking nothing by mouth (NPO), fingerstick glucose monitoring may be done every 4–6 hours with short-acting (e.g., insulin aspart, insulin lispro) supplemental insulin used to correct hyperglycemia
    - See Chapter 5: Glycemic Considerations for Tests and Procedures for more details about glycemic management
- On the day of the procedure, patients may take all other medications with a small sip of water 4 hours after capsule administration.
- If CE reveals a bleed in the small bowel and is associated with ongoing anemia or active bleeding, the patient should be managed with endoscopic therapy. Patients may be given somatostatin analogs (e.g., octreotide) or oral or intravenous iron therapy if indicated. If possible, anticoagulation and antiplatelet therapy should be discontinued in patients with small bowel hemorrhage.[26]
- If CE reveals celiac disease, patients should be referred to a registered dietician who can provide education on adherence to a lifelong gluten-free diet that includes avoidance of products containing proteins from wheat, barley, and rye. Oats should be introduced with caution and patients should be monitored for adverse reactions. Patients should undergo screening for possible micronutrient deficiencies such as iron, folic acid, vitamin D, and vitamin B12.[27]
- If CE reveals Crohn's disease, it should be treated according to current standards with medication therapy that delivers maximum efficacy with minimal toxicity and considers patient-specific factors. Some agents that may be considered include sulfasalazine, budesonide, thiopurines (azathioprine or 6-mercaptopurine), methotrexate, anti-tumor necrosis factor agents (infliximab, adalimumab, certolizumab pegol), natalizumab, vedolizumab, ustekinumab, or tacrolimus.[28]

References

1. Hosoe N, Naganuma M, Ogata H. Current status of capsule endoscopy through a whole digestive tract. *Dig Endosc.* 2015;27(2):205–215.
2. Enns RA, Hookey L, Armstrong D, et al. Clinical practice guidelines for the use of video capsule endoscopy. *Gastroenterology.* 2017;152(3):497–514.
3. Liu K, Kaffes AJ. Review article: the diagnosis and investigation of obscure gastrointestinal bleeding. *Aliment Pharmacol Ther.* 2011;34(4):416–423.
4. Keum B, Chun HJ. Capsule endoscopy and double balloon enteroscopy for obscure gastrointestinal bleeding: which is better? *J Gastroenterol Hepatol.* 2011;26(5):794–795.

5. Lepileur L, Drey X, Antonietti M, et al. Factors associated with diagnosis of obscure gastrointestinal bleeding by video capsule endoscopy. *Clin Gastroenterol Hepatol*. 2012;10(12):1376–1380.

6. D'Haens G, Löwenberg M, Samaan MA, et al. Safety and feasibility of using the second-generation Pill-Cam colon capsule to assess active colonic Crohn's disease. *Clin Gastroenterol Hepatol*. 2015;13(8):1480–1486.

7. Rubenstein JH, Inadomi JM, Brill JV, et al. Cost utility of screening for Barrett's esophagus with esophageal capsule endoscopy versus conventional upper endoscopy. *Clin Gastroenterol Hepatol*. 2007;5(3):312–318.

8. Kurien M, Evans KE, Aziz I, et al. Capsule endoscopy in adult celiac disease: a potential role in equivocal cases of celiac disease? *Gastrointest Endosc*. 2013;77(2):227–232.

9. Atlas DS, Rubio-Tapia A, Van Dyke CT, et al. Capsule endoscopy in nonresponsive celiac disease. *Gastrointest Endosc*. 2011;74(6):1315–1322.

10. Maiden L, Elliott T, McLaughlin SD, et al. A blinded pilot comparison of capsule endoscopy and small bowel histology in unresponsive celiac disease. *Dig Dis Sci*. 2009;54(6):1280–1283.

11. Flamant M, Trang C, Maillard O, et al. The prevalence and outcome of jejunal lesions visualized by small bowel capsule endoscopy in Crohn's Disease. *Inflamm Bowel Dis*. 2013;19(7):1390–1396.

12. Girelli CM, Porta P. Bulge or mass? A diagnostic dilemma of capsule endoscopy. *Endoscopy*. 2008;40(8):703–704.

13. Lim YJ, Chun HJ. Recent advances in NSAIDs-induced enteropathy therapeutics: new options, new challenges. *Gastroenterol Res Pract*. 2013;2013:761060.

14. Wallace JL. NSAID gastropathy and enteropathy: distinct pathogenesis likely necessitates distinct prevention strategies. *Br J Pharmacol*. 2012;165(1):67–74.

15. Van Weyenberg SJB, Van Turenhout ST, Bouma G, et al. Double-balloon endoscopy as the primary method for small-bowel video capsule endoscope retrieval. *Gastrointest Endosc*. 2010;71(3):535–541.

16. Kotwal VS, Attar BM, Gupta S, et al. Should bowel preparation, antifoaming agents, or prokinetics be used before video capsule endoscopy? A systematic review and meta-analysis. *Eur J Gastroenterol Hepatol*. 2014;26(2):137–145.

17. Rondonotti E, Spada C, Adler S, et al. Small-bowel capsule endoscopy and device-assisted enteroscopy for diagnosis and treatment of small-bowel disorders: European Society of Gastrointestinal Endoscopy (ESGE) technical review. *Endoscopy*. 2018;50(4):423–446.

18. Schoofs N, Deviere J, Van Gossum A. PillCam colon capsule endoscopy compared with colonoscopy for colorectal tumor diagnosis: a prospective pilot study. *Endoscopy*. 2006;38(10):971–977.

19. Van Gossum A, Munoz-Navas M, Fernandez-Urien I, et al. Capsule endoscopy versus colonoscopy for the detection of polyps and cancer. *N Engl J Med*. 2009;361:264–270.

20. Lee MM, Jacques A, Lam E, et al. Factors associated with incomplete small bowel capsule endoscopy studies. *World J Gastroenterol*. 2010;16(42):5329–5333.

21. Koulaoizidis A, Douglas S. Capsule endoscopy in clinical practice: concise up-to-date overview. *Clin Exp Gastroenterol*. 2009;2:111–116.

22. Meneghini LF. Perioperative management of diabetes: transitioning evidence into practice. *Cleve Clin J Med*. 2009;76(Suppl 4):S53–S59.

23. Sudhakaran S, Surani SR. Guidelines for perioperative management of the diabetic patient. *Surg Res Pract*. 2015:article ID 284063.

24. Cosson E, Catargi B, Cheisson G, et al. Practical management of diabetes patients before, during and after surgery: A joint French diabetology and anaesthesiology position statement. *Diabetes Metab*. 2018;44(3):200–216.

25. Hochberg I, Segol O, Shental R, et al. Antihyperglycemic therapy during colonoscopy preparation: a review and suggestions for practical recommendations. *United European Gastroenterol J*. 2019;7(6):735–740.

26. Gerson LB, Fidler JL, Cave DR, et al. ACG clinical guideline: diagnosis and management of small bowel bleeding. *Am J Gastroenterol*. 2015;110(9):1265–1287.

27. Rubio-Tapia A, Hill ID, Kelly C, et al. ACG clinical guidelines: diagnosis and management of celiac disease. *Am J Gastroenterol*. 2013;108(5):656–676.

28. Lichtenstein GR, Loftus EV, Isaacs KL, et al. ACG clinical guideline: management of Crohn's disease in adults. *Am J Gastroent*. 2018;113(4):481–517.

CHAPTER 31

Gastrointestinal Endoscopy - Lower

Julie A. Murphy, PharmD, FASHP, FCCP, BCPS ▪ Shahab Ud Din, MD
▪ Basil E. Akpunonu, MD, MSC, FACP

Background

Colonoscopy is an endoscopic technique used to visualize the colon for screening, diagnostic, and therapeutic purposes. A sigmoidoscopy allows for visualization of the distal part of the large intestine between the descending colon and rectum. The suffix "-scopy" is derived from "skopía" meaning "to view." Phillip Bozzini, an early 19th-century German physician, was the first to introduce a primitive scope ("Lichtleiter" or light conductor) to inspect internal anatomy of the larynx, urethra, bladder, and rectum. With time and technologic advancement, colonoscopes became available in the late 1960s with robust advancement noted especially in the last two decades.[1–4]

How to Use It

A screening colonoscopy is performed on asymptomatic patients for early identification of polyps or colorectal cancer. Exact recommendations for colorectal cancer screening vary among organizations like the American Cancer Society, United States Preventive Services Task Force, and American College of Physicians, but first colonoscopy is generally recommended at age 50 for an average-risk adult. A diagnostic colonoscopy may be performed when a patient is experiencing symptoms such as bleeding per rectum, abdominal pain, chronic diarrhea, melena, occult gastrointestinal (GI) bleeding (by positive fecal occult blood test), or iron deficiency anemia to identify the underlying pathology. Colonoscopy can help identify and treat diverticular bleeding, rectal or colonic neoplasm that may be benign or malignant, inflammatory bowel disease such as Crohn's or ulcerative colitis, arteriovenous malformations (AVM), anastomotic bleeding, hemorrhoids, ischemic colitis, or infectious colitis. Patients with inflammatory bowel disease or colonic polyposis syndrome may require repeated colonoscopies for both diagnostic and therapeutic purposes.[5–7]

How It Is Done

Colonoscopy/sigmoidoscopy is performed by a physician who has received specialized training in colonoscopy, such as a gastroenterologist or surgeon, after informed consent is obtained. Depending on who is performing the test, colonoscopy/sigmoidoscopy can be completed using general anesthesia, sedation/analgesia, or no sedation; therefore, the patient may be awake or asleep for the procedure. The procedure is usually performed in an outpatient endoscopy suite and takes approximately 30 minutes. Rarely, the procedure may be performed in the intensive care unit setting for an unstable patient with active bleeding. Colonoscopy may be performed presurgically to tattoo the diseased portion of the colon via colonoscope to aid in open surgical resection. Flexible sigmoidoscopy may be performed during an outpatient office visit without anesthesia or sedatives. A sigmoidoscopy usually takes approximately 20 minutes.

Bowel preparation (prep) is indicated prior to colonoscopy/sigmoidoscopy. The ideal prep should be simple to administer, tolerable to patients, and should not cause electrolyte disturbances or alterations in colonic mucosa. Patient-specific characteristics and comorbidities must be considered when choosing a regimen. Specific details about the various bowel preparation options are provided under "Medication Implications." After a light breakfast the morning prior to the colonoscopy, patients should follow a clear liquid diet. Data suggests that a low-residue diet may lead to improved preparation quality compared with a clear liquid diet. The day of the colonoscopy, patients should withhold liquids for at least 6 hours prior to the procedure.

Before the colonoscope or sigmoidoscope is inserted into the rectum, a visual inspection of the anus is followed by digital rectal exam to identify any local disease process. The colonoscope is advanced to the cecum, then slowly withdrawn as the colonic mucosa is inspected. The colonoscope has a small camera, with a light source, that transmits images to an external display monitor. The colonoscope has channels for instrument insertions required to remove polyps, cauterize bleeding vessels, or take biopsy samples from the colon. It also has openings to facilitate injection and suction of air/water to provide clearer images. Post procedure, the patient is briefly observed as they recover from anesthesia or sedative administration. The patient returns home or to the medical ward, if the procedure is completed while the patient is hospitalized. The endoscopist communicates recommendations to the patient and ordering physician based on findings. Histopathology reports for biopsies are usually available within 48–72 hours. A normal result is shared right away as "normal colonoscopy," which means the procedure showed normal appearing colonic mucosa with no polyps, cancer, ulcers, diverticula, hyperemia, or AVM.

General procedural complications ranging from anesthesia, cardiovascular, and respiratory morbidities to minimal risk of bacteremia or pneumonia may occur. Death within 30 days of colonoscopy is reported as <0.83%. The overall incidence of adverse events after colonoscopy is low, but risk increases with interventions (e.g., polypectomy), increasing patient age, or comorbid health conditions. Major complications related directly to colonoscopy like perforation, bleeding, post-polypectomy electrocoagulation syndrome, gas explosion, acute diverticulitis, and perineum infections occur at rates of <0.1%–0.63%. Minor self-limiting GI symptoms like nonspecific abdominal pain, paralytic ileus, nausea, and vomiting occur at higher rates than major complications. Colonoscopy should be avoided under conditions that may increase the risk of colon perforation like acute diverticulitis, toxic megacolon, or fulminant colitis. Colonoscopies are also avoided in complete or near-complete intestinal obstruction.[8-19]

Medication Implications

- Bowel preparation improves visualization.[8-10,12,13,20,21]
    - Most commonly used due to proven cleansing superiority: 4 L of polyethylene glycol-electrolyte lavage solution (PEG-ELS). However, 5%–15% of patients do not complete the prep, as it is the least palatable.
    - A more palatable alternative is 4 L of sulfate-free PEG-ELS.
    - Two liters of PEG-ELS with ascorbic acid is a low-volume prep that must be administered with an extra liter of clear fluid to maintain hydration. This regimen should be avoided in glucose-6-phosphate dehydrogenase deficiency due to risk of acute hemolysis.
    - Sodium phosphate tablets are not first line and have a black box warning of acute phosphate nephropathy, limiting their use in older patients or those with renal insufficiency. They should be avoided in patients with inflammatory bowel disease due to increased mucosal inflammation.
    - Split-dose prep (reserving half of the prep dose for the morning of the procedure) is recommended for ideal colon cleansing as in the hours following the initial prep consumption, chyme from the small intestine accumulates in the colon, obscuring visualization. The time between completion of the same-day prep dose and the start of the procedure should be no more than 3–4 hours.

- For sigmoidoscopy, enema bowel preparations (EBPs) were shown to be at least equivalent in bowel cleansing as oral preps. An EBP includes the administration of two phosphate enemas.
- Holding antiplatelets and anticoagulants prior to colonoscopy/sigmoidoscopy is based on procedure bleeding risk (e.g., with or without polypectomy)[22-25]:
  - Usually aspirin products should be held for 7–10 days. If the patient is considered high risk for cardiovascular disease, it is not recommended to stop (consult with cardiology). Aspirin can be resumed after colonoscopy/sigmoidoscopy.
  - Recommended time to hold $P2Y_{12}$ inhibitors depends on the agent (ticagrelor 3–5 days, clopidogrel 5–7 days, prasugrel 7–9 days, ticlopidine 10–14 days). Resuming antiplatelets within 5 days was not associated with an increase in delayed bleeding.
  - The recommended time to hold direct oral anticoagulants (DOACs) depends on the specific medication and the patient's creatinine clearance. See Chapter 13: Bronchoscopy and Chapter 4: Anticoagulation Management in the Periprocedural Period for more details about holding these medications in invasive procedures.
    - Agents may be resumed within 24 hours of colonoscopy/sigmoidoscopy
  - Dipyridamole and cilostazol should be held for 2 days prior to procedure.
  - Risk of thromboembolism must be considered. According to the American College of Chest Physicians, annual thromboembolism risk determines overall risk (i.e., high [>10%], moderate [5%–10%], or low [<5%]).
    - For low- to moderate-risk patients, stop warfarin 5 days prior to and check the international normalized ratio (INR) the morning of the procedure. Warfarin may be resumed 12–24 hours after colonoscopy/sigmoidoscopy.
    - For moderate- to high-risk patients, stop warfarin 5 days prior to procedure and bridge with therapeutic doses of low-molecular-weight heparin (LMWH) or unfractionated heparin (UH) when INR falls below the lower therapeutic goal limit. Stop LMWH 12 hours prior to procedure, and stop UH 4–6 hours prior to procedure. Warfarin may be resumed 12–24 hours after colonoscopy/sigmoidoscopy. Resume bridging therapy as soon as possible after colonoscopy/sigmoidoscopy. Therapeutic doses of LMWH or UH can be stopped 5 days after resuming warfarin and when the INR is above the lower therapeutic goal limit.
- Recommended time to hold nonsteroidal anti-inflammatory drugs (NSAIDs) is dependent on the half-life of the NSAID. NSAIDs can be resumed after colonoscopy/sigmoidoscopy[22,23]:
  - Ibuprofen, diclofenac, ketoprofen, indomethacin (1 day prior)
  - Naproxen, sulindac, celecoxib (2–3 days prior)
  - Meloxicam, piroxicam (10 days prior)
- Antihyperglycemic therapy[26]:
  - Metformin, meglitinides, acarbose, thiazolidinediones, dipeptidyl peptidase-4 inhibitors, glucagon-like peptide-1 (GLP-1) agonists: use as long as eating solid food; resume when eating regular meals.
  - Sulfonylureas and sodium-glucose cotransporter-2 inhibitors: do not take the day before or day of procedure; resume when eating regular meals.
  - Basal insulin, premixed rapid/short and medium insulin, or combined basal insulin and GLP-1 agonist:
    - Type 1 diabetes: inject 50%–80% of the usual dose in the 24 hours before colonoscopy; if usually inject in the morning, only inject 50%–80% of the usual dose; consult endocrinologist
    - Type 2 diabetes: inject 50% of the usual dose in the 24 hours before colonoscopy; resume when eating regular meals

- Rapid insulin in pens or insulin pump: once patient is no longer eating solid food, if glucose is > 200 mg/dL, give only corrections as in other fasting situations; resume when eating regular meals.
- Insulin pump (when discontinuing solid food):
  - Type 1 diabetes: reduce to 50%–80% of the usual dose; leave insulin pump on during procedure; give intravenous glucose if needed; resume usual dose when resuming regular meals; consult endocrinologist
  - Type 2 diabetes: reduce to 50% of the usual dose; leave insulin pump on during procedure; give intravenous glucose if needed; resume usual dose when resuming regular meals
- See Chapter 5: Glycemic Considerations for Tests and Procedures for more details.
- Stop iron supplements 7 days prior to colonoscopy/sigmoidoscopy; iron can turn the stool dark and tarry, hindering visualization of the colonic mucosa.[27]
- If colonoscopy/sigmoidoscopy reveals cancer (primary or metastatic), treat according to current standards and considering patient-specific factors and goals.
- If colonoscopy reveals ulcerative colitis, treat according to current standards with medication therapy that delivers maximum efficacy with minimal toxicity and considers patient-specific factors. Some agents that may be considered include 5-aminosalicylate, azathioprine, infliximab, adalimumab, golimumab, vedolizumab, tofacitinib, or ustekinumab. In hospitalized patients, intravenous methylprednisolone, infliximab, or cyclosporine may be used.[28]
- If colonoscopy reveals Crohn's disease, treat according to current standards with medication therapy that delivers maximum efficacy with minimal toxicity and considers patient-specific factors. Some agents that may be considered include sulfasalazine, budesonide, thiopurines (azathioprine or 6-mercaptopurine), methotrexate, anti-tumor necrosis factor agents (infliximab, adalimumab, certolizumab pegol), natalizumab, vedolizumab, ustekinumab, or tacrolimus.[29]
- If colonoscopy/sigmoidoscopy reveals diverticular bleeding, a combination of epinephrine injection and electrocautery therapy is indicated. Aspirin and NSAIDs should be avoided due to associated increased risk of bleeding. Patients should increase dietary fiber or begin fiber supplementation (32 g/day).[30–32]

References

1. "Colon." *The Merriam-Webster.com Dictionary*, Merriam-Webster. https://www.merriam-webster.com /dictionary/colon. Accessed 2 May. 2020.
2. "Scope." *The Merriam-Webster.com Dictionary*, Merriam-Webster. https://www.merriam-webster.com /dictionary/scope. Accessed 2 May. 2020.
3. Bush RB, Leonhardt H, Bush IV, et al. Dr. Bozzini's Lichtleiter. A translation of his original article (1806). *Urology*. 1974;3(1):119–123.
4. Wolff WI. Colonoscopy: history and development. *Am J Gastroenterol*. 1989;84(9):1017–1025.
5. Wolf AMD, Fontham ETH, Church TR, et al. Colorectal cancer screening for average-risk adults: 2018 guideline update from the American Cancer Society. *Ca Cancer J Clin*. 2018;68(4):250–281.
6. US Preventive Services Task Force. Screening for colorectal cancer: US preventive services task force recommendation statement. *JAMA*. 2016;315(23):2564–2575.
7. Qaseem A, Crandall CJ, Mustafa RA, et al. Screening for colorectal cancer in asymptomatic average-risk adults: a guidance statement from the American College of Physicians. *Ann Intern Med*. 2019;171(9):643–654.
8. ASGE Standards of Practice Committee, Saltzman JR, Cash BD, et al. Bowel preparation before colonoscopy. *Gastrointest Endosc*. 2015;81(4):781–794.
9. Hassan C, Bretthauer M, Kaminski MF, et al. Bowel preparation for colonoscopy: European Society of Gastrointestinal Endoscopy (ESGE) guideline. *Endoscopy*. 2013;45(2):142–150.
10. Rutherford CC, Calderwood AH. Update on bowel preparation for colonoscopy. *Curr Treat Options Gastro*. 2018;16(1):165–181.

11. Rex DK, Bond JH, Winawer S, et al. Quality in the technical performance of colonoscopy and the continuous quality improvement process for colonoscopy: recommendations of the U.S. Multi-Society Task Force on Colorectal Cancer. *Am J Gastroenterol.* 2002;97(6):1296–1308.

12. Johnson DA, Barkun AN, Cohen LB, et al. Optimizing adequacy of bowel cleansing for colonoscopy: recommendations from the U.S. Multi-Society Task Force on Colorectal Cancer. *Gastroenterology.* 2014;147(4):903–924.

13. Manoucheri M, Nakamura DY, Lukman RL. Bowel preparation for flexible sigmoidoscopy: which method yields the best results? *J Fam Pract.* 1999;48(4):272–274.

14. Nguyen DL, Jamal MM, Nguyen ET, et al. Low-residue versus clear liquid diet before colonoscopy: a meta-analysis of randomized, controlled trials. *Gastrointest Endosc.* 2016;83(3):499–507.

15. Warren JL, Klabunde CN, Mariotto AB, et al. Adverse events after outpatient colonoscopy in the Medicare population. *Ann Intern Med.* 2009;150(12):849–857.

16. ASGE Standards of Practice Committee, Fisher DA, Maple JT, et al. Complications of colonoscopy. *Gastrointest Endosc.* 2011;74(4):745–752.

17. Levin TR, Zhao W, Conell C, et al. Complications of colonoscopy in an integrated health care delivery system. *Ann Intern Med.* 2006;145(12):880–886.

18. Ladas SD, Karamanolis G, Ben-Soussan E. Colonic gas explosion during therapeutic colonoscopy with electrocautery. *World J Gastroenterol.* 2007;13(40):5295–5298.

19. Nelson DB, McQuaid KR, Bond JH, et al. Procedural success and complications of large-scale screening colonoscopy. *Gastrointest Endosc.* 2002;55(3):307–314.

20. Mehta JB, Singhal SB, Mehta BC. Ascorbic-acid-induced haemolysis in G-6-PD deficiency. *Lancet.* 1990;336(8720):944.

21. Sajid MS, Caswell JF, Abbas MAQ, et al. Improving the view during flexible sigmoidoscopy: a systematic review of published randomized, controlled trials comparing the use of oral bowel preparation versus enema bowel preparation. *Updates Surg.* 2015;67(3):247–256.

22. Feagins LA. Management of anticoagulants and antiplatelet agents during colonoscopy. *Am J Med.* 2017;130(7):786–795.

23. Beppu K, Osada T, Sakamoto N, et al. Optimal timing for resuming antithrombotic agents and risk factors for delayed bleeding after endoscopic resection of colorectal tumors. *Gastroenterol Res Pract.* 2014;2014:825179.

24. Douketis JD, Spyropoulos AC, Spencer FA, et al. Perioperative management of antithrombotic therapy: Antithrombotic therapy and prevention of thrombosis, 9th ed: American college of chest physicians evidence-based clinical practice guidelines. *Chest.* 2012;141(Suppl 2):e326S–e350S.

25. Baron TH, Kamath PS, McBane RD. Management of antithrombotic therapy in patients undergoing invasive procedures. *N Engl J Med.* 2013;368(22):2113–2124.

26. Hochberg I, Segol O, Shental R, et al. Antihyperglycemic therapy during colonoscopy preparation: a review and suggestions for practical recommendations. *United European Gastroenterol J.* 2019;7(6):735–740.

27. Ton L, Lee H, Taunk P, et al. Nationwide variability of colonoscopy preparation instructions. *Dig Dis Sci.* 2014;59(8):1726–1732.

28. Feuerstein JD, Isaacs KL, Schneider Y, et al. AGA clinical practice guidelines on the management of moderate to severe ulcerative colitis. *Gastroenterology.* 2020;158(5):1450–1461.

29. Lichtenstein GR, Loftus EV, Isaacs KL, et al. ACG clinical guideline: management of Crohn's disease in adults. *Am J Gastroent.* 2018;113(4):481–517.

30. Wilkins T, Baird C, Pearson AN, et al. Diverticular bleeding. *Am Fam Physician.* 2009;80(9):977–983.

31. Laine L, Smith R, Min K, et al. Systematic review: the lower gastrointestinal adverse effects of nonsteroidal anti-inflammatory drugs. *Aliment Pharmacol Ther.* 2006;24(5):751–767.

32. Aldoori WH, Giovannucci EL, Rockett HR, et al. A prospective study of dietary fiber types and symptomatic diverticular disease in men. *J Nutr.* 1998;128(4):714–719.

CHAPTER 32

Gastrointestinal Endoscopy - Upper

Gregory J. Hughes, PharmD, BCPS, BCGP

Background

Esophagogastroduodenoscopy (EGD) is a procedure that enables visualization and interaction with the upper gastrointestinal (GI) tract. It is called EGD because it uses a "scope" (an instrument for viewing; e.g., microscope, telescope) to access the esophagus (the "E"), stomach (gastric – the "G"), and duodenum (the "D"). It is also referred to as an upper endoscopy. EGD is one of the most common procedures performed by a gastroenterologist and can be used to diagnose and treat numerous conditions.[1]

How to Use It

For diagnostic purposes, EGD allows for direct viewing of the esophagus, stomach, and proximal duodenum. These views provide more information than a two-dimensional X-ray. By enabling access to the mucosa, a gastroenterologist can directly visualize, biopsy, photograph, and video record their findings. EGDs are also used to perform therapeutic interventions such as dilating strictures, placing stents, removing foreign bodies, placing gastrostomy tubes, treating GI bleeding, and treating intestinal metaplasia.[2]

EGD is indicated for both elective and urgent scenarios. Many elective indications include those that are extensions of the diagnostic process, such as the workup of abdominal pain, diarrhea, vomiting, dyspepsia, gastroesophageal reflux disease (GERD), peptic ulcers, dysphagia, anemia secondary to occult blood loss, and cancer staging. For many of these elective indications, EGD is not done as the first-line procedure. Rather, it is reserved for conditions that are recurring, have an unknown cause, or are refractory to other medical therapy (e.g., GERD symptoms refractory to acid suppression therapy, dyspepsia thought to be due to *Helicobacter pylori* that persists despite treatment). EGD is often indicated if complaints are concerning for structural disease, especially if occurring with alarm symptoms such as weight loss or anorexia. Other indications for elective EGD include confirming radiologically identified lesions with a tissue biopsy (e.g., neoplasia, ulcer, stricture, *H. pylori*) and surveilling premalignant conditions (e.g., Barrett's esophagus). Iron deficiency anemia can be worked up with EGD but may also involve lower or capsule endoscopies.[3] See Chapter 30: Gastrointestinal Endoscopy - Capsule and Chapter 31: Gastrointestinal Endoscopy - Lower for more details.

Indications for urgent EGD include acute GI hemorrhage (e.g., secondary to varices, ulcers, Mallory-Weiss tear), obstruction, and dilation of stenosis. Obstructions caused by food and foreign objects can be removed during EGD, and those caused by malignancies or stenosis can be treated with tube placement for gastric decompression and dilatation with stents.[3]

Of note, EGDs should not be performed when the results will not change medical management, to surveil for healed benign disease (e.g., esophagitis, gastric ulcer), or when perforated mucosa is known or suspected.[2]

How It Is Done

EGD can be done as an elective procedure in the outpatient setting. Though performed by a gastroenterologist, EGDs can be directly scheduled by a primary care physician when the indication is clear.[3] Urgent EGDs are often done in the inpatient setting in a GI/endoscopy suite but can be done at the bedside or in the operating room.[1]

At the time of the procedure, patients are usually administered sedation (e.g., midazolam, propofol) ranging from conscious sedation to general anesthesia to minimize patient discomfort and produce amnesia. Analgesia (e.g., fentanyl) is sometimes used if the patient experiences pain during the procedure.[4] The choice of sedation is dependent on a number of factors, including the risk of complications of sedation, ability to cooperate with instructions, and potential need for endotracheal intubation. See Chapter 6: Introductory to Anesthesia for more details about these choices. Reversal agents (i.e., flumazenil, naloxone) can be used if the patient experiences too much sedation, but are not routinely used.

When performing EGDs in an elective setting, it is necessary for the patient to fast in advance due to the increased risk of aspiration associated with the use of sedation in nonfasted states. The American Society of Anesthesiologists has specific recommendations for fasting prior to procedures requiring sedation. See Chapter 6: Introductory to Anesthesia for the timing requirements of the different types of foods. When EGD is performed urgently or when gastric emptying is impaired, it is necessary to consider the increased risk of aspiration. This risk affects the level of sedation chosen, the choice to consider delaying the procedure, and the use of endotracheal intubation to protect the airway.[1]

The endoscope is a flexible tube that is passed into the patient's mouth and advanced through the esophagus, stomach, and into the proximal duodenum.[3] Pictures and video are taken as the endoscope is advanced and certain structures (e.g., fundus of the stomach) are viewed when the endoscope is withdrawn. Images and histology results are generally uploaded into the medical record. Depending on the indication, EGDs may also involve the use of various accessories such as biopsy forceps, cytology brushes, needles for injection, hemostatic clips, polypectomy snares, foreign body retrieval instruments, and syringes for irrigation.[1]

Complications of EGD are those that are most commonly related to sedation (e.g., cardiopulmonary, aspiration).[1] See Chapter 6: Introduction to Anesthesia for details. Other complications include infections, bleeding, and perforation, although these events are rarely reported.

Bacteremia due to translocation of endogenous microbial flora is a common occurrence in the moments immediately following manipulation with the endoscope (with or without a biopsy). This bacteremia is usually brief (<30 minutes) and is not associated with clinical infections. It is noteworthy that transient episodes of bacteremia occur on a continual basis with daily events such as tooth brushing and flossing (20%–68%), using wooden toothpicks (20%–40%), and chewing food (7%–51%).[5] These frequencies are comparable or even exceed rates of transient bacteremia that occur with the highest-risk endoscopic procedures such as esophageal dilation and sclerotherapy of varices.[6] Despite the millions of EGDs that occur annually in the United States, infective endocarditis has only been reported in roughly 25 cases.[6] The role of antibiotics for prophylaxis is discussed in the "Medication Implications" section of this chapter. See Chapter 21: Culture - Blood for details about the workup of bacteremia.

A diagnostic EGD is considered a low-risk bleeding procedure whether or not a biopsy is performed. EGD techniques considered high risk for bleeding include dilatation for achalasia and the treatment of varices.[7] Recommendations on discontinuing and resuming antiplatelet and anticoagulant agents are discussed in the "Medication Implications" section of this chapter. See Chapter 4: Anticoagulation Management in the Periprocedural Period for a general overview about using these agents. During EGD, acute GI bleeding can be halted with several hemostatic techniques such as band ligation, clipping, or local injection of sclerosants such as epinephrine 1:10,000 which causes vasospasm.

Under optimal sedation conditions, EGD typically takes 5–10 minutes.[1] A normal EGD should reveal normal mucosa free from inflammation, ulceration, varices, masses, bleeding, or strictures.

Medication Implications

- Most medications can be taken with a small sip of water, despite recommendations to fast in the "How It Is Done" section. Medications that should be taken with food require special attention, particularly those that lower the blood glucose. Antihyperglycemic medications such as sulfonylureas and nonsulfonylurea secretagogues should be held the day of the procedure and possibly the day before the procedure. The Food and Drug Administration updated labeling for the sodium-glucose cotransporter-2 (SGLT2) inhibitors, stating that they should be held 3–4 days before fasting for EGD.[7] Basal insulin doses should be decreased by 20%–25% if taken the same day as the procedure. If basal insulin is used twice daily, the two doses prior to EGD should be similarly reduced.[8] See Chapter 5: Glycemic Considerations for Tests and Procedures for details about glycemic management.
    - When EGD is performed urgently, holding medications already administered is not an option, so the decision to perform the procedure will depend on numerous situational factors including indication, risk of delay, and stability of patient.
- When considering antiplatelet and anticoagulant agent use during EGD, one must balance the risk of bleeding (increased when continuing the medications) with the risk of undertreating conditions (by holding the medications). See Chapter 4: Anticoagulation Management in the Periprocedural Period for more details about balancing these risks.
    - Routine diagnostic EGDs are considered low risk from a bleeding standpoint, and antiplatelet and anticoagulants (e.g., warfarin, direct oral anticoagulants) should be continued through the periprocedural period.[7]
    - Balloon dilatation and treatment of varices during EGDs are high-risk bleeding procedures. When possible, they should be performed 5–7 days after cessation of $P2Y_{12}$ antagonists but aspirin should continue uninterrupted. Cessation of $P2Y_{12}$ antagonists should not occur within the first 30 days after a percutaneous coronary intervention with stent placement, and it may be reasonable to defer an elective EGD for at least 12 months following placement with a drug-eluting coronary stent. Dual antiplatelet therapy can be resumed following the procedure once hemostasis is confirmed.[7]
        - Anticoagulants should be held for the appropriate interval for these high-risk bleeding procedures. See Chapter 4: Anticoagulation Management in the Periprocedural Period for more details including dosing and half-life of specific agents. If the patient is also high risk for thromboembolic events, bridging therapy can be considered.
        - Following an EGD, warfarin can be restarted on the same day in patients who are not bleeding. Direct oral anticoagulants have a rapid onset and limited reversal options, so it is reasonable to delay restarting use until adequate hemostasis is confirmed.
- Several studies have been published evaluating patients receiving warfarin that are presenting with acute upper GI bleeding. These studies have found that the international normalized ratio (INR) was not a predictor of rebleeding, even when elevated. The data suggests that endoscopic hemostatic therapy is highly effective and that delaying an EGD to reverse the INR might not be worthwhile. Until more data are available, guidelines state that it is reasonable to perform EGD in bleeding patients with an INR <2.5.[7]
- As previously discussed in the "How It Is Done" section, bacteremia commonly occurs following EGD but is transient and does not result in clinical infections. As such, the guideline recommendations are against the routine administration of antibiotics to prevent infective endocarditis.[6] Specific patient population recommendations include:

- For patients with high-risk cardiac conditions who are already receiving antibiotics for another GI infection (e.g., cholangitis), antimicrobial coverage should include enterococci.[6]
- Patients with GI bleeding as a complication of cirrhosis often require EGD. Regardless if EGD is planned, these patients should receive antibiotics (e.g., ceftriaxone), as they are associated with several benefits, including reduced overall mortality.[6]
- Prophylactic antibiotics should not be added for patients with synthetic vascular grafts, nonvalvular cardiac devices (e.g., implantable cardioverter defibrillators), or orthopedic prostheses.[6]

- For patients undergoing EGD because of suspicion of GI bleeding, it is important to evaluate all medications. Identifying prescription medications, over-the-counter medications, and supplements that are ulcerogenic or could otherwise contribute to bleeding is essential (e.g., nonsteroidal anti-inflammatory drugs [including topical formulations], niacin [over-the-counter or prescription], and herbal supplements [e.g., ginger]). Bleeding identified during EGD would inherently be considered upper GI bleeding, so treatment frequently involves acid suppression therapy (e.g., proton pump inhibitor [PPI]) and discontinuation of the offending agent, if possible.
  - PPIs are highly effective at increasing the pH of the stomach, resulting in decreased rebleeding in some conditions. For example, though there is limited evidence comparing regimens, esomeprazole 80 mg intravenous bolus followed by 8 mg/hour for 72 hours has been suggested when managing bleeding secondary to peptic ulcer disease.[9] However, acute bleeding secondary to gastroesophageal varices responds to vasoactive medication, such as octreotide, but does not seem to benefit from the use of PPIs.[10]
- If the patient has a biopsy taken during EGD that returns positive for *H. pylori*, a three- to four-drug combination is necessary for treatment. Though numerous regimens are recommended, one first-line combination is a PPI, clarithromycin, and amoxicillin (or metronidazole) for 14 days. In choosing a regimen, it is necessary to consider factors such as allergies, drug interactions, side effects, patient adherence, *H. pylori* sensitivity, and dosing in renal dysfunction.[11]

References

1. Ahlawat R, Hoilat GJ, Ross AB. Esophagogastroduodenoscopy In: *StatPearls*: StatPearls Publishing; 2020. Accessed September 23, 2020. http://www.ncbi.nlm.nih.gov/books/NBK532268/.
2. Early DS, Ben-Menachem T, Decker GA, et al. Appropriate use of GI endoscopy. *Gastrointest Endosc.* 2012;75(6):1127–1131.
3. Gastrointestinal Endoscopy | Harrison's Principles of Internal Medicine, 19e | AccessPharmacy | McGraw-Hill Medical. Accessed September 23, 2020. https://accesspharmacy.mhmedical.com/Content.aspx?bookid=1130&sectionid=79747298.
4. Amornyotin S. Sedation and monitoring for gastrointestinal endoscopy. *World J Gastrointest Endosc.* 2013;5(2):47–55.
5. Wilson W, Taubert KA, Gewitz M, et al. Prevention of Infective Endocarditis: Guidelines From the American Heart Association: A Guideline From the American Heart Association Rheumatic Fever, Endocarditis, and Kawasaki Disease Committee, Council on Cardiovascular Disease in the Young, and the Council on Clinical Cardiology, Council on Cardiovascular Surgery and Anesthesia, and the Quality of Care and Outcomes Research Interdisciplinary Working Group. *Circulation.* 2007;116(15):1736–1754.
6. ASGE Standards of Practice CommitteeKhashab MA, Chithadi KV, et al. Antibiotic prophylaxis for GI endoscopy. *Gastrointest Endosc.* 2015;81(1):81–89.
7. Acosta RD, Abraham NS, Chandrasekhara V, et al. The management of antithrombotic agents for patients undergoing GI endoscopy. *Gastrointest Endosc.* 2016;83(1):3–16.
8. Dogra P, Jialal I. Diabetic Perioperative Management*StatPearls*: StatPearls Publishing; 2020. Accessed September 24, 2020. http://www.ncbi.nlm.nih.gov/books/NBK540965/.
9. Tarasconi A, Coccolini F, Biffl WL, et al. Perforated and bleeding peptic ulcer: WSES guidelines. *World J Emerg Surg.* 2020;15(1):3.

10. Lo EAG, Wilby KJ, Ensom MHH. Use of proton pump inhibitors in the management of gastroesopha-geal varices: a systematic review. *Ann Pharmacother*. 2015;49(2):207–219.
11. Chey WD, Leontiadis GI, Howden CW, et al. ACG clinical guideline: treatment of helicobacter pylori infection. *Am J Gastroenterol*. 2017;112(2):212–239.

CHAPTER 33

Hemodialysis

Yuriy Khanin, MD

Background

Hemodialysis (HD) is the process by which the solute composition of a solution (blood) is altered by exposing the solution to a second solution (dialysate) through a semipermeable membrane. Low-molecular-weight solutes easily interchange between the two solutions down a concentration gradient, but high-molecular-weight solutes will remain on either side of the membrane unchanged. Solutes pass through the membrane via two different mechanisms: diffusion and convection (ultrafiltration).[1]

How to Use It

HD is one of the modalities of renal replacement therapy that allows toxins and/or fluid to be removed from a patient's body and is performed under the care of a nephrologist. This procedure can be utilized in the management of acute kidney injury, toxin exposures, or end-stage kidney disease (ESKD). The preferred mathematical method for measuring the HD dose uses the pre- and post-HD serum urea nitrogen levels, duration of HD, and the patient's volume of distribution (Vd) of urea and is expressed as Kt/V.[2]

How It Is Done

HD is performed by combining a blood circuit, a dialysis fluid (dialysate) circuit, and a dialyzer (filter). Tubing generally referred to as the arterial line carries the blood from the vascular access through the dialyzer and then returns it to the patient via a venous line. See Chapter 34: Hemodialysis Access for details about vascular access options. No anesthesia or sedation is required to perform HD, though some patients who experience discomfort during cannulation of their arteriovenous fistula (AVF) can be given a lidocaine 2.5% cream or spray to apply to the AVF prior to HD. The dialyzer is a hollow fiber consisting of thousands of small tightly bound capillaries made of a synthetic polymer blend. The blood flows through these small capillaries, while the dialysate fluid runs outside the capillaries in a countercurrent direction. Dialyzers have varied membrane surface areas ranging from 0.8 to 2.5 m² to accommodate the treatment of patients of a range of sizes. HD for ESKD is generally performed thrice weekly, for 3–4 hours each session at an in-center unit, though nocturnal, home, and short daily HD modalities exist as well.[1] For certain toxin exposure or profound uremia, HD can be performed on consecutive days until no longer warranted.

Medication Implications

- The most common complications of HD are hypotension, cramps, nausea, vomiting, headache, chest pain, and itching.[1]
- Intradialytic hypotension (IDH) is associated with myocardial stunning, a higher mortality, and increased risk of access thrombosis. While various definitions exist, the most widely utilized is a systolic blood pressure <90 mmHg as it is most associated with mortality.[3–5]

- IDH can be reduced by giving antihypertensive medications after (not before) HD, changing therapy to shorter-acting agents, and dose-reducing medications.
- Eating during HD can precipitate or accentuate IDH due to dilation of splanchnic vessels which reduces total peripheral resistance. Patients should be advised to avoid eating during or right before HD.[6]
- Midodrine, an oral α-adrenergic agonist, reduces the frequency of IDH. A dose of 10 mg orally 1.5–2 hours before a HD session is typical, though higher doses have been reported.[1]
- Management of IDH is straightforward. If symptomatic, the patient should be placed in the Trendelenburg position, given a 0.9% sodium chloride bolus (100–250 mL) intravenously, and ultrafiltration should be stopped.[1]
- The pathogenesis of cramps during HD is unknown, but hypotension, hypovolemia, and high ultrafiltration rate appear to be risk factors as they cause vasoconstriction resulting in hypoperfusion of muscles.[1]
- Itching is a common problem with HD and is sometimes deemed to be secondary to hypersensitivity from the dialyzer. In this case, a different polymer membrane dialyzer should be utilized. Moisturizing and lubrication of the skin using emollients are recommended as first-line therapy.
  - At least one medication, a selective κ-opioid receptor agonist, is currently under investigation to improve itching in patients undergoing HD.[7]
- Disequilibrium syndrome is a set of systemic and neurologic symptoms that may occur following HD. Manifestations include nausea, vomiting, restlessness, and headache. More serious manifestations include seizures, obtundation, and coma. The cause of disequilibrium syndrome is thought to be secondary to an acute increase in brain water content as a result of highly uremic patients receiving a large amount of HD. Management is usually supportive; intravenous mannitol may provide benefit, but the data is mixed. Avoiding aggressive HD treatments in acutely uremic patients is key, and plasma urea ideally should not be lowered by more than 40%.[1]
- Dialyzer efficiency refers primarily to the ability of a dialyzer to remove small solutes (such as urea). The flux of a dialyzer refers to its ability to remove large molecules such as β2-microglobulin (molecular weight of 11,800 daltons). High-flux dialyzers will be able to remove medium-sized molecules with molecular weights of 500–20,000 daltons.
  - For patients undergoing HD thrice weekly, a higher HD dose (higher Kt/V) or use of a high-flux membrane did not show a statistically significant effect on survival, hospitalizations, or morbidity compared with lower dose or low-flux modalities. High-flux membranes were associated with roughly an 8% nonstatistically significant increased survival.[8]
- Nephrogenic systemic fibrosis (NSF) is characterized by thickening and hardening of the skin as well as fibrosis of the muscles, joints, and internal organs. NSF is only seen in patients with advanced kidney disease and gadolinium exposure (i.e., from magnetic resonance imaging studies). There is no proven effective medical therapy for NSF, though case reports exist supporting pentoxifylline and sodium thiosulfate as a treatment option.[9]
  - Using gadolinium-based contrast agents (GBCA) in patients with estimated glomerular filtration rates (eGFR) less than 30 mL/minute/1.73m² or HD-dependent patients should be considered on a case-by-case basis because of the risk of developing NSF. However, newer agents (group II and III) such as gadobutrol have not been associated with any cases of NSF. Patients undergoing HD should, however, be identified prior to GBCA administration to arrange timely HD (at the discretion of the nephrologist) to optimize gadolinium clearance, although there remains no evidence that HD reduces the risk of NSF.[10,11]
- Since HD consists of extracorporeal blood flow, some form of anticoagulation is required to prevent thrombosis in the circuit. Unfractionated heparin is the anticoagulant of choice in

the United States, while in the European Union, low-molecular-weight heparin (LMWH) is preferred. Heparin can be administered via the arterial line as a bolus followed by either a continuous infusion or by additional boluses as needed. No consensus exists on the optimal method of heparin dosing. Patients with moderate-high risk of bleeding or who have a heparin allergy can receive periodic saline flushes (250 mL) to prevent clotting; however, this is controversial, as some studies have suggested that a saline rinse can actually promote clotting.[1,12]

- The pharmacokinetics of medications may be altered by HD, and consulting a reference guide such as *The Renal Drug Handbook* or *Drug Prescribing in Renal Failure: Dosing Guidelines for Adults and Children* is recommended.[13,14] The main considerations that determine medication dosage in patients undergoing HD are renal clearance, therapeutic index, extent of protein binding, Vd, and the presence of comorbid hepatic dysfunction.[15]
  - Medications with a wide therapeutic index, such as cephalosporins, can often be given without a dose reduction; however, medications with narrow indices often need reduction and monitoring of levels, an example being lithium. The extent to which HD removes a particular medication from plasma is dependent on its water solubility, molecular weight, protein binding, and Vd. Knowing these properties will aid in estimating the clearance of the medication by HD. Medications with a low molecular weight, limited Vd, low protein binding, and high water solubility will be removed with HD and require supplemental dosing post-HD sessions.[1,3]
- Since many antibiotics used in patients undergoing HD require dose adjustments, a comprehensive reference guide is useful.
  - Vancomycin dosing in HD in particular often plagues physicians. The vancomycin trough should be checked prior to an HD session, and supplemental doses should be given during the last hour or immediately post treatment session. After consecutive target predialysis serum levels have been achieved, it is reasonable to transition to monitoring once-weekly predialysis troughs and supplement accordingly.[16]

References

1. Daugirdas JT, Blake PG, Ing TS. *Handbook of Dialysis*. 5th ed. Philadelphia, PA: Walters Kluwer Health; 2015.
2. Daugirdas JT, Depner TA. A nomogram approach to hemodialysis urea modeling. *Am J Kidney Dis*. 1994;23(1):33–40.
3. Flythe J, Xue H, Lynch KE, et al. Association of mortality risk with various definitions of intradialytic hypotension. *J Am Soc Nephrol*. 2015;26(3):724–734.
4. Chang TI, Paik J, Greene T, et al. Intradialytic hypotension and vascular access thrombosis. *J Am Soc Nephrol*. 2011;22(8):1526–1533.
5. McIntyre CW, Odudu A. Hemodialysis-associated cardiomyopathy: a newly defined disease entity. *Semin Dial*. 2014;27(2):87–97.
6. Sherman RA, Torres F, Cody RP. Postprandial blood pressure changes during hemodialysis. *Am J Kidney Dis*. 1988;12(1):37–39.
7. Fishbane S, Jamal A, Munera C, et al. A phase 3 trial of difelikefalin in hemodialysis patients with pruritus. *N Engl J Med*. 2020;382(3):222–232.
8. Eknoyan G, Beck GJ, Cheung AK, et al. Effect of dialysis dose and membrane flux in maintenance hemodialysis. *N Engl J Med*. 2002;347(25):2010–2019.
9. Abu-Alfa AK. Nephrogenic systemic fibrosis and gadolinium-based contrast agents. *Adv Chronic Kidney Dis*. 2011;18(3):188–198.
10. Schieda N, Maralani PJ, Hurrell C, et al. Updated clinical practice guideline on use of gadolinium-based contrast agents in kidney disease issued by the Canadian Association of Radiologists. *Can Assoc Radiol J*. 2019;70(3):226–232.
11. Michaely HJ, Aschauer M, Deutschmann H, et al. Gadobutrol in renally impaired patients: results of the GRIP study. *Invest Radiol*. 2017;52(1):55–60.

12. Sagedal S, Hartmann A, Osnes K, et al. Intermittent saline flushes during haemodialysis do not alleviate coagulation and clot formation in stable patients receiving reduced doses of dalteparin. *Nephrol Dial Transplant.* 2006;21(2):444–449.
13. Dunleavy A, Ashley C. *The Renal Drug Handbook: The Ultimate Prescribing Guide for Renal Practitioners.* 5th ed.: CRC Press; 2018.
14. Bennett WM, Aronoff GR, Morrison G, et al. *Drug Prescribing in Renal Failure: Dosing Guidelines for Adults and Children.* 5th ed. Philadelphia, PA: American College of Physicians; 2007.
15. Doogue MP, Polasek TM. Drug dosing in renal disease. *Clin Biochem Rev.* 2011;32(2):69–73.
16. Crew P, Heintz SJ, Heintz BH. Vancomycin dosing and monitoring for patients with end-stage renal disease receiving intermittent hemodialysis. *Am J Health Syst Pharm.* 2015;72:1856–1864.

CHAPTER 34

Hemodialysis Access

Yuriy Khanin, MD

Background

There are several means of vascular access through which hemodialysis (HD) can be performed, including catheters, arteriovenous fistulas (AVFs), and arteriovenous grafts (AVGs). These accesses provide the means for large-bore cannulas to be placed, usually in both an artery and a vein, thus facilitating a large volume of blood to exit and return to the patient after passing through a dialysis machine. HD access catheters are often abbreviated "permacath" or "Shiley"; however, this is incorrect nomenclature, as "Shiley" refers to a brand of tracheostomy tubes. Catheters should be referred to as non-tunneled or tunneled; however, as mentioned above, "Shiley" is often used in the hospital ward in reference to a non-tunneled HD catheter.[1] A tunneled catheter is placed via a subcutaneous tract, which facilitates fibrous ingrowth and prevents catheter migration or accidental removal.

How to Use It

HD access is the means through which a nephrologist can perform HD. The type of access that is used generally depends on the clinical situation. For instance, in emergent situations, a non-tunneled HD catheter is placed due to ease, convenience, and short-term need. Compared with a typical catheter used for central venous access, the lumen of an HD catheter has a larger diameter to provide a high rate of flow. AVF and AVG are the accesses to be placed when HD is not emergently needed and the patient will require indefinite HD. Tunneled HD catheters are primarily used for vascular access when HD is required for >1 week and the AVF/AVG are being planned. Under rare circumstances, a tunneled HD catheter can be a long-term access. AVFs are the preferred access for indefinite HD, as they have a lower incidence of infection, thrombosis, and overall better patient survival than AVGs and tunneled HD catheters.[1]

How It Is Done

HD catheters have two lumens attached to two colored ports (blue and red). By convention, the red port identifies the "arterial" lumen that draws blood from the body, and the blue port identifies the "venous" lumen for return of blood from the dialysis machine to the patient. Insertion sites for both non-tunneled and tunneled catheters include the right and left internal jugular veins, the femoral veins, and the subclavian veins. The right internal jugular vein is preferred because the pathway to the right atrium is short and straight. The catheter should be inserted via aseptic technique under ultrasound guidance to minimize complications.[2]

A tunneled HD catheter is placed subcutaneously between the catheterized vein and the skin exit site. They are generally placed surgically or percutaneously by interventional radiologists and, as such, cannot be performed in emergency situations. Hence, non-tunneled HD catheters are placed first and then can be "converted" to a tunneled HD catheter for long-term use.[2]

An AVF involves creating an anastomosis between an artery and a native vein, allowing blood to flow directly from the artery to the vein. An AVG is similar, except that the distance between the artery and vein is bridged by a tube made of prosthetic material such as polytetrafluoroethyl-ene polymer. AVF cannot be used immediately, as the fistula maturation process takes about 6–8 weeks to allow for pressure/flow remodeling to occur in the vein. AVG can be used earlier than AVF, generally within 1–3 weeks after placement. These types of HD access must be placed by trained vascular surgeons.[2]

Medication Implications

- HD access should ideally only be used for HD due to a high risk of infection when improper techniques are used. However, under certain situations, an access may be used by a trained HD nurse to gather blood specimens, administer medications, etc. In the event of a cardiac arrest, the HD access can be used to administer lifesaving medications such as epinephrine.
- Blood products and certain medications, mainly antibiotics, can be administered during an HD treatment via the HD access by a trained HD nurse. Due to the high risk of infection/thrombosis, an HD catheter should not be accessed by other staff.
- Non-tunneled HD catheters are often placed at the bedside and do not require the discontinuation of any dual antiplatelet therapy (DAPT), prophylactic, or full-dose anticoagulation.
- Desmopressin (DDAVP—a synthetic analog of antidiuretic hormone) leads to increased release of von Willebrand factor multimers and is often given prior to non-tunneled catheter placement to minimize bleeding due to uremia. The usual dose is 0.3 mcg/kg (maximum 20 mcg) intravenously over 15–30 minutes given one time 30 minutes prior to the procedure. Unfortunately, no study has shown reduced bleeding with DDAVP given pre-procedure. Other caveats include flushing, headache, and tachyphylaxis with repeated dosing (as von Willebrand factor stores are somewhat depleted as soon as a second dose is given on 2 consecutive days).[3] While DDAVP use can precipitate hyponatremia in certain patient populations, this risk is less likely to non-existent in those with advanced chronic kidney disease or acute kidney injury. The renal tubules of these patients do not function properly and therefore DDAVP cannot exert its effect of retaining low solute water, the mechanism which causes hyponatremia.
- Local anesthesia with lidocaine is often used to minimize pain and venous spasm for non-tunneled HD catheter placement. Placement of tunneled catheters and AVF/AVG are more invasive, requiring regional anesthesia, and in many cases AVF/AVG can even require general anesthesia with sedation.[1]
- Tunneled HD catheters and AVF/AVG are placed by surgeons and interventional radiologists. DAPT and anticoagulation will need to be held prior to the procedure, and the duration will be determined beforehand by individual patient characteristics, medication characteristics, and any institutional guidelines; thus communication is key.
- Complications from catheter placement include arterial puncture, hemothorax, pneumothorax, brachial plexus injury, arrhythmias, and air embolism. Prompt recognition is imperative, and intensive care unit level care may be required for treatment.[2]
- If stenosis develops (as suggested by a change in thrill or bruit), a vascular surgeon must be called to assess the AVF/AVG, a duplex study may be indicated, and percutaneous balloon angioplasty may successfully treat the lesion.[2]
- Prophylaxis against catheter thrombosis is important and needs to begin at the time of catheter usage. The three most common agents used are normal saline, heparin, and citrate. However, the majority of HD centers and hospitals will use heparin.[4]
  - Thrombosis is the most common complication of arteriovenous access and accounts for 80%–85% of access loss. Catheter thrombosis can often be treated with tissue plasminogen activator (tPA) 2 mg infused into each catheter lumen, but the management should be reserved for nephrologists and HD staff. As a last resort, the catheter can be replaced.[2]

- AVF/AVG thrombosis
  - Thrombosis of the AVF can occur either soon after its construction or as a late event. Treatment of thrombosis should be performed using either percutaneous methods or surgical thrombectomy, depending on the expertise of the institution.[2]
  - AVG thrombosis can be managed by surgical thrombectomy or by mechanical or pharmacomechanical thrombolysis, again depending on the expertise of the medical center.[2]
  - Anticoagulants and antiplatelet drugs may help prevent arteriovenous access thrombosis, but most studies published thus far do not support their routine use. However, if a systemic disease such as antiphospholipid syndrome is found to be the cause of recurrent arteriovenous access thrombosis, then full-dose anticoagulation may be warranted.[2]
- Infection of the access is usually manifested as erythema, pain, or purulent exudate. Fever may be the first and only sign. Blood cultures must be obtained in all cases of suspected access infections. Empiric antibiotics should include gram-negative and gram-positive coverage. See Chapter 21: Culture - Blood for more details.
  - The risk of infection is significantly reduced with tunneled catheters because of a cuff, which is usually positioned just proximal to the catheter exit site, which serves as a barrier to the migration of bacteria from the skin.[5]
  - There is conflicting evidence concerning the risk of infection based upon the site of insertion. General consensus has been that the highest risk is associated with femoral access.[5]
  - For non-tunneled catheters, the development of bacteremia requires prompt removal of the catheter and appropriate intravenous antibiotic therapy. Tunneled HD catheters are removed if suspicion is high and under infectious disease specialist guidance.
  - AVF infections are rare and are usually caused by staphylococci. They should be treated with 6 weeks of antibiotics.[2]
  - AVG infection occurs in 5%–20% of grafts placed, the majority of which are staphylococci as well. In addition to antibiotic coverage, an incision/resection of the graft may be required in certain situations. Infectious disease specialists should be consulted to help guide management.[2]

References

1. Vascular Access 2006. Work Group Clinical practice guidelines for vascular access. *Am J Kidney Dis.* 2006;48(Suppl 1):S176–S247.
2. Daugirdas JT, Blake PG, Ing TS. *Handbook of Dialysis.* 5th ed. Philidelphia, PA: Wolters Kluwer Health; 2015.
3. Mannucci PM, Bettega D, Cattaneo M. Patterns of development of tachyphylaxis in patients with haemophilia and von Willebrand disease after repeated doses of desmopressin (DDAVP). *Br J Haematol.* 1992;82(1):87–93.
4. Moran JE, Ash SR. ASDIN Clinical Practice Committee. Locking solutions for hemodialysis catheters; heparin and citrate—a position paper by ASDIN. *Semin Dial.* 2008;21:490.
5. Parienti JJ, Thirion M, Mégarbane B, et al. Femoral vs jugular venous catheterization and risk of nosocomial events in adults requiring acute renal replacement therapy: a randomized controlled trial. *JAMA.* 2008;299:2413–2422.

CHAPTER 35

Hepatobiliary Scintigraphy

Susan MK Lee, PharmD, BCPS, CDCES ▪ David Bernstein, MD, FAASLD, FACG, FACP, AGAF

Background

Hepatobiliary scintigraphy (hepatobiliary iminodiacetic acid or HIDA) is a noninvasive nuclear imaging test used to assess the patency of the extrahepatic biliary tree and gallbladder and the functionality of the liver and gallbladder. Radioactive tracer is injected into the bloodstream and transported to the liver where it is taken up and excreted into the biliary tree. The tracer is then taken up by the gallbladder and excreted into the small intestine. The radioactive tracer mimics the bile pathway (Fig. 35.1).

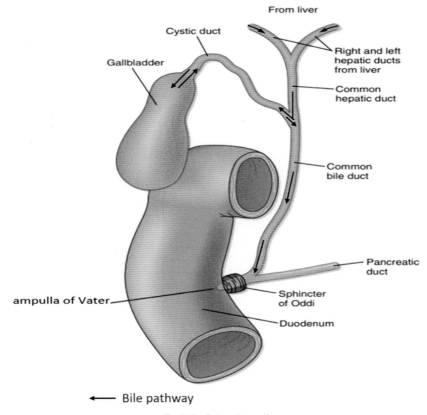

Fig. 35.1 Bile pathway.[18]

How to Use It

HIDA is typically obtained in patients complaining of right upper quadrant pain following completion of other abdominal imaging. In a normal HIDA scan, radioactive tracer is taken up by the liver and excreted into the biliary tree with visualization of the gallbladder and small intestine. The inability or delayed uptake by the liver is associated with chronic liver diseases such as cirrhosis of any etiology and/or the presence of cholestasis. Uptake of tracer without excretion or with delayed excretion may be caused by conditions such as primary biliary cholangitis, primary sclerosing cholangitis, drug-induced liver disease, post-liver transplantation cholestasis, biliary atresia, cholangiocarcinoma, common bile duct stones, and biliary strictures.[1]

Nonfilling of the gallbladder is consistent with acute gallbladder inflammation or acute cholecystitis (Fig. 35.2). The HIDA scan can also quantitatively measure the gallbladder ejection fraction, the rate at which the gallbladder excretes bile. A low ejection fraction may indicate functional abnormalities of the gallbladder, which may be a cause of chronic abdominal pain.[1]

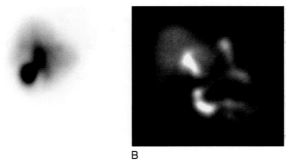

A   B

Fig. 35.2   Hepatobiliary scintigraphy scan radiologic imaging. (A) Tracer is excreted from the liver with visualization of the gallbladder. (B) Tracer is excreted into the biliary tree with non-visualization of the gallbladder.

The inability or delayed passage of tracer from the biliary tree into the small intestine is usually the result of an obstruction in the biliary tract such as cholangiocarcinoma, ampullary carcinoma, common bile duct stones, biliary strictures, or pancreatic cancer.[2]

The HIDA scan can diagnose complications of surgery, such as bile leaks or fistulas, when tracer is found outside the biliary tract.

How It Is Done

The HIDA scan can be performed in either an inpatient or outpatient setting. It must be performed in a radiology suite equipped with a gamma camera. In order to prepare for the test, the patient must not eat or drink for 4 hours prior to the test.[3] Essential medications may be taken with small sips of water.

Upon arrival at the radiology suite, the patient is asked to remove any jewelry or metal objects. The patient changes into a hospital gown and an intravenous line is placed into the hand or arm. The patient is asked to lie down on the table in the supine position and remain still for the testing period. A technician positions the gamma camera over the patient. The patient is awake during the procedure. A radioactive tracer is injected through the intravenous line. The most commonly used tracer is technetium (^{99m}Tc) mebrofenin. The HIDA scan usually takes about 60 minutes but can vary between 30 and 240 minutes.[3]

Following the procedure, most people should be able to go about their day as usual. If the results of the HIDA scan require no immediate action, the patient should be instructed to drink plenty of water to help quicken the movement of the tracer out of the body through the urine.

Radiation exposure is very low and can be safely used in adult and pediatric patients. Pregnant women should not undergo HIDA scan due to the unknown potential risk to the fetus unless the benefits of the test outweigh the risks. Breastfeeding should be avoided for at least 1 day following the scan.[4]

Medication Implications

- ^{99m}Tc mebrofenin (also referred to as BrIDA) is a type of iminodiacetic acid used as a radioactive tracer during the HIDA scan. It has high liver uptake, rapid biliary clearance, and less renal excretion than previously used tracers.[5,6] Urticaria and rash are the most common side effects, although they occur infrequently.
- In preparation for the HIDA scan, certain medications should be avoided.
    - Opioid analgesics may delay biliary-to-bowel transit time by causing the sphincter of Oddi to contract. Opioids should be withheld for at least 6 hours prior to the HIDA scan.[7]
    - Radiology exams with barium should not be performed 24–48 hours before the HIDA scan as retained barium can interfere with the HIDA scan results.
    - Medications that decrease gallbladder emptying, either directly or indirectly (i.e., by affecting sphincter of Oddi function), should be avoided if possible prior to performing the HIDA scan (Box 35.1).[8–10]
        - Medications that can affect the sphincter of Oddi should be avoided. The sphincter of Oddi is a smooth muscle valve that regulates the biliary and pancreatic flow into the duodenum. Opioids such as morphine and codeine may cause spasm of the sphincter of Oddi, leading to decreased biliary clearance. Octreotide, a somatostatin analog, can also increase the contractility of the sphincter of Oddi and therefore should be avoided prior to the scan.[11]
- Pharmacologic interventions used during the HIDA scan may increase the quality of the scan.[9,10]
    - If a patient had nothing by mouth for more than 12 hours, including patients on total parenteral nutrition, the gallbladder may fill with viscous bile that inhibits the uptake of radioactive tracer into the gallbladder. In this circumstance, sincalide is administered at a dosage of 0.02 mcg/kg in 50 mL normal saline over 30 minutes, followed by the radiotracer.[12] Sincalide mimics cholecystokinin, a hormone released in the small intestine after a meal, which causes contraction of the gallbladder and relaxation of the sphincter

---

BOX 35.1 ■ Medications That Decrease Gallbladder Emptying

Atropine
Benzodiazepines
Histamine-2 receptor antagonists
Indomethacin
Octreotide
Opioids
Nicotine
Nifedipine
Progesterone
Theophylline

of Oddi, allowing for uptake and visualization of the radioactive tracer in the gallbladder. Side effects of abdominal discomfort may occur if sincalide is administered too rapidly. Biliary obstruction is a likely diagnosis if there is absent or poor biliary flow into the duodenum despite sincalide infusion.[12,13]

- If the HIDA scan is being performed to assess the gallbladder ejection fraction, a patient will be given sincalide injection over 1 hour beginning 60 minutes after the administration of the radioactive tracer. This leads to gallbladder contraction and the release of bile, which facilitates the calculation of the gallbladder ejection fraction.
- If, after tracer administration, the gallbladder is visualized but not the small bowel, sincalide should be given. If bowel visualization occurs without visualization of the gallbladder, a second dose of radioactive tracer should be given followed by morphine.[14,15]
- A sub-analgesic dose of morphine 0.04 mg/kg or a standard dose of 2 mg per dose is used to shorten the procedure time from 4 hours to approximately 1.5 hours.[9,16] Morphine contracts the sphincter of Oddi, allowing for bile flow into the gallbladder.
  - This method is appropriate for use when the gallbladder is not visualized within 60 minutes and there is no presence of biliary obstruction.
  - Morphine should not be used for patients with morphine allergy, respiratory depression, or pediatric patients with increased intracranial pressure.[9]
  - Since an intact sphincter of Oddi is required for this intervention to be effective, morphine should not be used to shorten the procedure time if the patient had a sphincterotomy.[8]
- For infants, the HIDA scan can evaluate for the presence of biliary atresia. Phenobarbital is used for 5 days prior to the scan. Phenobarbital is given orally at 5 mg/kg/day, divided into two doses daily. Phenobarbital enhances biliary excretion of the radiotracer and increases the specificity of the test.[17]
- Recommendations following completion of the HIDA scan:
  - If the gallbladder fails to fill with radioactive tracer, a cholecystectomy (surgical removal of the gallbladder) may be indicated
  - Delayed passage of tracer through the biliary tract may require additional tests such as endoscopic ultrasound or endoscopic retrograde cholangiopancreatography (ERCP). See Chapter 28: Endoscopic Retrograde Cholangiopancreatography for more details

References

1. Diseases of the Gallbladder and Bile Ducts | Harrison's Principles of Internal Medicine, 20e. |Access-Medicine |McGraw-Hill. https://accessmedicine.mhmedical.com/content.aspx?sectionid=192284017&bookid=2129&Resultclick=2. Accessed August 28, 2020.
2. Liver, Biliary Tract, and Pancreas | Basic Radiology, 2e. |AccessMedicine |McGraw-Hill. https://access-medicine.mhmedical.com/content.aspx?bookid=360&sectionid=39669020. Accessed August 28, 2020.
3. Ziessman HA. Hepatobiliary scintigraphy in 2014. *J Nucl Med*. 2014;55(6):967–975.
4. Imaging Agents | Nuclear Hepatology | Springer Link. https://link.springer.com/book/10.1007%2F978-3-642-00648-7 Accessed August 28, 2020.
5. Choletec (Technetium Tc 99m Mebrofenin) [package insert]. Monroe Township, NJ: Bracco Diagnostics Inc; 2018.
6. Gupta M, Choudhury PS, Singh S, et al. Liver functional volumetry by TC-99m mebrofenin hepatobiliary scintigraphy before major liver resection: a game changer. *Indian J Nucl Med*. 2018;33:277–283.
7. Low CS, Ahmed H, Notghi A. Pitfalls and limitations of radionuclide hepatobiliary and gastrointestinal system imaging. *Semin Nucl Med*. 45:513-29.
8. Afghani E, Lo SK, Covington P, et al. Sphincter of Oddi function and risk factors for dysfunction. *Front Nutri*. 2017;4(1):1–18.
9. Tulchinsky M, Ciak BW, Delbeke D, et al. SNM practice guideline for hepatobiliary scintigraphy 4.0*. *J Nucl Med Tech*. 2010;38(4):210–218.
10. Ziessman HA. Interventions used with cholescintigraphy for the diagnosis of hepatobiliary disease. *Semin Nucl Med*. 2009;39(3):174–185.

11. Imaging and Quantification of Hepatobiliary Function | Nuclear Hepatology | Springer Link. https://link.springer.com/book/10.1007%2F978-3-642-00648-7 Accessed August 28, 2020.

12. Kinevac (sincalide) [package insert]. Monroe Township, NJ: Bracco Diagnostics Inc; 2018.

13. DiBaise JK, Richmond BK, Ziessman HA, et al. Cholecystokinin-cholescintigraphy in adults: consensus recommendations of an interdisciplinary panel. *Clin Gastroenterol Hepatol*. 2011;9:376–384.

14. Solomon RW, Harari AA, Dragotti R, et al. Morphine-modified hepatobiliary scanning protocol for the diagnosis of acute cholecystitis. *Am J Roentgenology*. 2016;207:865–870.

15. Kim CK. Pharmacologic intervention for the diagnosis of acute cholecystitis: cholecystokinin pretreatment or morphine, or both? *J Nucl Med*. 1997;38:647–649.

16. Kim CK, Tse KK, Juweid M, et al. Cholescintigraphy in the diagnosis of acute cholecystitis: morphine augmentation is superior to delayed imaging. *J Nucl Med*. 1993;34:1866–1870.

17. Kwatra N, Shalaby-Rana E, Narayanan S, et al. Phenobarbital-enhanced hepatobiliary scintigraphy in the diagnosis of biliary atresia: two decades of experience at a tertiary center. *Ped Rad*. 2013;43:1265–1375 May.

18. Transport and Metabolic Functions of the Liver. In: Koeppen B, Stanton B, eds. *Berne & Levy Physiology*. 7th ed.: Philadelphia: Elsevier; 2017.

CHAPTER 36

Implantable Cardiac Devices

Amit Alam, MD ▦ Ali Seyar Rahyab, MD

Background

The most common implantable cardiac devices are permanent pacemakers (PPMs) and implantable cardioverter defibrillators (ICD). PPM is placed in a patient with complete heart block or sinus node dysfunction leading to bradycardia. It takes over the "timekeeping" function of the sinoatrial node (located in the right atrium) and provides the necessary electrical impulses to maintain a normal heart rate. ICD is placed in a patient who is at high risk for lethal ventricular tachycardia or ventricular fibrillation. It can be used in primary prevention (in a patient who has never had a ventricular arrhythmia) or in secondary prevention (after a patient has had an episode of ventricular tachycardia or ventricular fibrillation) to provide a potentially lifesaving "shock" should a ventricular arrhythmia occur. It may be used in patients with a prior cardiac arrest, heart failure, or with congenital cardiac disease.[1]

For patients with advanced heart failure, a left ventricular assist device (LVAD) may be implanted to deliver continuous blood flow through the weak left ventricle. This may be done as destination therapy (DT) for patients who are not heart transplant candidates and patients may live with an LVAD for years. Alternatively, patients may have an LVAD placed for a bridge to transplant (BTT) indication and the device will provide support while the patient awaits a heart transplant. Patients with heart failure may also have an implantable device for monitoring pulmonary artery systolic pressure via an implanted pulmonary artery sensor. This device is typically used for patients with chronic heart failure, multiple heart failure hospitalizations, and significant heart failure symptoms. The device provides real-time pulmonary artery systolic pressure readings that can be used to predict if a patient will have a heart failure exacerbation.[1]

How to Use It

PERMANENT PACEMAKER

A PPM may have as few as one lead or as many as three leads. A lead is a specialized wire that conducts electrical impulses. A one-lead device is connected to the right atrium of the heart and provides electrical impulses to pace the heart at a set rate. This device would be used in the subset of patients who have sinus node disease without any other conduction disease from the atria to the ventricles. A two-lead device will have both a right atrial and right ventricular lead, which allows for more complex management. The right atrial lead can sense atrial activity and use that to cause pacing in the ventricles via the right ventricular lead. This would be helpful in a patient with heart block in which the native impulse does not reach the ventricles. In a patient with sinus node dysfunction and lack of intrinsic atrial activity, along with disease in the conduction system, the PPM can send an impulse to the atria via the right atrial lead and then send an impulse to the ventricles via the right ventricular lead. A PPM with three leads is usually referred to as a cardiac resynchronization therapy (CRT) device. It has a right atrial lead, a right ventricular lead, and a coronary sinus lead on the left side. Overall, it functions similarly to a two-lead PPM with the additional benefit being that the coronary sinus lead will send an impulse to the left ventricle, while the right ventricular lead also activates the right ventricle thereby allowing both ventricles to contract simultaneously. A CRT device is typically used in patients with heart failure who also have abnormal conduction to the ventricles.[1,2]

IMPLANTABLE CARDIOVERTER DEFIBRILLATOR

An ICD may also have one, two, or three leads, which are progressively in the right atrium, right ventricle, and coronary sinus, respectively. The main function of ICD is to detect ventricular tachycardia or ventricular fibrillation and deliver a lifesaving "shock" or "defibrillation" to reset the electrical rhythm of the heart back into normal sinus rhythm. A "shock" is a high-energy electrical impulse generated by the battery and discharged by the capacitor in the device. For ventricular tachycardia, the device may attempt what is referred to as anti-tachycardia pacing in an effort to terminate the arrhythmia without delivering a shock. The anti-tachycardia pacing function delivers a rapid heart rate that can overtake the ventricular arrhythmia. If anti-tachycardia pacing is not effective and the ventricular tachycardia persists, the device will deliver a "shock." Newer-generation ICD devices with the appropriate leads may also function as a PPM or a CRT device.[2,3]

Both PPM and ICD can be interrogated by the electrophysiologist to evaluate the device's health, including its battery life, and to review any abnormal cardiac rhythms that were detected. In the hospital or clinic, the interrogation is done with an external computer that uses a wireless wand peripheral that is placed over the device to obtain information. Newer devices can be remotely interrogated as they first sync to a remote monitor that the patient has in his/her possession, which subsequently transmits data to the physician's office. A typical battery life for a device is up to 10 years, and when it runs low, the device is replaced entirely with the battery (the leads, which are implanted in the heart, stay in place and are reattached to the new device).[3]

LEFT VENTRICULAR ASSIST DEVICE

LVAD is an advanced therapy for chronic severe heart failure. There are several manufacturers and models. LVAD functions by pumping blood it receives from the left ventricular apex via an external pump into the aorta directly. LVAD can provide enough cardiac output for the patient to perform activities of daily life. It contains battery packs that are externally located and connected to the device via a driveline. The LVAD controller monitors blood flow through the device, and the cardiologist may interrogate the device to ensure it is functioning appropriately.[1]

PULMONARY ARTERY (SYSTOLIC) PRESSURE SENSOR

A pulmonary artery (systolic) pressure sensor monitors the blood pressure in the pulmonary artery. This device allows the cardiologist to ascertain when a patient may have worsening of his/her volume status. If the patient's pulmonary artery (systolic) pressures are rising, it may signal that the patient is retaining fluid and may need increased medication, a renewed focus on dietary habits, or admission to the hospital. The device data is uploaded and can be remotely monitored by the cardiologist.[1,3]

How It Is Done

PERMANENT PACEMAKER/IMPLANTABLE CARDIOVERTER DEFIBRILLATOR

An electrophysiologist is a cardiologist who specializes in treating cardiac rhythm disorders. The electrophysiologist will implant the PPM or ICD in the electrophysiology laboratory, which is very similar to a cardiac catheterization laboratory. The procedure is performed via a minimally invasive approach. The electrophysiologist will obtain access to the heart via the venous system from the femoral vein to place the leads in the appropriate location. Subsequently, a subcutaneous pocket is created, typically on the left chest, where the PPM or ICD is placed. The generator is the part of the device that contains the battery and electronics. The generator is then connected to the leads placed in the heart.[3]

LEFT VENTRICULAR ASSIST DEVICE

LVAD is implanted in the operating room by a cardiothoracic surgeon. It is an open surgical procedure that requires a median sternotomy, just like coronary artery bypass grafting, or through a minimally invasive lateral thoracotomy approach. During this procedure the patient is placed on the heart-lung machine and the LVAD device is attached to the apex of the heart. A conduit is connected from the LVAD to the ascending aorta, which allows blood to be pumped out of the left ventricular apex into the aorta and directly into the systemic circulation. A driveline is connected to the external controller that houses the battery packs. The recovery from this procedure is similar to coronary artery bypass grafting.[3]

PULMONARY ARTERY (SYSTOLIC) PRESSURE SENSOR

The pulmonary artery (systolic) pressure sensor is placed by an interventional or advanced heart failure cardiologist in the cardiac catheterization laboratory. It is implanted via a minimally invasive procedure in which the right side of the heart is accessed via the venous system from the femoral vein. The sensor is typically placed in a branch of the left pulmonary artery. The procedure is typically brief.[3,4]

Medication Implications
BEFORE THE PROCEDURE

- PPM/ICD
  - Anticoagulants are not necessarily stopped.
    - Warfarin is typically continued uninterrupted for most patients; however, direct oral anticoagulants may be held or continued depending on a particular patient's bleeding versus thrombophilic risks. For the direct oral anticoagulants, they may be held approximately 1–2 days prior to the procedure depending on the agent and renal function.[5]
  - Aspirin should be continued.
    - Continuing dual antiplatelet agents (DAPTs), aspirin plus a $P2Y_{12}$ inhibitor, depends on the indication[5]
    - If used for a bare metal stent placed within 4 weeks or for a newer-generation drug-eluting stent placed within 3 months, it is recommended to continue DAPT.
    - If the procedure is after this window, it should be considered to discontinue the $P2Y_{12}$ inhibitor 5–7 days before the procedure, as their use is also associated with bleeding complications.
- LVADs
  - Oral anticoagulants and DAPTs are stopped prior to the procedure
  - Intravenous heparin may be continued
- Pulmonary artery (systolic) pressure sensor
  - No restrictions are generally observed, and the device may be inserted if a patient is using anticoagulation and/or antiplatelet agents

TABLE 36.1 ■ **Characteristics of Beta Blockers Used in Patients With Heart Failure With Reduced Ejection Fraction**

Beta Blocker[6]	Mechanism[6]	Initial Dose[6]	Average Dose Achieved in Trials[6]	Adverse Effects or Special Considerations
Bisoprolol[7]	Selective beta1 antagonist	1.25 mg daily	8.6 mg daily	Cardioselective and is a preferred choice in individuals with chronic obstructive pulmonary disease or asthma
Carvedilol[8]	Nonselective beta and alpha1 antagonist	3.125 mg twice daily	37 mg daily	Preferred choice for concomitant blood pressure control
Metoprolol succinate[9]	Selective beta1 antagonist	12.5–25 mg daily	159 mg daily	Cardioselective and is a preferred choice in individuals with chronic obstructive pulmonary disease or asthma

DURING THE PROCEDURE

- PPM/ICD
    - The procedure may be performed using general anesthesia or conscious sedation in the electrophysiology laboratory
- LVADs
    - The procedure is performed in the operating room using general anesthesia
- Pulmonary artery (systolic) pressure sensor
    - Conscious sedation is typically used for the procedure in the cardiac catheterization laboratory

AFTER THE PROCEDURE

- PPM/ICD
    - Anticoagulants/DAPTs are generally resumed 24–48 hours after the procedure if there was no evidence of bleeding or complications
- LVADs
    - Patients are required to continue lifelong warfarin (targeting an international normalized ratio [INR] 2–3; typically around 2.5) with an LVAD. See Chapter 38: Lower Extremity Venous Duplex Ultrasound for more details about using warfarin
- Pulmonary artery (systolic) pressure sensor
    - No medication changes are necessary for the device. Patients must take DAPT or remain on any form of anticoagulation for 30 days post procedure
- Selected patients with heart failure with reduced ejection fraction are treated with neuro-hormonal blockade with the following guideline-directed medications to reduce morbidity and mortality.[6]
    - Beta blocker: See Table 36.1
    - Angiotensin-converting enzyme inhibitor (ACE-I) or angiotensin-II receptor blocker (ARB) or angiotensin receptor-neprilysin inhibitor (ARNI): See Table 36.2
    - Aldosterone antagonist: See Table 36.3

TABLE 36.2 ■ **Characteristics of ACE-I/ARB/ARNI Used in Patients With Heart Failure With Reduced Ejection Fraction**

ACE-I/ARB/ARNI[6]	Mechanism[6]	Initial Dose[6]	Average Dose Achieved In Trials[6]	Adverse Effects or Special Considerations
Enalapril[10]	ACE-I	2.5 mg twice daily	16.6 mg daily	General side effects for ACE-I: Angioedema is an uncommon but serious side effect. Hyperkalemia, elevated creatinine, or cough may occur.
Lisinopril[11]	ACE-I	2.5–5 mg daily	32.5–35 mg daily	General side effects for ACE-I as noted above
Losartan[12]	ARB	25–50 mg daily	129 mg daily	General side effects for ARB: Hyperkalemia or elevated creatinine may occur. Cough or angioedema occur less frequently than with ACE-I.
Valsartan[13]	ARB	20–40 mg twice daily	254 mg daily	General side effects for ARBs as noted above.
Sacubitril/ valsartan[14]	ARNI	24/26 mg twice daily	Target dose: 24/26 mg, 49/51 mg OR 97/103 mg twice daily	Contraindicated if there is a history of angioedema from a prior ACE-I or ARB. Side effects also include hyperkalemia, elevated creatinine, and cough.

ACE-I, angiotensin-converting enzyme inhibitor; *ARB,* angiotensin-II receptor blocker; *ARNI,* angiotensin receptor-neprilysin inhibitor.

TABLE 36.3 ■ **Characteristics of Aldosterone Antagonists Used in Patients With Heart Failure With Reduced Ejection Fraction**

Aldosterone Antagonist[6]	Mechanism[6]	Initial Dose[6]	Average Dose Achieved In Trials[6]	Adverse Effects or Special Considerations
Spironolactone[15]	Antagonist at aldosterone-dependent sodium-potassium channels in the distal convoluted renal tubule	12.5–25 mg daily	26 mg daily	Side effects include hyperkalemia, elevated creatinine, and gynecomastia.

Continued

TABLE 36.3 ▪ Characteristics of Aldosterone Antagonists Used in Patients With Heart Failure With Reduced Ejection Fraction—cont'd

Aldosterone Antagonist[6]	Mechanism[6]	Initial Dose[6]	Average Dose Achieved In Trials[6]	Adverse Effects or Special Considerations
Eplerenone[16]	Blocks aldosterone binding to the mineralocorticoid receptor	25 mg daily	42.6 mg daily	Contraindications for all patients: Serum potassium >5.5 mEq/L at initiation, creatinine clearance ≤30 mL/minute, or use with a strong cytochrome P450 3A inhibitor. Contraindications for the treatment of hypertension: type 2 diabetes with microalbuminuria, serum creatinine >2.0 mg/dL in males or >1.8 mg/dL in females, creatinine clearance <50 mL/minute, or concomitant use of potassium supplements or potassium-sparing diuretics.

References

1. Zipes DP, Libby P. *Braunwald's Heart Disease: A Textbook of Cardiovascular Medicine.* 11th ed.: Amsterdam, published by Elsevier. Chapters; 2019; 27, 28, 29, 41.
2. Kusumoto FM, Schoenfeld MH, Barrett C, et al. 2018 ACC/AHA/HRS guideline on the evaluation and management of patients with bradycardia and cardiac conduction delay: a report of the American College of Cardiology/American Heart Association Task Force on Clinical Practice Guidelines, and the Heart Rhythm Society. *J Am Coll Cardiol.* 2018;140(8):e333–e381.
3. Antman E. *Cardiovascular Therapeutics: A Companion to Braunwald's Heart Disease.* 4th ed.: Amsterdam, published by Elsevier. Chapters; 2012; 13, 15, 22.
4. Abraham WT, Adamson PB, Bourge RC, et al. Wireless pulmonary artery haemodynamic monitoring in chronic heart failure: a randomised controlled trial. *Lancet.* 2011;377(9766):658–666.
5. Sticherling C, Marin F, Birnie D, et al. Antithrombotic management in patients undergoing electrophysiological procedures: a European Heart Rhythm Association (EHRA) position document endorsed by the ESC Working Group Thrombosis, Heart Rhythm Society (HRS), and Asia Pacific Heart Rhythm Society (APHRS). *Europace.* 2015;17(8):1197–1214.
6. Yancy CW, Jessup M, Bozkurt B, et al. 2017 ACC/AHA/HFSA Focused Update of the 2013 ACCF/AHA Guideline for the Management of Heart Failure. *J Am Coll Cardiol.* 2017;70(6):776–803.
7. Bisoprolol [package insert]. Quebec, Canada: Sandoz; 2009.
8. Carvedilol [package insert]. Triangle Park, NC: GlaxoSmithKline; 2017.
9. Metoprolol Succinate [package insert]. Morgantown, WV: Mylan Pharmaceuticals Inc; 2019.
10. Enalapril [package insert]. Morgantown, WV: Mylan Pharmaceuticals Inc; 2017.
11. Lisinopril [package insert]. Whitehouse Station, NJ: Merck & Co., Inc; 2019.
12. Losartan [package insert]. Whitehouse Station, NJ: Merck & Co., Inc; 2019.
13. Valsartan [package insert]. East Hanover, NJ: Novartis Pharmaceuticals Corporation; 2019.
14. Sacubitril/Valsartan [package insert]. East Hanover, NJ: Novartis Pharmaceuticals Corporation; 2019.
15. Spironolactone [package insert]. New York, NY: G.D.Searle LLC; 2018.
16. Eplerenone [package insert]. New York, NY: G.D. Searle LLC; 2018.

CHAPTER 37

Intravenous Access

Daniel Putterman, MD

Background

Venous access is something that is often taken for granted. Establishing reliable venous access will facilitate a wide array of medical therapies and diagnostic exams. Currently, there are numerous types of intravenous (IV) access available, including peripheral IV (PIV), midline catheters, peripherally inserted central catheters (PICCs), non-tunneled and tunneled central venous catheters (CVCs), and completely implantable devices known as "ports." Selecting the appropriate type of venous access may not always be easy. The type of access needed depends on a number of factors, mainly the type of therapy and duration.

Probably the most important initial consideration when selecting venous access is the type of therapy planned. Some medications and fluids are nontoxic and can be administered safely through any type of access. However, there are many medications that are toxic and should only be administered through specific types of access. It is critical to know the safety profile of the planned therapy.

Irritants are medications and fluids that can cause localized inflammation of the vein called phlebitis. If the vein is disrupted, the medication can leak into the surrounding tissues, termed "infiltration." There is a spectrum of severity ranging from slight pain and erythema to severe pain, induration, and fever. Inflammation can be associated with thrombus formation, called thrombophlebitis. Mild reactions can be managed by discontinuing the IV and elevation. More severe cases may also require anti-inflammatory medication, compression, and potentially anticoagulation if there is extensive thrombus.

Vesicants are medications that can cause severe tissue damage or necrosis if infused into the tissue surrounding the vein, called "extravasation." Complications of extravasation can be severe leading to tissue loss and potentially requiring surgical management. The safety profile of certain vesicants precludes them from ever being administered peripherally, and are thus often referred to as "non-peripherally compatible" in much of the literature. Some examples of vesicants and their mechanism of injury are listed in Table 37.1.

How to Use It

IV access has several benefits and is frequently used in the hospital setting. Certain medications and fluids can only be given IV. Other medications have significantly improved efficacy when delivered IV. Certain diagnostic studies involving radiographic imaging also often require IV medication and contrast agent administration. Central venous access may be required for medications and fluids that cannot be given peripherally if they are damaging to the blood vessel or surrounding tissues if extravasation occurs. The frequent phlebotomy necessary in many hospitalized patients may also occasionally necessitate specialized venous access when it cannot be performed conventionally.

How It Is Done

PIVs are short catheters that are placed into and terminate in superficial palpable veins. They are usually placed in the upper extremities and come in a range of sizes, typically from 24 to 16 gauge. They are the most common form of venous access, and greater than 90% of hospitalized patients

TABLE 37.1 ■ **Examples of Vesicants**[4,15]

Drug Type	Category	Examples	Mechanism of Action
	Alkylating agents	Carboplatin	Keep cells from replicating by damaging DNA
		Cisplatin	
	Antimetabolites	5-Fluorouracil (5-FU)	Interfere with DNA/RNA replication
		Gemcitabine	
Antineoplastic drugs		Methotrexate	
	Antitumor Antibiotics	Daunorubicin	Anthracyclines: interfere with DNA replicating enzyme
		Doxorubicin	
		Paclitaxel	Mitotic inhibitors: keep cells from dividing
		Cabazitaxel	
Antimicrobials		Acyclovir	Tissue necrosis
		Vancomycin	
		Dobutamine	Vasoconstrictive
Adrenergics		Norepinephrine	
		Phenylephrine	
		Vasopressin	
		Parenteral nutrition	High osmolarity
Fluids/Electrolytes		Sodium bicarbonate	Hypertonic
		Sodium chloride >3%	Hypertonic
		Contrast media	Nonionic media: directly related to volume
Other		Amiodarone	High osmolarity
		Mannitol >20%	High osmolarity

will have one. They can be placed by many types of practitioners and do not require imaging equipment or an advanced skill set. PIVs are limited by low durability, often only for 2–3 days. Many facilities have policies for IV dwell times. To reduce the likelihood of catheter-related infections, the Centers for Disease Control and Prevention recommends using another type of venous catheter if the anticipated duration of therapy exceeds 6 days.[1]

Midline catheters are peripheral venous access devices between 3 and 10 inches in length (8–25 cm). They are placed in an upper arm vein, such as the brachial or cephalic, usually using ultrasound guidance. Midlines terminate below the level of the axillary vein. They are approved for therapy for up to 29 days.[2]

PICCs are small-gauge (3–5 French), variable length (typically 30–50 cm), flexible catheters placed into an upper extremity vein, terminating in the superior vena cava. PICC utilization has increased significantly, as they offer several advantages over other catheters. PICCs can be placed at the patient's bedside by trained staff. They are durable and can be maintained for an indefinite period of time. Patients can be trained to use them, allowing for care both inside and outside of the hospital. PICCs are appropriate for peripherally compatible infusants if the duration anticipated is >6 days (however, if the duration anticipated is <30 days, consider midline). PICCs are appropriate for non-peripherally compatible infusants for any duration of therapy.

Non-tunneled CVCs are placed to provide short-term access to the central venous circulation. They come in a variety of lengths and sizes, typically ranging 15–30 cm in length and 5–11 French in diameter, as well as a wide variety of lumens. Large single-lumen catheters or vascular sheaths are often referred to as Cordis catheters; however, that is a brand name and may not reflect the actual device used. They are recommended for both peripherally and non-peripherally compatible infusants for short durations (<14 days) in critically ill patients or if invasive hemodynamic monitoring is needed. PICCs, tunneled catheters, and ports should be considered when >14-day access is needed. Non-tunneled CVCs are commonly placed into the jugular, subclavian, or femoral vein. Access site selection depends on the clinical status of the patient and operator expertise. Subclavian access has a lower risk of infection than either jugular or femoral access, but a higher incidence of other complications including pneumothorax and bleeding. Femoral access sites have a higher incidence of thrombosis and infection, and are only recommended for short-term access when other sites are unavailable.[3]

Implanted catheters are intended for long-term use and are often considered to be semi-permanent. They include both tunneled CVCs and ports. Tunneled CVCs are often referred to by brand names such as Hickman, Broviac, or Hohn catheters. They are available in different sizes and number of lumens. They exit the skin a distance away from the venous access site and are often anchored to the skin by a cuff of fabric bonded to the catheter. While the cuff is primarily intended to prevent dislodgement, there may be some benefit of infection reduction.[4]

Ports, often referred to by the brand names Mediport or Port-a-Cath, comprise two components that are completely buried under the skin. They come in different shapes and sizes, and are single or double lumen. Ports consist of a palpable reservoir, usually implanted in a subcutaneous chest pocket, connected to a catheter that extends through a subcutaneous tunnel into a venous access site. They terminate in the central venous system. They are intended only for intermittent infusions >30 days.

Table 37.2 summarizes characteristics of the IV access options.

Medication Implications

- The easiest way to determine if a planned medication is a vesicant or an irritant is to consult with a hospital's pharmacy department. Other resources include the Infusion Nurses Society and Oncology Nursing Society guidelines for chemotherapy and immunotherapy.[5]
- Knowledge of the properties of the planned medication often determine status. Many chemotherapeutic medications are cytotoxic and are therefore the most commonly encountered vesicants.
- Noncytotoxic medications can also be classified as vesicants and irritants.
  - Direct mechanism of action can determine classification. Vasopressors such as norepinephrine and vasopressin cause vasoconstriction, and tissue necrosis can result from ischemia if extravasation occurs
  - pH is a contributing factor when considering peripheral compatibility. Until recently, if an infusant had a pH <5 or >9, it was considered inappropriate for peripheral infusion. In 2016, the Infusion Nurses Society revised their recommendation based on evidence review and omitted pH as a sole factor for determining appropriateness. However, extreme pH values should be considered and examined further[6]

TABLE 37.2 ■ Characteristics of Intravenous Access Options

		Vesicant/Irritant Acceptable	Non-Peripheral Compatible	Phlebotomy Acceptable	Duration (Days)	In/ Outpatient	Other Considerations
Peripheral access	PIV	Short-term only	No	No	<7	Inpatient	Phlebotomy only at time of insertion
	Midline	Short-term only	No	No	7–29	Either	Phlebotomy only at time of insertion
	PICC	Yes	Yes	Conditional	Indefinite	Either	PICCs should only be used for phlebotomy if other options are exhausted
Central access	Non-tunneled	Yes	Yes	Yes	<14	Inpatient	
	Tunneled	Yes	Yes	Yes	>15	Either	
	Ports	Yes	Yes	Conditional	>30	Outpatient	Phlebotomy can be performed by trained staff

PICCs, peripherally inserted central catheters; PIV, peripheral intravenous.

- High osmolarity (>900 mOsm/L) may cause chemical phlebitis. Concentrated formulations of commonly administered fluids such as 3% sodium chloride or 8.4% sodium bicarbonate are considered vesicants

PERIPHERAL INTRAVENOUS AND MIDLINE CATHETERS

- PIVs and midline catheters can be used only for infusion of peripherally compatible agents.
  - PIVs are not recommended for continuous infusion of irritants or vesicants. Some vesicants may be given peripherally for a short duration (a few hours) until central venous access is established. For instance, vasopressors can be administered peripherally during emergent resuscitation prior to or during placement of a CVC. Others such as most chemotherapeutic agents and total parenteral nutrition (TPN) should never be given peripherally
  - While classified as a vesicant, computed tomography (CT) contrast agents can be administered peripherally with an established PIV of at least 20 gauge
  - Risk factors for developing phlebitis/thrombophlebitis include extended IV duration, location, poor placement technique, multiple prior IVs, and type of infusion. A study by Maki et al.[7] demonstrated a risk of 50% phlebitis by day 4 of catheter dwell time
  - Prevention is generally considered the best way to prevent these complications. In general, select the smallest gauge access that will accommodate the patient and intended therapy. IVs of 20–24 gauge function for infusions. Veins in the forearm and hand should be used before using veins near the wrist and other joints. Extremities that have had prior trauma, venous thrombosis, and surgery including dialysis access should not be used
  - Removal of the PIV should be performed when infiltration/extravasation has been identified. Cold compresses are recommended in most cases to reduce local inflammation. Warm compresses are recommended for vasopressor extravasation to improve circulation
  - Where available, ultrasound guidance can be used to place PIVs in patients with limited access. These ultrasound-guided PIVs should be treated as a PIV after placement
  - TPN is also a commonly encountered vesicant and should never be administered by PIV
- Midline catheters
  - As with PIVs, midlines are not recommended for continuous vesicant infusion
  - Benefits include a lower risk of mechanical or chemical phlebitis and greater durability than PIVs. Midlines have been reported to be durable to completion of therapy on inpatients 79%–89% of the time.[8] Midlines are also approved for home infusions
  - Midline catheters have a lower incidence of infection than CVCs, including PICCs. An analysis of midline catheters reported an incidence of 0.2 infections per 1000 catheter days.[9] The same analysis reported 1.0–3.2 blood stream infections per 1000 catheter days for PICCs and 2.4–4.7 blood stream infections per 1000 catheter days for non-tunneled CVCs. As they are not CVCs, infections are not considered central line-associated blood stream infections (CLABSIs), which has important implications for Centers for Medicare and Medicaid Services reimbursement
  - Midline thrombosis rate is low (<2%); however, this is potentially underestimated as many are asymptomatic. Midlines are contraindicated in patients with end-stage renal disease (ESRD) on hemodialysis (HD) or chronic kidney disease (CKD) stage 3b or worse (estimated glomerular filtration rate <45 mL/minute)
  - Other infrequent complications include occlusion, dislodgement, and leakage
  - Midline catheters are contraindicated in patients who have had upper extremity deep vein thrombosis (DVT)
  - Midlines are also not recommended for phlebotomy

PERIPHERALLY INSERTED CENTRAL CATHETERS AND CENTRAL VENOUS CATHETERS

- These catheters provide access to the central venous system and can be used for peripherally and non-peripherally compatible infusions. The main consideration when placing one of these catheters is the timing and duration of therapy.
- The Michigan Appropriateness Guide for Intravenous Catheters (MAGIC) provides an excellent algorithm for selecting the appropriate access.[10] The main focus is PICC appropriateness, but other catheter types are included. A MAGIC mobile app is available to assist catheter selection.
  - There is no limit to how long a PICC can stay in place. However, PICCs should not be used indefinitely out of convenience. PICCs and all central lines should never remain in place unless they meet appropriateness guidelines because of the risk of infection
  - PICCs can also be used for transfusions and phlebotomy for patients with difficult access if the anticipated need is >6 days
  - Severe complications including thrombosis and infection can occur. Studies demonstrated venous thrombosis in 6%–10% of patients, central venous stenosis in 4.8%, and central venous occlusion in 2%.[11] One study reported a DVT rate as high as 27%.[12] Thrombosis is often asymptomatic; however, it can have significant implications for future venous access. PICCs are therefore contraindicated for patients with ESRD on HD or with renal disease (CKD 3b or worse). These patients require patent upper extremity veins for arteriovenous fistulas and grafts that serve as dialysis access sites. Upper extremity DVT prevent these types of access from being established, limiting therapeutic options and potentially life expectancy as a result. See Chapter 34: Hemodialysis Access for details about the various accesses used for HD
  - Incidence of PICC-related CLABSI among hospitalized patients was 5.2%. Among outpatients, the risk of CLABSI was 0.5% in patients who received PICCs[13]
  - Many PICCs are "power-rated" and can be used for CT contrast administration
  - Complications increase with the greater size of catheter and number of lumens. As a rule, select the smallest usable PICC with the least number of lumens

IMPLANTABLE CATHETERS

- Tunneled CVCs
  - They can be used for infusion of peripherally and non-peripherally compatible infusants. They are generally reserved for access with anticipated duration >15 days. As they are often implanted in the chest, they may be better tolerated by patients and should be considered when therapy is continuous and indefinite, such as cardiac inotrope agent administration
  - They have a lower thrombosis rate than PICCs and should be considered for patients contraindicated for PICCs due to CKD
- Implantable ports (commonly just "ports") can be used for both peripherally and non-peripherally compatible infusants
  - They are ideal for long-term chemotherapy access. They should never be used for continuous infusions or phlebotomy and are generally reserved only for outpatient care
  - After placement, ports are accessed by placing a special needle through the skin into the reservoir for each dose and removing the needle when the dose is complete. Access typically requires special training and certification
  - Port placement is a procedure typically requiring sedation performed by either an interventional radiologist or surgeon

- There is no limit on how long a port can be maintained, but they should be removed when therapy is concluded
- Ports can have complications including infection, thrombosis, fracture, and occlusion. Infection rates for ports are considerably lower than the other types of CVC, including tunneled[14]

References

1. O'Grady NP, Alexander M, Burns LA, et al. *Guidelines for the prevention of intravascular catheter-related infections, 2011*: Centers for Disease Control and Prevention; 2011. Accessed September 3, 2020. https://www.cdc.gov/infectioncontrol/pdf/guidelines/bsi-guidelines-H.pdf.
2. Bard Poly Midline Instructions for use. BD website. 2017. Accessed September 3, 2020. https://www.bd.com/en-us/offerings/capabilities/vascular-access/vascular-iv-catheters/midline-iv-catheters/bard-poly-midline-catheters.
3. Merrer J, De Jonghe B, Golliot F, et al. Complications of femoral and subclavian venous catheterization in critically ill patients: a randomized controlled trial. *JAMA*. 2001;286(6):700–707.
4. Groeger JS, Lucas AB, Thaler HT, et al. Infectious morbidity associated with long-term use of venous access devices in patients with cancer. *Ann Intern Med*. 1993;119(12):1168–1174.
5. Gorski LA, Stranz M, Cook LS, et al. Development of an evidence-based list of noncytotoxic vesicant medications and solutions. *J Infus Nurs*. 2017;40(1):26–40.
6. Gorski LA, Hagle ME, et al. Intermittently delivered IV medication and pH: reevaluating the evidence. *J Infus Nurs*. 2015;38(1):27–46.
7. Maki DG, Ringer M. Risk factors for infusion-related phlebitis with small peripheral venous catheters. A randomized controlled trial. *Ann Intern Med*. 1991;114(10):845–854.
8. Dawson RB, Moureau NL. Midlines: an essential tool in CLABSI reduction. *Infect Control Today*. 2013;17:42–45.
9. Maki DG, Kluger DM, Crinch CJ. The risk of bloodstream infection in adults with different intravascular devices: a systematic review of 200 published prospective studies. *Mayo Clin Proc*. 2006;81(9):1159–1171.
10. Chopra V, Flanders SA, Saint S, et al. The Michigan Appropriateness Guide for Intravenous Catheters (MAGIC): results from a multispecialty panel using the RAND/UCLA appropriateness method. *Ann Intern Med*. 2015;163(6 Suppl):S1–40.
11. Chopra V, Anand S, Hickner A, et al. Risk of venous thromboembolism associated with peripherally inserted central catheters: a systematic review and meta-analysis. *Lancet*. 2013;382(9889):311–325.
12. Bonizzoli M, Batacchi S, Cianchi G, et al. Peripherally inserted central venous catheters and central venous catheters related thrombosis in post-critical patients. *Intensive Care Med*. 2011;37(2):284–289.
13. Chopra V, O'Horo JC, Rogers MA, et al. The risk of bloodstream infection associated with peripherally inserted central catheters compared with central venous catheters in adults: a systematic review and meta-analysis. *Infect Control Hosp Epidemiol*. 2013;34(9):908–918.
14. Barbetakis N, Asteriou C, Kleontas A, et al. Totally implantable central venous access ports. Analysis of 700 cases. *J Surg Oncol*. 2011;104(6):654–656.
15. Jackson-Rose J, Del Monte J, Groman A, et al. Chemotherapy extravasation: establishing a national benchmark for incidence among cancer centers. *Clin J Oncol Nurs*. 2017;21(4):438–445.

CHAPTER 38

Lower Extremity Venous Duplex Ultrasound

Kimberly E. Ng, PharmD, BCPS ■ Jonathan S. Ruan, MD, FACC, RPVI

Background

Diagnostic ultrasonography is the use of ultrasound to image anatomical structures. Ultrasound is sound waves that have a frequency above what the human ear can hear, or higher than 20×10^4 Hz. Diagnostic ultrasound is usually on the order of MHz, or 10^6 Hz. These sound waves are generated from an ultrasound probe, which houses a piezoelectric element that vibrates in response to electric current. Ultrasound waves, if aimed at a structure, may be reflected back toward the probe. The received sound waves are transmitted to a computer, which processes them and generates an image. Clinical ultrasonography uses images that are generated by the computer in different modes, including 2-D, M-mode, spectral Doppler, and color Doppler imaging. 2-D imaging is the standard representation of a structure in a two-dimensional view. Spectral Doppler displays velocities of red blood cells in a specified area on a graph over time. Color Doppler imaging displays the direction and speed of blood flow across a displayed area using a color map.[1] A lower extremity venous duplex ultrasound is the application of clinical ultrasonography to the veins of the lower extremity using a combination of 2-D, spectral Doppler, and color Doppler imaging, otherwise known as "duplex" imaging.

How to Use It

Ultrasonography of the lower extremities is imaging that can be used to evaluate venous diseases of the lower extremities. According to the 2019 ACR-AIUM-SPR-SRU Practice Parameter for the Performance of Peripheral Venous Ultrasound Examination, venous ultrasound exams can be used to evaluate for suspected deep venous thrombosis (DVT) or venous obstruction. For patients who are at high risk for DVT, venous ultrasound can be applied for serial DVT evaluation despite a negative initial exam. Venous ultrasound can also be used for the assessment of venous insufficiency, reflux, and varicosities as well as postprocedural assessment of venous ablation. Ultrasound can be used for patient follow-up in those with known venous thrombosis on therapy who undergo a clinical change where a change in thrombus burden will alter treatment. Visualization via ultrasound can also determine a potential source for known pulmonary embolism.[2] In addition, lower extremity venous duplex ultrasound may be used to monitor patients with distal, or infrapopliteal, DVTs to help guide whether they should receive anticoagulation.[3]

How It Is Done

The full lower extremity venous duplex ultrasound exam is done from the inguinal ligament to the ankle. It can be performed either in the inpatient or outpatient setting and requires no sedation or analgesia and no meal restrictions. The common femoral vein, deep femoral vein at the confluence of the femoral vein, great saphenous vein at the sapheno-femoral junction, femoral, popliteal, posterior tibial, and peroneal veins are imaged. When testing for DVT, the veins are tested every

2 cm for compressibility by pressing down on the skin with the ultrasound transducer. Spectral Doppler and color Doppler are used to assess blood flow.[2]

When testing for venous insufficiency, the patient should be standing. If the patient cannot stand, he or she should be placed in >45 degree reverse Trendelenburg position. The leg that is being imaged should not be weight bearing. Reflux should be elicited by using several maneuvers including a calf squeeze then release, manual compression of the vein clusters, pneumatic calf cuff deflation, active foot dorsiflexion and relaxation, and the Valsalva maneuver. The vein should then be imaged in the longitudinal axis using 2-D and spectral Doppler to look for venous flow in the opposite physiologic direction lasting greater than 0.5 seconds.[4,5]

Medication Implications

While the lower extremity venous duplex ultrasound is noninvasive and requires no pre- or peri-procedural medication to be administered, there are many medication implications to consider when a DVT is diagnosed. Anticoagulation for acute symptomatic proximal DVTs is generally indicated because it reduces the incidence of pulmonary emboli and mortality. There are many anticoagulants to choose from and many situations influencing the choice and duration of the anticoagulant.[3]

Patients without cancer who have proximal DVTs should receive anticoagulation for 3 months, preferably using a direct oral anticoagulant (DOAC) such as dabigatran, rivaroxaban, apixaban, or edoxaban over warfarin. In patients with a proximal DVT and cancer, low-molecular-weight heparin (LMWH) is preferred. In patients with DVTs that are provoked, treatment should last for 3 months, assuming the provoking risk factor is no longer present. In patients with DVTs that are not provoked, treatment may need to be longer, to be determined clinically based on bleeding risk. In cancer patients who have a proximal DVT, treatment should be longer than 3 months.[3]

While anticoagulation for acute symptomatic proximal DVTs is clearly indicated to reduce pulmonary emboli and mortality, treatment for distal DVTs is not as clear. Approximately 15% of isolated distal DVTs subsequently extend into the popliteal veins. Therefore, the benefit of anticoagulation must be weighed against the risk of bleeding. In patients with certain risk factors such as having a previous history of venous thromboembolism (VTE), cancer history, or having extensive thrombosis, anticoagulation is indicated. If anticoagulation is not chosen, surveillance with ultrasound should be performed after initial diagnosis of distal DVT. Choosing to neither initiate anticoagulation nor surveil a known distal DVT should not occur. Upon surveillance, if the distal DVT has not extended, the patient should not receive anticoagulation. If the distal DVT has extended, the patient should receive anticoagulation.[3]

ORAL ANTICOAGULANTS

Warfarin

Warfarin, a vitamin K antagonist, is the oldest oral anticoagulant that has been used to treat proximal DVTs. Its therapeutic effects were studied in a randomized controlled trial of placebo versus intravenous unfractionated heparin (UH) followed by warfarin for 14 days in 35 patients with DVT. Patients who received heparin followed by warfarin had less pulmonary emboli and mortality than patients who received placebo.[6] Due to ethical concerns, since this study, there have been no further studies examining the effects of anticoagulation versus placebo in patients who have DVTs. All subsequent studies in this patient population compare anticoagulants to other anticoagulants. When using warfarin, its use must be overlapped with intravenous UH or LMWH during an initial period of hypercoagulability. When initiated without intravenous UH or LMWH for DVTs, patients have an increased early incidence of asymptomatic DVT extension (nearly 40% of patients in landmark study).[7] Warfarin can be reversed with vitamin K and/or prothrombin complex concentrate (human) in the setting of acute major bleeding or the need for an urgent surgery or invasive procedure.[8] See Chapter 4: Anticoagulation Management in the Periprocedural Period for more details.

Warfarin has a food-drug interaction with foods that contain large amounts of vitamin K. Ingestion of larger than usual amounts of vitamin K–containing foods (commonly thought of as green leafy vegetables, but there are many others) will cause an international normalized ratio (INR) decrease and subsequent potential for subtherapeutic warfarin levels. Warfarin also has the potential for many drug interactions due to metabolism via multiple cytochrome P450 enzymes. Over-the-counter medications such as aspirin and other nonsteroidal anti-inflammatory drugs (NSAIDs) have potential to increase bleeding risk. Prior to initiating or discontinuing medications while a patient is using warfarin, one should consult an appropriate drug information resource to ensure no interactions exist.

DABIGATRAN

Dabigatran is a direct thrombin inhibitor indicated for the treatment of DVT in patients who have first been treated with a parenteral anticoagulant for 5–10 days as well as for prevention of DVT recurrence.[9] Dabigatran was found to be comparable to warfarin for prevention of recurrent VTE or VTE-related death and had comparable major bleeding reported for DVT treatment and prevention of recurrence.[10] For patients with a creatinine clearance (CrCl) > 30 mL/minute, 150 mg twice daily is recommended.[8] Concomitant use with P-glycoprotein inducers reduces exposure to dabigatran and should be avoided. In patients with CrCl 30–50 mL/minute, a dose reduction of 75 mg twice daily is recommended when administered with P-glycoprotein inhibitors dronedarone or ketoconazole. Use with P-glycoprotein inhibitors in severe renal impairment should be avoided.[9] Dabigatran can be reversed in the setting of major bleeding with idarucizumab 5 g intravenously divided as two consecutive doses.[11] See Chapter 4: Anticoagulation Management in the Periprocedural Period for more details.

RIVAROXABAN

Rivaroxaban is a factor Xa inhibitor indicated for the treatment of DVT and reduction in the risk of recurrence of DVT.[12] Rivaroxaban was found to be comparable to enoxaparin/warfarin for prevention of recurrent VTE and had comparable major bleeding or clinically relevant nonmajor bleeding events.[10] If being used to treat a DVT, rivaroxaban 15 mg twice daily should be taken with food for the first 21 days, followed by 20 mg once daily with food for the remaining days of treatment. If being used for the reduction in risk of recurrence, 10 mg once daily with or without food can be used after at least 6 months of standard anticoagulation treatment. For patients with a CrCl < 15 mL/minute, use is not recommended for these indications. Rivaroxaban should not be used in patients with a CrCl 15–<80 mL/minute when combined with moderate inhibitors of P-glycoprotein and cytochrome P450 3A.[12] Coagulation factor Xa (recombinant), inactivated-zhzo (Andexxa) is indicated for the reversal of life-threatening or uncontrolled bleeding due to rivaroxaban.[13] See Chapter 4: Anticoagulation Management in the Periprocedural Period for more details.

APIXABAN

Apixaban is a factor Xa inhibitor indicated for treatment of DVT and reduction in the risk of recurrent DVT. The recommended dose is 10 mg twice daily for 7 days, followed by 5 mg twice daily. Following initial therapy for at least 6 months, for the reduction in the risk of recurrent DVT, 2.5 mg twice daily is recommended. There is no dose adjustment recommended in renal impairment. Apixaban dose should be decreased by 50% when administered with combined strong inhibitors of P-glycoprotein and cytochrome P450 3A4. If a patient is receiving 2.5 mg twice daily, use should be avoided. Use should also be avoided with combined strong inducers of P-glycoprotein and cytochrome P450 3A4.[14] Apixaban was found to be comparable to LMWH and warfarin for prevention of the combined endpoint of recurrent VTE or VTE-related death and was found to have less bleeding.[9] Coagulation factor Xa (recombinant), inactivated-zhzo (Andexxa) is indicated for the reversal of life-threatening or uncontrolled bleeding due to apixaban.[13] See Chapter 4: Anticoagulation Management in the Periprocedural Period for more details.

EDOXABAN

Edoxaban is a factor Xa inhibitor indicated for the treatment of DVT.[15] Compared to warfarin, edoxaban shows no significant differences in mortality, recurrent DVTs, or major bleeding.[3] The recommended dose is 60 mg once daily. A dose reduction to 30 mg once daily is recommended for patients with CrCl 15–50 mL/minute or body weight ≤60 kg or who use certain P-glycoprotein inhibitors.[15] There is no approved reversal agent for edoxaban; however, coagulation factor Xa (recombinant), inactivated-zhzo (Andexxa) is potentially effective based on its mechanism of action. See Chapter 4: Anticoagulation Management in the Periprocedural Period for more details.

PARENTERAL ANTICOAGULANTS

Unfractionated heparin

UH can be administered parenterally as an intravenous or subcutaneous injection. Treatment with UH, followed by warfarin, decreases the incidence of VTE and mortality in patients with DVTs compared with patients who received placebo.[6] Use of intravenous UH is monitored for therapeutic efficacy using a laboratory test known as the activated partial thromboplastin time (aPTT). The goal aPTT is calibrated by individual institutions but is generally around 1.5 to 2 times the normal aPTT based on its equivalence to a goal anti–factor Xa concentration range (which is usually less readily available).[16] UH is usually administered as a bolus dose of 5000 units followed by a continuous intravenous infusion. Based upon laboratory-specific aPTT values and cutoffs, dosing can then be adjusted to ensure that a patient maintains safe and appropriate anticoagulation. If a patient experiences bleeding secondary to heparin use, it can be reversed with protamine sulfate. Dosing for protamine is based on heparin exposure as 1 mg of protamine can neutralize 80–100 units of UH when administered within 15 minutes of UH dose. Less protamine is required if administered after a longer period due to the short half-life of UH. Besides bleeding risk associated with UH, it also has the potential to cause heparin-induced thrombocytopenia with thrombosis (HITT).[17]

LOW-MOLECULAR-WEIGHT HEPARIN

LMWHs including enoxaparin, dalteparin, and tinzaparin are derived from standard UH. LMWHs have a longer half-life than UH. Subcutaneous UH has a half-life of only 1–2 hours, whereas LMWH half-life is up to 6 hours (or longer with renal impairment). Onset of anticoagulation with LMWH is immediate and offers a predictable anticoagulant response that does not require blood monitoring. LMWH is also less likely to cause thrombocytopenia. LMWHs have been found to be at least as safe and effective as UH for the treatment of VTE. As LMWH is subcutaneously administered, it allows patients to be treated at home when an injectable preparation is needed.[18]

References

1. Armstrong WF, Ryan T. Physics and instrumentation. In: *Feigenbaum's Echocardiography*. 8th ed. Philadelphia, PA: Wolters Kluwer; 2019:9–37.
2. AIUM Practice Guideline for the Performance of Peripheral Venous Ultrasound Examinations. *J Ultrasound Med.* 2015;34(8):1–9.

3. Kearon C, Akl EA, Ornelas J, et al. Antithrombotic therapy for VTE disease: CHEST Guideline and Expert Panel Report. *Chest*. 2016;149(2):315–352.
4. Cavezzi A, Labropoulos N, Partsch H, et al. Duplex ultrasound investigation of the veins in chronic venous disease of the lower limbs – UIP consensus document. Part II. Anatomy. *Eur J Vasc Endovascular Surg*. 2006;31(3):288–299.
5. Coleridge-Smith P, Labropoulos N, Partsch H, et al. Duplex ultrasound investigation of the veins in chronic venous disease of the lower limbs – UIP consensus document. Part I. Basic Principles. *Eur J Vasc Endovascular Surg*. 2006;21(4):83–92.
6. Barritt DW, Jordan SC. Anticoagulant drugs in the treatment of pulmonary embolism. A controlled trial. *Lancet*. 1960;1(7138):1309–1312.
7. Brandjes DPM, Heijboer H, Büller HR, et al. Acenocoumarol and heparin compared with acenocoumarol alone in the initial treatment of proximal-vein thrombosis. *N Engl J Med*. 1992;327(21):1485–1489.
8. Kcentra (Prothrombin Complex Concentrate (Human)) prescribing information. Kankakee, IL: CSL Behring LLC; 2018 October.
9. Pradaxa (dabigatran) prescribing information. Ridgefield, CT: Boehringer Ingelheim Pharmaceuticals, Inc.; 2019 November.
10. Clinical Resource, Comparison of Oral Anticoagulants. Pharmacist's Letter/Prescriber's Letter. December 2019.
11. Praxbind (idarucizumab) prescribing information. Ridgefield, CT: Boehringer Ingelheim Pharmaceuticals, Inc; 2018 April.
12. Xarelto (rivaroxaban) prescribing information. Titusville, NJ: Janssen Pharmaceuticals, Inc; 2019 November.
13. Andexxa (coagulation factor Xa (recombinant), inactivated-zhzo) prescribing information. South San Francisco, CA: Portola Pharmaceuticals, Inc; 2018 December.
14. Eliquis (apixaban) prescribing information. Princeton, NJ: Bristol-Myers Squibb Company; 2019 November.
15. Savaysa (edoxaban) prescribing information. Parsippany, NJ: Daiichi Sankyo, Inc.; 2015 January.
16. Heparin Sodium Injection prescribing information. Deerfield, IL: Baxter Healthcare Corporation.
17. Baglin T, Barrowcliffe TW, Cohen A, et al. Guidelines on the use and monitoring of heparin. *Br J Haematol*. 2006;133(1):19–34 Apr.
18. Hauer KE. Low-molecular-weight heparin in the treatment of deep venous thrombosis. *West J Med*. 1998;169(4):240–244.

CHAPTER 39

Lumbar Puncture

Hira Shafeeq, PharmD, BCPS

Background

Lumbar puncture (LP), also called a "spinal tap," is an invasive procedure performed to obtain cerebrospinal fluid (CSF) from the subarachnoid space in the spinal column. It requires the percutaneous insertion of a spinal needle between two lumbar vertebrae located in the lower back. LP is performed for two primary purposes: diagnostic and therapeutic. Most commonly, LPs are performed for suspected central nervous system infection (e.g., bacterial meningitis, viral encephalitis). Occasionally, LPs can also be performed therapeutically to remove CSF in order to alleviate discomfort associated with elevated intracranial pressure (ICP).[1]

How to Use It

CSF obtained from LP is sent for analysis based on the suspected condition. LP is essential for establishing the diagnosis of CSF infection. Complications associated with the procedure include: postprocedural headaches and backaches, bleeding (including spinal hematoma or epidural bleeding), and rarely brain herniation.[1] Additional imaging such as magnetic resonance imaging or computed tomography may be helpful to rule out conditions associated with high ICP in order to minimize the chance of brain herniation. It may not be possible to obtain an LP until an underlying coagulopathy has been resolved in order to reduce complications associated with postprocedural bleeding. Patients with a history of liver dysfunction and underlying coagulopathy will also need additional laboratory testing before an LP can be performed. Generally, a platelet count of $\geq 50 \times 10^9$/L and international normalized ratio (INR) of ≤ 1.4 is recommended for an LP to be considered a safe procedure.[2,3]

Components of CSF analysis include: opening pressure, appearance, cell count and differential, protein, and glucose. A high white blood cell (WBC) count is indicative of infection. Opening pressure is measured when the needle is initially inserted into the spinal column.[4] A normal opening pressure can range from 10 to 200 mm H_2O, depending on the patient's body habitus.[5] Higher opening pressure (typically in the range of 200–500 mm H_2O) is indicative of bacterial meningitis.[6] Gram stain, culture, and viral polymerase chain reaction (PCR) can also be sent for laboratory analysis based on the physical presentation of the patient with a high suspicion of infection.[6,7] A high WBC count with neutrophil predominance is indicative of bacterial meningitis, while lymphocyte predominance is associated with viral encephalitis. A low concentration of glucose and high protein concentration are also concomitant features of bacterial meningitis.[6] Cryptococcal antigen, India ink stain, fungal cultures, and acid-fast bacilli cultures are usually sent for specific suspected infections, often in immunocompromised patients. CSF culture has a low yield; therefore, the CSF analysis rather than the CSF culture is used to guide diagnosis and treatment for a suspected infection.[6,7]

How It Is Done

LP is typically performed by a physician, medical student, or a physician assistant. It generally requires informed consent to be obtained from the patient or their representative. LP is an invasive procedure that is typically done in an inpatient setting, although it can also be performed in certain controlled outpatient settings such as a neurology outpatient clinic. The patient may be given an anxiolytic (e.g., alprazolam 0.25–0.5 mg or lorazepam 0.5–2 mg orally 30–60 minutes before procedure) for relaxation prior to the procedure. The patient is instructed to lie down in a fetal position in order to create space between the spinal processes for needle insertion. The needle is typically inserted between the spinal processes of L3–L5. This area is marked by palpating for the superior aspect of the iliac crest and drawing a line to the spinal column. The point crossing the spinal cord corresponds to the L4 spinal column, clearly marking the usual target for the LP (between L3 and L4 or L4 and L5, Fig. 39.1).[8] An aseptic technique is used to clean the area before needle insertion. A topical anesthetic such as lidocaine is injected subcutaneously to numb the area of needle insertion prior to the procedure. Once the spinal needle is inserted, the opening pressure is measured using a manometer and CSF is collected to send for analysis, culture, and PCR.[4]

Medication Implications

- Lidocaine is injected subcutaneously to numb the area prior to needle insertion. A usual dose is lidocaine 1% 1 mL injected at the site of needle insertion just before the procedure.
- It is recommended to administer anti-infectives for suspected meningitis or encephalitis as soon as possible, after the completion of the diagnostic LP.

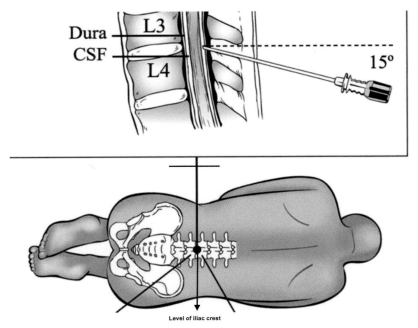

Fig. 39.1 The point crossing the spinal cord corresponds to the L4 spinal column, clearly marking the usual target for the lumbar puncture (between L3 and L4 or L4 and L5). *CSF,* cerebrospinal fluid.

- Patients are administered a combination of empiric anti-infectives for suspected bacterial meningitis based on their risk factors (i.e., age, past medical history) and typically includes two or more antibacterial agents such as ceftriaxone, vancomycin, and ampicillin.[5]
- Patients will need to be initiated on acyclovir 10 mg/kg intravenously every 8 hours if viral encephalitis is suspected.[6] Renal adjustment of the dose is recommended in patients with moderate renal insufficiency with a creatinine clearance ≤50 mL/minute.
- Refer to corresponding Infectious Diseases Society of America (IDSA) guidelines for appropriate empiric anti-infectives if fungal or cryptococcus meningitis is suspected in an immunocompromised patient.[9,10]
- Specific guidelines for periprocedural management of anticoagulation related to LP are not available. Most of the recommendations are inferred from recommendations related to neuraxial anesthesia.[3,11,12] Table 39.1 identifies for how long antiplatelet and anticoagulant medications should be withheld before and after LP. The time interval for reinitiating these antithrombotic therapies may be extended due to a traumatic LP (an LP that resulted in vascular injury, typically resulting with a high red blood cell count in the CSF analysis).
  - The risks of stent thrombosis leading to myocardial infarction or death may be too high to discontinue $P2Y_{12}$ inhibitors (e.g., clopidogrel, prasugrel, ticagrelor) in certain patients, specifically those with drug-eluting coronary artery stents placed within the previous 12 months (especially the first 6 months) and bare metal coronary artery stents placed within the previous 1 month. Physicians may decide to forego obtaining an LP in these patients or bridging with low-dose aspirin depending on the benefit-risk ratio.[3] See Chapter 20: Coronary Artery Bypass Grafting for more details about $P2Y_{12}$ inhibitors. See Chapter 46: Percutaneous Coronary Intervention for more details about stents and dual antiplatelet therapy.
  - Consider parenteral bridge therapy in high-risk patients receiving chronic anticoagulation therapy with warfarin. Bridge therapy describes administration of a parenteral anticoagulant when warfarin is held and the patient's INR is below the recommended therapeutic range (i.e., <2 or <2.5). This includes: patients with venous thromboembolism within the previous 3 months, previous venous thromboembolism while on therapeutic anticoagulation, those with mechanical heart valves, those with atrial fibrillation and previous stroke/transient ischemic attack in the past 3 months, or previous stroke/transient ischemic attack with a CHA_2DS_2-VASc score of ≥3.[2,3,11]
  - Anticoagulation reversal agents can be used for patients receiving anticoagulation therapy when simply withholding therapy and waiting to perform LP is not an option due to the urgency of a given situation. For example:
    - Warfarin can be reversed with fresh frozen plasma, intravenous vitamin K, or prothrombin complex concentrates
    - Dabigatran can be reversed with idarucizumab
    - Anti-Xa inhibitors can be reversed with andexanet alfa[2,3,10,11]
  - See Chapter 38: Lower Extremity Venous Duplex Ultrasound and Chapter 4: Anticoagulation Management in the Periprocedural Period for more details about anticoagulants.
- Postprocedural headache is a common complication associated with the procedure (10%–30%). A classic symptom of post-LP headache is the positional nature of the headache (i.e., worsening symptoms with an upright position and symptom resolution or improvement with resuming the recumbent position). The patient should be instructed to maintain a comfortable supine position. If prolonged, analgesics (e.g., acetaminophen, nonsteroidal anti-inflammatory agents) or fluids can be used to treat the headaches; however, these therapies have not been proven to be beneficial.
  - Specific therapeutic measures, such as injecting 20–30 mL of the patient's own blood (a "blood patch") or epidural saline into the epidural space, are usually reserved for patients with unresolved headaches 72 hours post symptom onset.[13]

TABLE 39.1 ▪ Periprocedural Management of Antithrombotics for Lumbar Puncture in Patients With Normal Renal Function[a]

Medication	Time to Withhold Prior to Procedure	Time to Reinitiation After Procedure
Antiplatelets		
Aspirin low dose (81 mg)	Not recommended to withhold during procedure	N/A
Aspirin high dose (325 mg)[b]	Limited evidence	Limited evidence
Clopidogrel	7 days	Immediately after the procedure
Ticagrelor	5 days	6 hours
Ticlopidine	10–14 days	Immediately after the procedure
Prasugrel	7 days	6 hours
Anticoagulants		
Apixaban (5 mg/day)	26–30 hours	6 hours
Apixaban (20 mg/day)	24–48 hours	6–24 hours
Dabigatran[b]	48–72 hours	6 hours
Fondaparinux prophylaxis	36–42 hours	6–12 hours
Fondaparinux treatment	Avoid LP	Avoid LP
LMWH prophylaxis	12 hours	4 hours
LMWH treatment	24 hours	4 hours
Rivaroxaban	24 hours	6 hours
Unfractionated heparin prophylaxis (dose ≤ 15,000 IU/day)	4–6 hours	1 hour
Unfractionated heparin treatment (intravenous)	4–6 hours or normalized aPTT	1 hour
Warfarin	4–5 days, check INR on day of procedure, target INR ≤ 1.4, consider bridging for high-risk patients with LMWH	12 hours

aPTT, activated partial thromboplastin time; INR, international normalized ratio; *LMWH,* low-molecular-weight heparin; *LP,* lumbar puncture.
[a]Patients with reduced renal function may need a longer wait time prior to procedure depending on their renal function and renally dependent medication clearance.
[b]Evidence is limited to make a recommendation at this time.

References

1. Colvin MO, Shiloh AL, Eisen LA. Lumbar Puncture. In: Oropello JM, Pastores SM, Kvetan V, eds. *Critical Care.* New York, NY: McGraw-Hill Education; 1. https://accessmedicine.mhmedical.com/content.aspx?bookid=1944&sectionid=143522877 (Accessed April 6, 2020).
2. Dodd KC, Emsley HCA, Desborough MJR, et al. Periprocedural antithrombotic management for lumbar puncture: Association of British Neurologists clinical guideline. *Pract Neurol.* 2018;18(6):436–446.

3. Horlocker TT, Vandermeuelen E, Kopp SL, et al. Regional anesthesia in the patient receiving antithrombotic or thrombolytic therapy: American Society of Regional Anesthesia and Pain Medicine Evidence-Based Guidelines (Fourth Edition). *Reg Anesth Pain Med.* 2018;43(3):263–309.

4. Robbins E, Hauser SL, et al. Technique of Lumbar Puncture. In: Jameson JL, Fauci AS, Kasper DL et al, eds. *Harrison's Principles of Internal Medicine.* 20th ed. New York, NY: McGraw-Hill Education; 2018. accessmedicine.mhmedical.com/content.aspx?aid=1164035665 (accessed April 6, 2020).

5. Seehusen DA, Reeves MM, Fomin DA. Cerebrospinal fluid analysis. *Am Fam Physician.* 2003;68(6):1103–1108.

6. Tunkel AR, Hartman BJ, Kaplan SL, et al. Practice guidelines for the management of bacterial meningitis. *Clin Infect Dis.* 2004;39(9):1267–1284.

7. Tunkel AR, Glaser CA, Bloch KC, et al. The management of encephalitis: clinical practice guidelines by the Infectious Diseases Society of America. *Clin Infect Dis.* 2008;47(3):303–327.

8. Engelborghs S, Niemantsverdriet E, Struyfs H, et al. Consensus guidelines for lumbar puncture in patients with neurological diseases. *Alzheimers Dement (Amst).* 2017;8:111–126.

9. Pappas PG, Kauffman CA, Andes DR, et al. Clinical practice guideline for the management of candidiasis: 2016 Update by the Infectious Diseases Society of America. *Clin Infect Dis.* 2016;62(4):e1–50.

10. Perfect JR, Dismukes WE, Dromer F, et al. Clinical practice guidelines for the management of cryptococcal disease: 2010 Update by the Infectious Diseases Society of America. *Clin Infect Dis.* 2010;50(3):291–322.

11. Douketis JD, Spyropoulos AC, Spencer FA, et al. Perioperative management of antithrombotic therapy. *Chest.* 2012;141(2):e326S–e350S.

12. Layton KF, Kallmes DF, Horlocker TT. Recommendations for anticoagulated patients undergoing image-guided spinal procedures. *AJNR Am J Neuroradiol.* 2006;27(3):468–470.

13. Ahmed SV, Jayawarna C, Jude E. Post lumbar puncture headache: diagnosis and management. *Postgrad Med J.* 2006;82(973):713–716.

Magnetic Resonance Cholangiopancreatography

Julie A. Murphy, PharmD, FASHP, FCCP, BCPS ▪ Shahab Ud Din, MD
▪ Basil E. Akpunonu, MD, MSC, FACP

Background

Magnetic resonance cholangiopancreatography (MRCP) is a noninvasive special type of magnetic resonance imaging (MRI) that utilizes a powerful magnetic field and radio waves to produce detailed pictures of the hepatobiliary and pancreatic systems, including the liver, gallbladder, bile ducts, pancreas, and pancreatic duct. The word "cholangiopancreatography" is derived from Greek by combining "chole" (bile), "angio" (vessel), "pancreato" (pancreas), and "graphy" (write). MRCP was first described in 1991 by Wallner and colleagues and over time has evolved into a desirable imaging study in the diagnosis of pancreaticobiliary pathologies, especially for patients allergic to iodine-based contrast materials or in patients with failed or incomplete endoscopic retrograde cholangiopancreatography (ERCP).[1-4] See Chapter 41: Magnetic Resonance Imaging and Chapter 28: Endoscopic Retrograde Cholangiopancreatography for more details about these tests.

How to Use It

MRCP is used to identify the presence of stones/calculi, strictures, tumors, infection, or inflammation involving the gallbladder, bile ducts, liver, pancreas, and pancreatic duct. In general, it has been used in the assessment of unexplained abdominal pain. More specifically, it has utility in evaluating the underlying cause of pancreatitis and to assess for long-term scarring and determining the amount of healthy pancreatic function. MRCP is helpful in diagnosing choledocholithiasis in patients with obstructive jaundice or patients with dilated common bile duct (CBD) disease. MRCP is better at detecting CBD disease compared with ultrasound or computed tomography scan. MRCP has an aggregated sensitivity of 85%, specificity of 93%, positive predictive value of 87%, and negative predictive value of 82% for the detection of choledocholithiasis. In the identification of the site and extent of a stricture, MRCP has a sensitivity of 91%–100%. Strictures may be benign or malignant. Benign strictures are due to previous hepatobiliary/gallbladder surgeries, trauma, infection/inflammation due to choledocholithiasis, or primary sclerosing cholangitis. Malignant strictures may indicate cholangiocarcinoma. Among pancreatic cancers, pancreatic ductal adenocarcinomas (PDACs) account for 95% of exocrine pancreatic cancers. Up to 75% of PDACs are located in the head of the pancreas, and at times it is imaged as "double duct" sign, which refers to simultaneous dilatation of both the pancreatic duct and CBD from distal obstruction of these ducts producing a Y-shaped contrast ductal image that may extend to the central biliary trees. This sign can also be seen in other pathologies such as ampullary tumors and an impacted gallstone in the distal duct with surrounding inflammation causing obstruction of the pancreatic duct.

Secretin-stimulated MRCP (s-MRCP) is a special type of MRCP performed after intravenous administration of secretin, an endogenous duodenal enzyme that causes the release of pancreatic enzymes that fill the pancreatic duct and makes it more prominent within 3–5 minutes of administration with return to normal in 10 minutes. In addition, it causes sphincter of Oddi constriction. This helps assess pancreatic ductal anatomy/congenital anomalies and abnormalities such as strictures or communication between pancreatic duct and pseudocyst/pancreatic fistulas. It also helps in assessment of pancreatic exocrine function and sphincter of Oddi dysfunction. These features of s-MRCP are especially helpful in assessing patients with chronic pancreatitis.

Functional magnetic resonance cholangiography is another variation of MRCP using an intravenous lipophilic paramagnetic contrast agent that is excreted into bile. Contrast agents include gadobenate dimeglumine (Gd-BOPTA), gadolinium ethoxybenzyl diethylenetriamine penta-acetic acid (Gd-EOB-DTPA), and mangafodipir trisodium. Functional MRCP better demonstrates communication between cystic lesions and draining bile ducts aiding in diagnosis of Caroli disease, helps differentiate true biliary duct obstruction from pseudo-obstruction, documents biliary anatomy in right-lobe living donors, and helps localize bile leaks postsurgery.[2,5-13]

How It Is Done

MRCP is conducted by a radiologist and may be performed in an inpatient or outpatient setting in a radiology unit or center, respectively. A magnetic field is produced by passing an electric current through wire coils that send and receive radio waves. Radio waves realign hydrogen atoms that exist naturally in the body, without causing any chemical changes in the tissues. As hydrogen atoms realign, they emit different amounts of energy depending on the type of body tissue. This energy is captured to create an image. Body fluids, such as bile and pancreatic secretions, have high signal intensity on heavily T2-weighted magnetic resonance sequences (they appear white). Background tissues generate little signal (they appear dark).

Oral contrast agents may be used to decrease fluid signals from the upper gastrointestinal tract and allow for better visualization of the pancreatobiliary duct system. While ferumoxsil improves MRCP image quality, its metallic taste is a hindrance to routine use. Alternatives include iron- and manganese-rich fruit juices (e.g., blueberry, acai, or pineapple juice), although image quality is dependent on iron or manganese content and type of juice.

In general, MRCP takes 10–30 minutes to complete. If contrast material is used, MRCP may take up to 1 hour to complete. Patients should not eat or drink for at least 4–6 hours prior to the procedure to improve imaging quality and diagnostic yield by promoting gastric emptying and allowing for gallbladder filling unbold. A typical MRI machine looks like a long cylinder with a central donut hole opening where the exam table slides into the center of the magnet. Variants of the MRI machine include a short-bore system designed not to surround the patient and an "open MRI" unit that is open on the sides to fit larger patients. Patients who suffer from claustrophobia may experience an anxiety attack during MRI scanning. Absolute contraindications to MRCP include presence of cardiac pacemaker/defibrillator, intracranial metal clips, and ocular or cochlear implants. Relative contraindications include presence of cardiac prosthetic valves, neurostimulators, penile implants, and metal prosthesis. Metal objects used in orthopedic surgery generally pose no risk during MRI. Patients should inform the radiologist of the presence of any bullet, shrapnel, or other metal in their body, as it may move or heat up during the procedure. Patients wear a gown or personal loose clothing with no metal fasteners. All jewelry and other accessories (e.g., watches, hearing aids, eyeglasses, body piercings, removable dental work) should be removed, as the MRI unit may make them into projectiles and potentially cause injuries. During the exam, patients may experience increased body warmth in the area being imaged. The coils within the machine make loud tapping or thumping sounds when images are taken, so patients may be provided with headphones or ear plugs. The technologist can see and communicate with the patient throughout the procedure. The advantages of MRCP include it being noninvasive, not needing contrast (although usually given), wide availability, and being well tolerated. MRCP may be a valuable and safe technique for the evaluation of pregnant patients with acute pancreaticobiliary disease but should preferably be done in the second or third trimester.[14–19] See Chapter 41: Magnetic Resonance Imaging for more details.

Medication Implications

- Morphine or fentanyl may be used to cause sphincter of Oddi constriction and help improve visualization of the biliary duct in upstream segmental nondilated biliary ducts.[20]
- A mild sedative medication before procedure or conscious sedation (benzodiazepines [e.g., midazolam]) may be required for patients who suffer from claustrophobia and experience an anxiety attack during MRI scanning.
- Glycemic control:
  - For blood glucose control in patients with type 1 diabetes:
    - See Chapter 30: Gastrointestinal Endoscopy - Capsule
  - For blood glucose control in patients with type 2 diabetes:[21,22]
    - See Chapter 30: Gastrointestinal Endoscopy - Capsule; a few differences are noted here
    - Sodium-glucose cotransporter-2 (SGLT2) inhibitors: avoid morning of MRCP
    - Thiazolidinediones: avoid several days before MRCP
  - See Chapter 5: Glycemic Considerations for Tests and Procedures for more details about glycemic management.
- If gallstones are small (5 mm or smaller) or if a patient is not a candidate for surgery, ursodiol 8–10 mg/kg/day in two to three divided doses may be used to promote dissolution of the stones. Use beyond 24 months is not established.[23]
- If acute pancreatitis is identified, goal-directed therapy for fluid management is indicated. Options include normal saline and lactated Ringer's.[24]
- There are a few aspects to the treatment of chronic pancreatitis[25–30]:
  - Pain: No matter the cause of chronic pancreatitis, patients experience pain. The goal is to reduce, not eliminate, pain. Reversible causes of pain should be treated. Tramadol 200–400 mg oral daily is commonly used initially. More potent narcotics (e.g., morphine, oxycodone) are often required. Adjunctive agents (e.g., tricyclic antidepressants, selective serotonin reuptake inhibitors, serotonin-norepinephrine reuptake inhibitors, and gabapentinoids) may be administered with opioids. Use of pregabalin has been shown to reduce pain and opioid use. Patients with autoimmune pancreatitis may benefit from corticosteroids. Alcohol abstinence may reduce pain.
  - Exocrine insufficiency: Providing pancreatic enzyme replacement therapy (PERT) during the prandial and postprandial periods is necessary to prevent long-term malnutrition. PERT is available as enteric-coated capsules (formulated as microbeads, microtablets, or microspheres that should not be crushed or chewed) and non-enteric-coated tablets. Of note, studies present lipase units as either international units (IU) or United States Pharmacopeia (USP units). Products in the United States are identified by the amount of lipase (USP units) they contain (1 IU = 3 USP units). PERT should be initiated with at least 40,000 to 50,000 USP units of lipase with each meal and half that amount with snacks. In most PERT studies, patients consumed a diet consisting of ~100 g of fat per day. PERT should be administered during the early and late portion of the meal (e.g., one-half of the pills after a few bites, and the rest of the pills as the final few bites are ingested). If the response is inadequate (persistent steatorrhea):
    - Ensure proper administration during meals and snacks.
    - Consider dosage adjustment up to 90,000 USP units with each meal, or more if needed.

- Consider simultaneous administration of acid-reducing agents (e.g., proton pump inhibitors, sodium bicarbonate). This allows lipase to be released from the pH-sensitive delivery systems in the small intestine, where fat absorption normally occurs. (Note: non-enteric-coated PERT preparations require simultaneous acid-reducing agent administration.)
  - Ensure the patient can afford PERT. Insurers may only pay for certain products. In the United States, the cost per capsule/tablet ranges from $1 to $6. Depending on the formulation and dosage that the patient requires, PERT may cost more than $100 per day.
- Endocrine insufficiency: Patients with chronic pancreatitis should be evaluated yearly for the presence of diabetes. Insulin may be beneficial, but there is a risk for hypoglycemia. Metformin may reduce the long-term cancer risk but may be insufficient as monotherapy to treat diabetes.
- If MRCP indicates pancreatic, biliary tract, or ampullary carcinomas, treat according to current standards and considering patient-specific factors and goals. Chemotherapy may be indicated for those with unresectable, locally advanced disease or distant metastasis, or for those with recurrence after resection.[31,32]
- Some transdermal formulations of medications include metal components and may not be suitable for use during tests that involve MRI. See Chapter 41: Magnetic Resonance Imaging for more details.

References

1. Wallner BK, Schumacher KA, Weisenmaier W, et al. Dilated biliary tract: evaluation with MR cholangiography with a T2-weighted contrast-enhanced fast sequence. *Radiology*. 1991;181(3):805–808.
2. Manfredi R, Costamagna G, Brizi M, et al. Severe chronic pancreatitis versus suspected pancreatic disease: dynamic MR cholangiopancreatography after secretin stimulation. *Radiology*. 2000;214(3):849–855.
3. Varghese JC, Farrell MA, Courtney G, et al. Role of MR cholangiopancreatography in patients with failed or inadequate ERCP. *AJR Am J Roentgenol*. 1999;173(6):1527–1533.
4. Soto JA, Yucel EK, Barish MA, et al. MR cholangiopancreatography after unsuccessful or incomplete ERCP. *Radiology*. 1996;199(1):91–98.
5. Reimer P, Schneider G, Schima W. Hepatobiliary contrast agents for contrast-enhanced MRI of the liver: properties, clinical development and applications. *Eur Radiol*. 2004;14(4):559–578.
6. Griffin N, Charles-Edwards G, Grant LA. Magnetic resonance cholangiopancreatography: the ABC of MRCP. *Insights Imaging*. 2012;3(1):11–21.
7. Verma D, Kapadia A, Eisen GM, et al. EUS vs MRCP for detection of choledocholithiasis. *Gastrointest Endosc*. 2006;64(2):248–254.
8. Geenen JE, Hogan WJ, Dodds WJ, et al. Intraluminal pressure recording from the human sphincter of Oddi. *Gastroenterology*. 1980;78(2):317–324.
9. Park MS, Yu JS, Lee JH, et al. Value of manganese-enhanced T1- and T2-weighted MR cholangiography for differentiating cystic parenchymal lesions from cystic abnormalities which communicate with bile ducts. *Yonsei Med J*. 2007;48(6):1072–1074.
10. Fayad LM, Holland GA, Bergin D, et al. Functional magnetic resonance cholangiography (fMRC) of the gallbladder and biliary tree with contrast-enhanced magnetic resonance cholangiography. *J Magn Reson Imaging*. 2003;18(4):449–460.
11. Aduna M, Larena JA, Martín D, et al. Bile duct leaks after laparoscopic cholecystectomy: value of contrast-enhanced MRCP. *Abdom Imaging*. 2005;30(4):480–487.
12. Thurley PD, Dhingsa R. Laparoscopic cholecystectomy: postoperative imaging. *AJR Am J Roentgenol*. 2008;191(3):794–801.
13. Lee MG, Lee HJ, Kim MH, et al. Extrahepatic biliary diseases: 3D MR cholangiopancreatography compared with endoscopic retrograde cholangiopancreatography. *Radiology*. 1997;202(3):663–669.
14. Hirohashi S, Hirohashi R, Uchida H, et al. MR cholangiopancreatography and MR urography: improved enhancement with a negative oral contrast agent. *Radiology*. 1997;203(1):281–285.

15. Barish MA, Yucel EK, Ferrucci JT. Magnetic resonance cholangiopancreatography. *New Engl J Med.* 1999;341(4):258–264.
16. Riordan RD, Khonsari M, Jeffries J, et al. Pineapple juice as negative oral contrast in magnetic resonance cholangiopancreatography: a preliminary evaluation. *Br J Radiol.* 2004;77(924):991–999.
17. Frisch A, Walter TC, Hamm B, et al. Efficacy of oral contrast agents for upper gastrointestinal signal suppression in MRCP: a systematic review of the literature. *Acta Radiologica Open.* 2017;6(9):1–7.
18. Bittman ME, Callahan MJ. The effective use of acai juice, blueberry juice and pineapple juice as negative contrast agents for magnetic resonance cholangiopancreatography in children. *Pediatr Radiol.* 2014;44(7):883–887.
19. Oto A, Ernst R, Ghulmiyyah L, et al. The role of MR cholangiopancreatography in the evaluation of pregnant patients with acute pancreaticobiliary disease. *Br J Radiol.* 2009;82(976):279–285.
20. Sahni VA, Mortele KJ. Magnetic resonance cholangiopancreatography: current use and future applications. *Clin Gastroenterol Hepatol.* 2008;6:967–977.
21. Sudhakaran S, Surani SR. Guidelines for perioperative management of the diabetic patient. *Surg Res Pract.* 2015:2015 article ID 284063.
22. Cosson E, Catargi B, Cheisson G, et al. Practical management of diabetes patients before, during and after surgery: a joint French diabetology and anaesthesiology position statement. *Diabetes Metab.* 2018;44(3):200–216.
23. Abraham S, Rivero HG, Erlikh IV, et al. Surgical and nonsurgical management of gallstones. *Am Fam Physician.* 2014;89(10):795–802.
24. Crockett SD, Wani S, Gardner TB, et al. American gastroenterological association institute guideline on initial management of acute pancreatitis. *Gastroenterology.* 2018;154(4):1096–1101.
25. Forsmark CE. Management of chronic pancreatitis. *Gastroenterology.* 2013;144(6):1282–1291.
26. Olesen SS, Bouwense SA, Wilder-Smith OHG, et al. Pregabalin reduces pain in patients with chronic pancreatitis in a randomized controlled trial. *Gastroenterology.* 2011;141(2):536–543.
27. Trang T, Chan J, Graha DY. Pancreatic enzyme replacement therapy for pancreatic exocrine insufficiency in the 21(st) century. *World J Gastroenterol.* 2014;20(33):11467–11485.
28. de la Iglesia-García D, Huang W, Szatmary P, et al. Efficacy of pancreatic enzyme replacement therapy in chronic pancreatitis: systematic review and meta-analysis. *Gut.* 2017;66(8):1474–1486.
29. Pham A, Forsmark C. Chronic pancreatitis: review and update of etiology, risk factors, and management. *F1000Res.* 2018;7 F1000 Faculty Rev-607.
30. Perbtani Y, Forsmark CE. Update on the diagnosis and management of exocrine pancreatic insufficiency. *F1000Res.* 2019;8 F1000 Faculty Rev-1991.
31. Furuse J, Takada T, Miyazaki M, et al. Guidelines for chemotherapy of biliary tract and ampullary carcinomas. *J Hepatobiliary Pancreat Surg.* 2008;15(1):55–62.
32. O'Reilly D, Fou L, Hasler E, et al. Diagnosis and management of pancreatic cancer in adults: a summary of guidelines from the UK national institute for health and care excellence. *Pancreatology.* 2018;18(8):962–970.

CHAPTER 41

Magnetic Resonance Imaging

Samantha Moore, PharmD, BCCCP

Background

Magnetic resonance imaging (MRI) is an imaging technique that uses a strong magnetic field, radiofrequency waves, and nuclear resonance to produce highly detailed images of the body.[1]

How to Use It

MRI provides high-quality cross-sectional images of the body in any anatomic plane (i.e., axial, sagittal, coronal). It provides superior differentiation of the fat and water content of various tissues, including the brain, muscles, ligaments, and tendons.[1,2] As a result, it is the preferred imaging modality for the musculoskeletal system and is used to evaluate shoulder and knee injuries, various soft-tissue conditions, and osteomyelitis. Spine MRI is used to assess for disk herniation, infection, metastatic disease, and degenerative changes. A brain MRI provides more detailed imaging than a head computed tomography (CT) scan and can detect smaller and more subtle abnormalities, including brain tumors, acute ischemia, and infection. Cardiac MRI has multiple applications and is useful in evaluating cardiac function, cardiac structures, and myocardial viability. MRI can be used to characterize renal masses, stage renal cell carcinoma, diagnose hepatocellular carcinoma, and further assess hepatic lesions. It is also commonly used in cancer staging, including head, neck, cervical, and rectal cancer.[2] MRI does not require ionizing radiation exposure like CT scans. As a result, it is the preferred alternative to CT scans in pregnant patients.[3]

While MRI has many advantages, there are limitations to its use. In most emergency scenarios, MRI is not the preferred initial imaging modality given its lengthy acquisition time. Patients who are critically ill are poor candidates for MRI given the inherent difficulties in ventilation and monitoring while the patient is isolated in a narrow scanner. However, in some scenarios, the potential benefit of an MRI study in a critically ill patient may outweigh the risks.[4]

How It Is Done

The physics of MRI are complex and beyond the scope of this chapter. In brief, the human body is made of mostly water, with each water molecule containing two hydrogen ions. MRI takes advantage of this by using a strong static magnetic force to interact with the body's numerous hydrogen ions. The magnet will cause the hydrogen nuclei to align with the magnetic field. Then, a weaker oscillating magnetic field in the radiofrequency range (known as the "RF pulse") is applied to the patient, which causes their hydrogen nuclei to be thrown out of alignment and resonate. When the RF pulse is turned off, the hydrogen nuclei will realign with the strong magnetic field and release energy. The amount of energy released is recorded by MRI receiver coils and reconstructed into images by a computer.[1]

Image contrast depends on several factors. Intrinsic factors include the density of the hydrogen protons in the tissues and the interaction of protons with surrounding tissues (T1 relaxation) and with other protons (T2 relaxation). Additionally, different RF pulse sequences can be used to

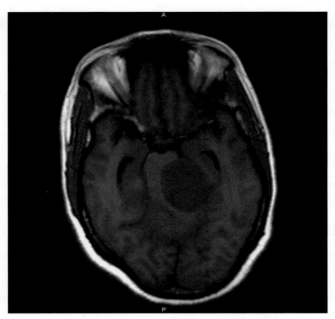

Fig. 41.1 Diagnostic image of a T1-weighted brain magnetic resonance imaging scan without intravenous gadolinium-based contrast in the axial view. This patient has a visible left cerebellopontine angle mass.

create images that highlight different tissue characteristics. Two of the most commonly used MRI pulse sequences are referred to as T1-weighted (water appears dark, fat is bright; Fig. 41.1) and T2-weighted (water appears bright, fat is slightly less bright than water; Fig. 41.2).[1] Unlike X-rays or CT scans, the term "radiodensity" should not be used to describe tissue appearance on MRI. To describe the grayscale of tissues, the term "intensity" is used (i.e., high signal intensity = white; intermediate signal intensity = gray; low signal intensity = black).[1]

The MRI scan itself is noninvasive and painless, although it can cause anxiety in claustro-phobic patients. It is performed in an MRI suite in an inpatient and outpatient setting. For most indications, patients do not need to fast before the MRI scan. The exceptions are patients who require sedation for the procedure or are undergoing an abdominal or pelvic MRI.[5]

The MRI machine consists of a large and powerful cylindrical magnet with a relatively narrow opening that the patient is advanced through as they lie supine on a sliding table. This narrow opening can preclude the use of MRI in morbidly obese patients. The MRI study generally lasts between 20 and 60 minutes, which is significantly longer than an X-ray or a CT scan. See Chapter 16: Chest X-Ray and Chapter 17: Computed Tomography Scan for more details about these tests. During the image acquisition periods, patients will be told to remain completely still, as even small movements can result in motion artifacts.[1] Once the imaging study is complete, the radiologist will interpret the results and provide a written report to the ordering provider.

While there is no ionizing radiation exposure with MRI, there are many safety concerns with the MRI machine due to the powerful magnetic force that is always active, even when it is not in use. Standard medical equipment that contains ferromagnetic metal (e.g., a wheelchair, oxy-gen tank, infusion pump pole) can become a dangerous projectile if brought too close to the MRI machine.[6] Indwelling ferromagnetic implants or foreign material (e.g., older intracranial aneurysm clips, metallic fragments in the eye) can become displaced and damage adjacent tis-sue. Mechanical and electrical medical devices (e.g., pacemakers, defibrillators, cochlear implants,

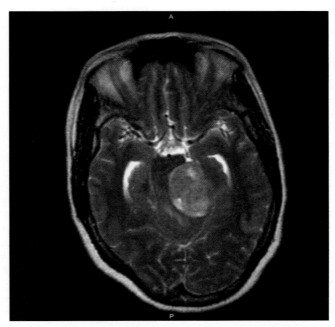

Fig. 41.2   Diagnostic image of a T2-weighted brain magnetic resonance imaging (MRI) scan in the axial view. This patient has a visible left cerebellopontine angle mass. Note the hyperintensity of the cerebral spinal fluid and the mass on the T2-weighted MRI compared with the T1-weighted MRI (Fig. 41.1).

infusion pumps, glucose monitors) can be damaged and malfunction if brought too close to the scanner. During the MRI scan, ferromagnetic metal that is in contact with the patient (e.g., metal jewelry, tattoos, electrocardiography leads, medication patches) can become hot and cause burns.[7] To improve MRI safety, modern medical devices are classified as MRI safe, MRI conditional, or MRI unsafe (Table 41.1).[8] Additionally, the MRI suite is divided into four safety zones (I–IV) based on the proximity to the scanner, with zone I being farthest away and zone IV being the room where the scanner is located. No source of ferromagnetic metal or any medical device or object classified as MRI unsafe should be brought into zone IV.[8]

During an MRI, the scanner produces loud clicking and knocking noises, which can be bothersome to patients. Additionally, patients who are claustrophobic may have difficulty tolerating an MRI scan and require procedural sedation to remain calm and still. Low-dose oral or intravenous (IV) benzodiazepines are most commonly used. Patients who are hemodynamically unstable or

TABLE 41.1 ■ The Food and Drug Administration Magnetic Resonance Imaging (MRI) Safety Labeling Criteria for Objects and Devices[8]

MRI safe	The object or device is safe in all MRI environments, including zone IV (nonmetal and nonmagnetic objects)
MRI conditional	The object or device is safe in all MRI zones (including zone IV) **ONLY IF it is under the exact conditions and MRI setting described in the object or device labeling**
MRI unsafe	The object or device is not safe in the MRI environment. Avoid bringing into zone III and **NEVER bring into zone IV**

at risk of respiratory depression from procedural sedation may require closer monitoring and/or intubation and general anesthesia.[5]

Medication Implications

- Standard hospital infusion pumps are not MRI safe. If a patient requires a continuous medication infusion throughout the MRI scan (e.g., propofol infusion for anesthesia), it must be administered through a pump that is MRI compatible. If an institution does not have MRI safe/compatible infusion pumps, very long IV tubing can be used with the standard infusion pump kept outside the zone IV area.[6]

- Before undergoing MRI, patients should be screened for the presence of implanted infusion pumps that are used to deliver opioid analgesia, intrathecal baclofen, chemotherapy in the treatment of liver cancer, or other medications. If the pump is confirmed MRI compatible, the patient can undergo MRI strictly under the specified conditions of safe use, which may be found with the device's approved product information or from the manufacturer's hotline or website. Patients with implanted infusion pumps classified as MRI unsafe cannot routinely undergo MRI, as it may result in pump dysfunction and overdosing, underdosing, or mechanical pump failure. If an MRI is required, the pump may need to be emptied of medication before the scan and then reprogrammed after the scan before it can be safely used.[9]

- Similarly, patients with external portable infusion pumps (e.g., insulin pumps) that are not MRI compatible or MRI safe must remove their pump and metal infusion set prior to the MRI scan.[10] Patients with an insulin pump can usually disconnect from their pump for an hour or less without adverse consequences. If there is concern about briefly stopping the insulin infusion or if the scan is going to be longer than an hour, the patient can receive a bolus dose of short-acting insulin or be switched to an insulin infusion. Other medication infusions that cannot be safely stopped will need to be switched to an alternative delivery method.

- Transdermal medication patches often include ferromagnetic metal and have been reported to cause burns if kept on the patient during an MRI scan. As a result, the Food and Drug Administration issued a safety warning to remove medication patches prior to MRI (even clear patches), unless the manufacturer clearly states the patches are MRI safe. A new patch should be applied as soon as the MRI scan is complete to avoid interruption in the therapeutic effects of the medication.[11]

- Depending on the indication for MRI, patients may receive IV contrast media with magnetic properties to improve the visibility of the vasculature or enhance contrast between pathologic (e.g., areas of inflammation, infection, infarction, tumors) and normal tissue (Fig. 41.3). The most commonly used class of contrast is gadolinium-based contrast agents (GBCAs), which causes T1 shortening and appears hyperintense (bright) on T1-weighted imaging.[1]

- Acute reactions to GBCAs are extremely rare. Most reactions that do occur are physiologic and mild, with symptoms of coldness, warmth, pain at the injection site, headache, paresthesias, nausea, or dizziness.[12]

- GBCAs undergo renal elimination. At standard doses, GBCA is not considered nephrotoxic.[12] However, patients with stage 4 or 5 chronic kidney disease (CKD) (estimated glomerular filtration rate [eGFR] <30 mL/minute/1.73 m^2) or acute kidney injury (AKI) who receive a GBCA are at risk of developing nephrogenic systemic fibrosis (NSF). Patients with CKD on hemodialysis (HD) are at the highest risk. NSF is a rare but devastating disorder that occurs from a gadolinium complex precipitating in tissues with resultant fibrosis. Fibrosis most commonly occurs in the skin and subcutaneous tissue. However, it may occur

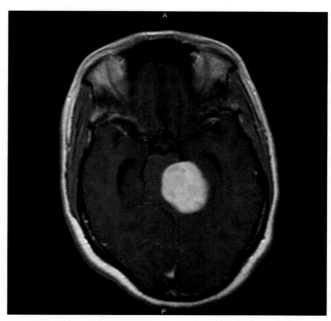

Fig. 41.3 Diagnostic image of a T1-weighted brain magnetic resonance imaging scan with intravenous gadolinium-based contrast (GBCA) in the axial view. This patient has a visible left cerebellopontine angle mass. Note the hyperintensity of the mass after GBCA compared with that before contrast (Fig. 41.1).

anywhere in the body, including the periarticular space and the diaphragmatic muscle resulting in irreversible contractures and respiratory failure, respectively.[1,13,14]

- GBCAs are classified by the American College of Radiology into three groups based on their known risk of causing NSF (Table 41.2).[13,14]
  - Group I GBCAs have the highest risk of causing NSF, and almost all known cases of NSF have been caused by group I agents. The use of group I GBCAs in patients with CKD 4 or 5 (eGFR <30 mL/minute/1.73 m²) or AKI is contraindicated.[14]

TABLE 41.2 ■ American College of Radiology Group Classification of Gadolinium-Based Contrast Agents Based on Nephrogenic Systemic Fibrosis (NSF) Risk[14]

Group I[a] (High NSF risk)	Gadodiamide (Omniscan®)
	Gadopentetate dimeglumine (Magnevist®)
	Gadoversetamide (OptiMARK®)
Group II (Low NSF risk)	Gadobenate dimeglumine (MultiHance®)
	Gadobutrol (Gadavist®)
	Gadoteric acid (Dotarem®)
	Gadoteridol (ProHancev®)
Group III[a] (Unknown NSF risk)	Gadoxetate disodium (Eovist®)

[a]Patients at risk of NSF (e.g., acute kidney injury, chronic kidney disease stage 4 or 5, on hemodialysis) should not receive group I or III agents.

- Group II GBCAs used at standard doses have been associated with few or no unconfounded cases of NSF and are considered to have an extremely low risk of causing NSF. Group II agents may be used in patients with CKD 4 or 5 (eGFR <30 mL /minute/1.73 m²) or AKI.[14]
- Group III GBCAs are believed to have a low NSF risk, but there is insufficient data to demonstrate safety in high-risk patients. As a result, use of group III GBCAs should be avoided in patients with CKD stage 4 or 5 (eGFR <30 mL/minute/1.73 m²) or AKI.[14]

- Depending on the indication for imaging, providers may consider a CT scan with iodinated contrast medium (ICM) as an alternative in patients with CKD who are anuric and dependent on HD as they are not at risk of contrast-induced nephropathy from ICM. If an MRI scan with GBCA is required, a group II agent should be used.[14]

References

1. Zaer N, Amini B, Elsayes K. Overview of diagnostic modalities and contrast agents. In: Elsayes K, Oldham S, eds. *Introduction to Diagnostic Radiology*: McGraw-Hill; 2014. https://accessmedicine.mhmedical .com/content.aspx?sectionid=95875179&bookid=1562.
2. Chen M, Whitlow C. Scope of diagnostic imaging. In: Chen M, Pope T, Ott D, eds. *Basic Radiology*. 2nd ed.; McGraw-Hill; 2011. Accessed June 18, 2020. https://accessmedicine.mhmedical.com/content .aspx?sectionid=39669007&bookid=360.
3. American College of Obstetricians and Gynecologists' Committee on Obstetric Practice. Guidelines for diagnostic imaging during pregnancy and lactation. *Obstet Gynecol*. 2017;130(4):e210–e216.
4. Qadir N, Matthew R. Imaging of the critically ill patient: radiology. In: Oropello J, Pastores S, Kvetan V, eds. *Critical Care*: McGraw-Hill; 2017. Accessed June 17, 2020. https://accessmedicine.mhmedical.com /content.aspx?sectionid=143516056&bookid=1944.
5. Apfelbaum JL, Gross JB, Connis RT, et al. Practice guidelines for moderate procedural sedation and analgesia 2018. *Anesthesiology*. 2018;128(3):437–479.
6. Wynnychenko T, Szokol J, Murphy G. Infusion pump use in the MRI. *Anesth Analg*. 2000;91:249–250.
7. Sammet S. Magnetic resonance safety. *Abdom Radiol (NY)*. 2016;41(3):444–451.
8. Kanal E, Barkovich AJ, Bell C, et al. ACR guidance document on MR safe practices: 2013. *J Magn Reson Imaging*. 2013;37(3):501–530.
9. Safety concerns with implantable infusion pumps in the magnetic resonance (MR) environment: FDA safety communication. Published 2017. https://www.fda.gov/medical-devices/safety-communications /safety-concerns-implantable-infusion-pumps-magnetic-resonance-mr-environment-fda-safety.
10. Umpierrez GE, Klonoff DC. Diabetes technology update: use of insulin pumps and continuous glucose monitoring in the hospital. *Diabetes Care*. 2018;41(8):1579–1589.
11. Kuehn B. FDA warning: remove drug patches before MRI to prevent burns to skin. *JAMA*. 2009;301(13):1328.
12. ACR Committee on Drugs and Contrast Media. Adverse reactions to gadolinium-based contrast media. ACR Manual on Contrast Media. Published 2020. Accessed May 20, 2020. https://www.acr.org /-/media/ACR/files/clinical-resources/contrast_media.pdf.
13. Mathur M, Jones JR, Weinreb JC. Gadolinium deposition and nephrogenic systemic fibrosis: a radiologist's primer. *Radiographics*. 2020;40(1):153–162.
14. ACR Committee on Drugs and Contrast Media. Nephrogenic systemic fibrosis. ACR Manual on Contrast Media. Published 2020. Accessed May 20, 2020. https://www.acr.org/-/media/ACR/files/clinical -resources/contrast_media.pdf.

CHAPTER 42

Nasogastric Tubes

Kimberly Means, PharmD, BCCCP

Background

Nasogastric (NG) tubes are commonly called Salem sumps™ or abbreviated and called NG tubes. These tubes vary in diameter and length and can serve many purposes. NG tubes are inserted through the nare, down through the oropharynx, to terminate in the stomach. Hieronymus Fabricius ab Aquapendente, a 16th-century Italian professor of anatomy and surgery, is thought to be the first to use a silver tube as an NG tube for enteral feeding.[1]

How to Use It

NG tubes can be used for medication administration, enteral feeding, aspiration and measurement of gastric contents, lavage in suspected poisonings or drug overdoses, preventing aspiration or vomiting, or decompression of the stomach.[2] There are many considerations regarding administration of medications through NG tube, including dosage form, dose, and frequency. Enteral feedings can be given through these tubes as boluses, intermittent feedings, or continuous feedings. These tubes can be used in the case of suspected or confirmed gastrointestinal bleeding to enable visualization of the gastrointestinal tract.[3]

How It Is Done

NG tubes are typically used in an inpatient setting and can be placed at the patient's bedside by a nurse, advanced practice provider, or physician. NG tubes are made of acid-resistant polymer and are measured in French (Fr) units and can be classified as small bore (5–12 Fr) or large bore (≥14 Fr).[4,5] Larger-bore tubes can be less comfortable for the patient but clog less easily. Patients may cough, gag, or vomit during placement, so providers must be alert to these potential complications. To decrease the risk of epistaxis upon insertion, the provider may nasally administer oxymetazoline or phenylephrine.[3] To decrease potential pain during the procedure, the provider may administer viscous lidocaine or 4% lidocaine via atomizer or nebulizer.[3] Before insertion, the practitioner should estimate how deep the NG tube will need to be inserted to safely terminate in the stomach. To determine this distance, the practitioner should measure, with NG tube, from the xiphoid process to the angle of the mandible and then the nostril.[3] The length should be marked on the tube as a reminder of how far to insert the tube. The distal tip of the tube has holes to allow passage of enteral nutrition, medications, or removal of gastric contents.

NG tubes are placed by lubricating the tip of the tube, having the patient positioned in the "sniffing" position with the neck flexed and the head extended.[3] The tube is then inserted through the nare, into the nasal cavity, advanced through the posterior oropharynx, through the esophagus, to finally terminate in the stomach.[3] The patient may be asked to take sips of liquid to help guide the passage of NG tube through the nose and into the stomach.[6] Once placed in the proper position, the tube needs to be secured, typically with tape, to ensure that it remains in proper position. Patients do not necessarily need to be awake for an NG tube to be placed. Comatose patients may also have an NG tube placed using the same procedure without having the patient take sips of liquid. Proper placement of the distal tip of the tube in the stomach must be confirmed before being used to administer medications or tube feeding. Placement can be verified by auscultation of the abdomen or aspiration of gastric contents; however, the more reliable method of confirmation is a chest X-ray.[1,6] To auscultate, air may be injected into the tube using a catheter-tip syringe and listening for borborygmus over the epigastrium.[3] If the NG tube is not in the correct position, it needs to be promptly removed and replaced, if necessary. The patient may have a change in respiratory rate or effort or may be unable to speak if the tube is not in the correct place.[1]

Patients suffering from facial or neck trauma may not be appropriate for the placement of an NG tube due to altered anatomy and risk of additional trauma. Potential complications of NG tube placement include epistaxis, sore throat, mucosal bleeding, or perforation.[2] Prolonged use of an NG tube can lead to mucosal damage, swallowing difficulties, and possible sinusitis.[1] NG tubes can also be mistakenly placed in the lung and cause atelectasis, pneumothorax, pneumonia, lung abscess, and pulmonary hemorrhage.[1,2] Additional potential injuries from misplacement are vascular injuries and intracranial injuries.[2] Enteral complications of NG tubes include breaking of the tube, kinking or knotting of the tube, or perforation of the esophagus, stomach, or intestines.[2]

Medication Implications

- If the NG tube is being used to suction and medication must be administered via the NG tube, the tube should be clamped for 30 minutes before and after administering the medication.[7]
- If administering medications that should be given on an empty stomach, enteral feedings should be discontinued for 1 hour before medication administration and should not be re-initiated until 2 hours after medication administration.[8]
- To avoid incompatibility issues with enteral feedings, the tube should be flushed with 15–30 mL of water before and after medications are administered.[7]
  - Ideally, multiple medications should be given separately and the tube flushed with at least 5 mL of water in between each individual medication.[5]
- NG tubes should be flushed routinely (i.e., every 4 hours or after each enteral feeding or medication administration) to aid in maintaining patency.[7]
- Medications and enteral feedings should not be mixed together due to compatibility concerns.[7]
- NG tubes should not be used to deliver enteral feedings for longer than 4 weeks.[2]
- Liquid formulations
  - Liquid medication formulations are preferred over solid dosage forms, as liquid preparations are more readily absorbed and are less likely to clog the NG tube.[7]
  - Of the liquid dosage forms, elixirs or suspensions are preferred over syrups, especially if the pH is ≤4, as this can result in clumping if the syrup comes in contact with enteral nutrition formulas.[7,9]
  - Use caution with liquid dosage forms, as some can contain sorbitol, potentially causing gastrointestinal distress.[7]
  - Viscous or highly concentrated liquid preparations should be diluted further with water before administration through an NG tube.[7]
  - Liquid medications for enteral administration should be dispensed in an oral syringe, as opposed to a syringe with a Luer lock to prevent accidental parenteral administration.[8]
- Solid formulations
  - Some immediate-release tablets, if simple and compressed, may be crushed into a fine powder and administered via an NG tube and flushed with 15–30 mL of water after administration.[7]

- Extended-release, enteric-coated, cytotoxic, teratogenic, carcinogenic, buccal, or sublingual medications should not be crushed and administered through an NG tube.[5,7]
  - Enteric-coated tablets are formulated to prevent gastritis and break down by gastric acid before absorption occurs; therefore, crushing these tablets would decrease these protective properties[8]
  - A note of caution: if an extended-release tablet is scored and able to be divided, it does not necessarily mean that it should be crushed or chewed (e.g., metoprolol succinate)[10]
- Dosing and frequency of medications may need to be changed when converting from extended-release or other inappropriate dosage forms to dosage forms appropriate for NG tube administration.
- Several references exist to guide providers regarding appropriate medications and dosage forms that can be administered through an NG tube. The Institute for Safe Medication Practices' (ISMP) "Do Not Crush" list, medication prescribing information, and common drug information references are very helpful resources to determine the appropriateness of dosage forms for crushing.
- Absorption of medications may be altered due to administration into the stomach, as most medications are best absorbed in the small intestine.[7]
- Smaller-bore tubes are more likely to become occluded than larger-bore tubes.
- Several methods have been published recommending various flushing strategies to unclog feeding tubes.
  - Typically, warm water is used first line to unclog an NG tube.[4]
  - If warm water is not successful, carbonated beverages have also been used to unclog tubes.[4]
  - One published method recommends crushing a pancrelipase tablet (authors used Viokase brand) and a sodium bicarbonate tablet (324 mg) into a fine powder and combining with 5 mL of water, which can then be instilled into the clogged tube.[11]

References

1. Rajbhandari R. and Wright SC. Chapter 119. Placement of nasogastric tube. In: McKean SC, Ross JJ, Dressler DD, et al., eds. *Principles and Practice of Hospital Medicine.* 1st ed. New York, NY: McGraw-Hill; 2012.
2. McKean SC. Chapter 123. Feeding tube placement. In: McKean SC, Ross JJ, Dressler DD, et al., eds. *Principles and Practice of Hospital Medicine.* 2nd ed. New York, NY: McGraw-Hill; 2017.
3. Thomsen TW, Shaffer RW, Setnik GS. Nasogastric intubation. *N Engl J Med.* 2006;354(17):e16.
4. Bandy KS, Albrecht S, Parag B, et al. Practices involved in the enteral delivery of drugs. *Curr Nutr Rep.* 2019;8(4):356–362.
5. Gora ML, Tschampel MM, Visconti JA. Considerations of drug therapy in patients receiving enteral nutrition. *Nutr Clin Pract.* 1989;4(3):105–110.
6. DeLegge MH. Enteral access and associated complications. *Gastroenterol Clin North Am.* 2018;47(1):23–37.
7. Williams NT. Medication administration through enteral feeding tubes. *Am J Health Syst Pharm.* 2008;65(24):2347–2357.
8. Magnuson BL, Clifford TM, Hoskins LA, et al. Enteral nutrition and drug administration, interactions, and complications. *Nutr Clin Pract.* 2005;20(6):618–624.
9. Williams PJ. How do you keep medicines from clogging feeding tubes? *Am J Nurs.* 1989;89(2):181–182.
10. Metoprolol Succinate [package insert]. Corona, CA: Watson Laboratories, Inc.; 2014.
11. Marcuard SP, Stegall KL, Trogdon S. Clearing obstructed feeding tubes. *JPEN J Parenter Enteral Nutr.* 1989;13(1):81–83.

CHAPTER 43

Nephrostomy Tubes

Yuriy Khanin, MD

Background

Percutaneous nephrostomy tubes (PCNs) are placed through the skin directly into a portion of the kidney, hence the name (percutaneous = pertaining to through the skin; nephrostomy = making an opening in the kidney). This procedure has four broad indications: relief of urinary obstruction, diagnostic testing, access for therapeutic interventions, and urinary diversion. In the hospital setting, the most common scenario related to PCN that a general medicine service experiences is a patient presenting with obstructive uropathy with or without kidney injury.

How to Use It

While PCN placement is often indicated for decompression of the renal collecting system, the cause of obstructions vary from relatively benign renal calculi to a malignancy-associated obstruction. In addition, PCNs can be used as a temporary diversion to facilitate healing of the renal collecting system in conditions such as hemorrhagic cystitis, complex infections, malignant fistulas, or urinary leaks. PCNs can be a diagnostic test; for instance, they can be used to diagnose a ureteropelvic junction obstruction, called the Whitaker test, or relieving said obstruction, called endopyelotomy. Lastly, PCNs can be used to safely instill chemotherapy and other medications directly into the upper urinary tract.[1,2]

How It Is Done

PCN was first described in 1955 as a needle decompression for hydronephrosis.[3] The technique and the indications for PCN have greatly evolved since then. Now the procedure is performed under ultrasound, fluoroscopic, or computed tomography (CT) guidance in an inpatient or outpatient setting. The patient is placed in the prone position and local anesthesia with lidocaine 1% is injected. Then, a needle is inserted into the selected renal collecting site, and if this needle relieves an obstructed system, spontaneous urine efflux will immediately occur. A guidewire is then inserted upon which the nephrostomy tube (generally 12–14 French) is advanced. Confirmation can be performed with injection of contrast material. The catheter is then secured with sutures and adhesive dressings.[1]

Medication Implications

- Minor complications that require no specific therapy may be seen in 15%–25% of patients who undergo a nephrostomy procedure.[4] Major complications can be divided into procedural and postprocedural.
    - Injury to adjacent structures, such as the pleura or bowel, is uncommon. The overall reported incidence of colonic perforation is less than 0.2% of cases.[5] If unrecognized, it can

lead to fistula formation and associated abscess. If occurring, conservative management with bowel rest and broad-spectrum antibiotics for 7 days is generally successful.[6]
- The reported incidence of pleural complications in PCN placement is 0.1% to 0.2%.[5] The management involves treating the resulting pneumothorax or pleural fluid with chest tube placement. See Chapter 15: Chest Tube for more details about this procedure.
- Bleeding is the most common complication, followed by infection; hydro-/hemo-/urothorax.[4]
  - Hematuria occurs in up to 95% of all PCN cases, though it should resolve within 24–48 hours. Unstable vital signs or a decrease in hematocrit is unusual and should be investigated, as severe postoperative bleeding requiring intervention is reported to occur in 1%–4%.[5] If no hematuria is noted, then retroperitoneal bleeding should be suspected and evaluated with CT imaging. Small retroperitoneal hematomas form a tamponade on their own and generally only require supportive care with blood transfusions. A rapidly enlarging hematoma or decreasing hematocrit requires intervention.
  - When significant bleeding occurs, angiographic studies are indicated for evaluation of bleeding vessels and embolization can be performed; surgical intervention is rarely necessary.[7]
- Low-grade temperature elevation and chills are common postoperative findings with an incidence noted to be as high as 100%.[8] Therefore, an infectious workup can generally be deferred as long as the patient is asymptomatic and clinically stable. Profound sepsis or septic shock is rare, reported to occur in 1%–3% of all patients.[9] The most common organisms isolated are gram-negative bacilli; therefore, empiric coverage with a third-generation antipseudomonal cephalosporin (e.g., ceftazidime) or carbapenem is indicated until cultures result.[10]
  - A single dose of ceftriaxone or vancomycin in patients with penicillin allergy can be administered preprocedure for prophylactic coverage. If purulent-appearing urine is unexpectedly discovered during PCN placement, the urine should be sent for culture and sensitivity, and empiric antibiotics should be continued.[11]
- Coagulation studies and a complete blood count should be obtained before PCN placement, as it is deemed a procedure with a high risk of bleeding. Correction of coagulation abnormalities is recommended to a goal international normalized ratio (INR) <1.5, an activated partial thromboplastin time (aPTT) value <1.5 times control (for those using heparin), and platelet counts >50,000.[12] However, individual institutions may have their own thresholds, and it is best to discuss this with the performing physician.
  - Aspirin and clopidogrel should be held 5 days prior to elective PCN placement to allow for some platelet activity recovery. Warfarin should also be held 5 days preprocedure, as this should allow for the INR to reach the procedural target <1.5. When holding anticoagulation (i.e., with warfarin), the decision to bridge using unfractionated heparin is at the discretion of the physician and depends on the patient's thromboembolic risk. Low-molecular-weight heparin should be held 24 hours prior to procedure. Direct oral anticoagulants (DOACs) can be held 2–4 days prior to procedure depending on the individual agent and the patient's creatinine clearance. See Chapter 13: Bronchoscopy and Chapter 4: Anticoagulation Management in the Periprocedural Period for details about the timing of discontinuing DOACs. DOAC reintroduction is often delayed for 1–2 days as PCN is a high bleeding risk procedure. Therapeutic doses of unfractionated heparin should be held 2–3 hours preprocedure, as this should allow enough time for the aPTT to reach the target <1.5 times control. Individual institutions and departments may have their own guidelines, and it is always best to discuss these issues well in advance.[11,13]
- There are no absolute contraindications to PCN. That being said, when a patient presents with renal obstruction and severe electrolyte abnormalities such as hyperkalemia, emergent

hemodialysis prior to PCN may be quicker and more dependable in correcting the abnormalities.[11]

- Tube dislodgement is a frequent complication post-PCN with a reported incidence of 1.6%–29%, which is why the majority of PCN have self-retaining loops and are further secured with sutures and dressings.
  - If tube dislodgement occurs within 1 week of placement of PCN, a new puncture with a new tract is required. If the dislodgement occurs more than 1 week after placement, then a mature tract may exist and the nephrostomy tube may be replaced.[14]
- To prevent silent tube obstruction, routine PCN exchange every 3–6 months is recommended.[11]
- In patients with acute kidney injury and urinary obstruction, relieving the obstruction with PCN generally yields improvement in kidney function within 1 week. However, this is influenced by the kidney injury degree, level, duration, and presence of an infection.[6] Medications that were previously adjusted to reduced dosing because of acute kidney injury should have their dosing readjusted as the injury resolves.
- Unilateral obstruction does not routinely cause kidney injury because hypertrophy and hyperfiltration compensates in the contralateral kidney. However, if the contralateral kidney is atrophic or the patient has underlying kidney disease, a unilateral obstruction can present with acute renal failure. At times, a furosemide renal scan may be requested by a nephrologist to determine whether PCN in unilateral obstruction may be beneficial.

References

1. Dyer RB, Regan JD, Kavanagh PV, et al. Percutaneous nephrostomy with extensions of the technique: step by step. *Radiographics*. 2002;22:503–525.
2. Karlin GS, Badlani GH, Smith AD. Endopyelotomy versus open pyeloplasty: comparison in 88 patients. *J Urol*. 1988;140:476–478.
3. Goodwin WE, Casey WC, Woolf W. Percutaneous trocar (needle) nephrostomy in hydronephrosis. *J Am Med Assoc*. 1955;157:891–894.
4. Bjarnason H, Ferral H, Stackhouse DJ, et al. Complications related to percutaneous nephrolithotomy. *Semin Intervent Radiol*. 1994;11:213–225.
5. Ramchandani P, Cardella J F, Grassi C J, et al. Society of Interventional Radiology Standards of Practice Committee Quality improvement guidelines for percutaneous nephrostomy. *J Vasc Interv Radiol*. 2003;14(9 Pt 2):S277–S281.
6. Gerspach JM, Bellman GC, Stoller ML, et al. Conservative management of colon injury following percutaneous renal surgery. *Urology*. 1997;49(6):831–836.
7. Farrell TA, Hicks ME. A review of radiologically guided percutaneous nephrostomies in 303 patients. *J Vasc Interv Radiol*. 1997;8:769–774.
8. Lee WJ, Patel U, Patel S, et al. Emergency percutaneous nephrostomy: results and complications. *J Vasc Interv Radiol*. 1994;5(1):135–139.
9. Ramchandani P, Cardella J F, Grassi C J, et al. SCVIR Standards of Practice Committee Quality improvement guidelines for percutaneous nephrostomy. *J Vasc Interv Radiol*. 2001;12(11):1247–1251.
10. Wagenlehner FM, Weidner W, Naber KG. Optimal management of urosepsis from the urological perspective. *Int J Antimicrob Agents*. 2007;30(5):390–397.
11. Dagli M, Ramchandani P. Percutaneous nephrostomy: technical aspects and indications. *Semin Intervent Radiol*. 2011;28:424–437.
12. Patel IJ, Davidson JC, Nikolic B, et al. Consensus guidelines for periprocedural management of coagulation status and hemostasis risk in percutaneous image-guided interventions. *J Vasc Interv Radiol*. 2012;23:727–736.
13. Bell BR, Spyropoulos AC, Douketis JD. Perioperative management of the direct oral anticoagulants: a case-based review. *Hematol Oncol Clin North Am*. 2016;30:1073.
14. Stables DP. Percutaneous nephrostomy: technique, indications, and results. *Urol Clin North Am*. 1982;9:15–29.

CHAPTER 44

Oxygen Supplementation

Sameer Khanijo, MD, FACP, FCCP

Background

The practice of oxygen supplementation for hospitalized patients generally does not follow any standardized protocols. It is often a hospital norm that patients are provided supplemental oxygen regardless of their blood oxygen saturations (SaO_2). Until recently, many healthcare professionals believed that oxygen had little or no deleterious effects. However, recent publications indicate that supplemental oxygen use in patients with normal SaO_2 increases mortality.[1]

It is widely recognized that severe hypoxemia leads to rapid organ failure and death. Supplemental oxygen, when used appropriately to treat hypoxemia, is an essential aspect of resuscitation and will improve mortality. However, there is little clinical evidence that hyperoxia, or supraphysiologic levels of oxygen, has any clinical benefit.[2]

Supplemental oxygen is widely available and frequently used in the hospital setting, and as such, there is some terminology that is important to be aware of when discussing oxygen use. The purpose of oxygen supplementation is to maintain global oxygen delivery. Oxygen delivery describes the amount of oxygen delivered to tissues in each minute and is a product of the cardiac output and arterial oxygen content. Oxygen content of arterial blood is the sum of the oxygen bound to hemoglobin and the oxygen dissolved in plasma in each 100 mL of blood.[3] Oxygen extraction is the fraction of oxygen delivered to the tissues that is actually utilized by those tissues. It is the ratio of oxygen consumption to oxygen delivery. In a healthy adult, about 20%–30% of oxygen delivered is utilized by the tissues and can be noted in the difference in pressure of oxygen present in an arterial blood gas (ABG) compared with a central venous blood gas. A full understanding of oxygen delivery, consumption, and extraction is important for pulmonary physiology but too vast a topic for this chapter and can be found in pulmonary physiology textbooks such as *West's Respiratory Physiology: The Essentials*. Lastly, oxygen supplementation is used to treat hypoxia. Hypoxia is defined as low oxygen content and pressure within cells. It is caused by dysregulated oxygen delivery, poor cellular oxygen utilization, and hypoxemia, which is a low partial pressure of oxygen within the blood.[4]

Hypoxia is evaluated by the partial pressure of dissolved oxygen in arterial blood (PaO_2) and is measured via an ABG. However, repeated arterial blood draws are often not feasible due to difficulty of blood draw, pain and discomfort, and lack of an arterial line for continuous blood monitoring outside of an intensive care unit setting. Therefore, pulse oximetry can provide oxygen saturation via absorption of specific wavelengths of light to compare oxyhemoglobin with deoxyhemoglobin. Oxygen saturation is the ratio of oxygenated hemoglobin to total hemoglobin and thereby provides an indirect measure of PaO_2. This is less invasive and easier to follow. Pulse oximetry has the added benefit of being immediate, continuous (if necessary), inexpensive, and does not cause the patient any pain. In addition, these devices can be purchased easily and be used at the point of care both by physicians in the hospital and patients at home.

How to Use It

The Centers for Medicare and Medicaid Services (CMS) guidelines for initial oxygen certification require SaO_2 ≤88% on room air or ABG with PaO_2 ≤55 mmHg. These values may be obtained either with the patient at rest or with exertion. Without these criteria, patients will not be eligible for financial coverage of home oxygen supplementation upon discharge from the hospital.

In the hospital setting, the exact targets for oxygenation are not as clear. The British Thoracic Society recommends that oxygen should be prescribed to maintain SaO_2 at 94%–98% for most acutely ill patients or 88%–92% for those patients at risk for hypercapnic respiratory failure.[5] A subsequent expert panel recommendation from the *British Medical Journal* (BMJ) *Rapid Recommendations Series* made strong recommendations that for patients who are provided oxygen therapy, the goal SaO_2 should be no higher than 96%. They also recommended a lower target range of SaO_2 between 90% and 94% for most patients, and specifically made a strong recommendation against initiating supplemental oxygen therapy in patients with acute myocardial infarction or stroke whose SaO_2 is greater than 92%.[6]

There is a belief that supplemental oxygen relieves dyspnea in the absence of hypoxemia. Dyspnea is defined by the American Thoracic Society as a "subjective experience of breathing discomfort that consists of qualitatively distinct sensations that vary in intensity." Furthermore, they assert that the sensation of dyspnea is derived from multiple social, psychological, physiologic, and environmental factors and elicits distinct physiologic and behavioral responses in each person.[7] Dyspnea is a subjective feeling and is not necessarily tied to hypoxia. In patients with normal SaO_2, there is evidence that supplemental oxygen does not appear to benefit subjective breathlessness scores when compared with room air administered via nasal cannula.[8]

There may be a role for noninvasive positive pressure ventilation both in the hospital and in an outpatient setting for a variety of indications including hypoxemia, hypercapnia, hypoventilation, and obstructive sleep apnea. See Chapter 51: Sleep Study for more details about noninvasive therapies.

How It Is Done

Oxygen supplementation can be provided through low-, intermediate-, and high-flow systems. Conventional low-flow systems provide a relatively stable fraction of inspired oxygen (FiO_2) as long as the respiratory rate and pattern are stable. These systems can be set to deliver a high FiO_2, but the actual amount received will vary from breath to breath. Some examples of low-flow systems include nasal cannula, face mask, face tent, and non-rebreather mask. Intermediate-flow systems are used in patients with a variable respiratory rate and pattern to provide a consistent FiO_2 to meet a patient's respiratory demands. An example of an intermediate-flow system is a Venturi mask. Venturi masks provide higher-flow rates than conventional low-flow devices and provide a predictable FiO_2 by regulating the ratio of supplemental oxygen to room air. Both low- and intermediate-flow systems are limited by an increase in entrained room air, thereby reducing the provided FiO_2 with increased respiratory demand. As patients breathe faster and/or deeper, they inspire more room air oxygen from the environment, and thereby dilute the percentage of oxygen that they receive from low- and intermediate-flow devices. High-flow devices overcome this limitation by delivering up to 60 L/minute of precisely titrated FiO_2 up to 100%. High-flow nasal cannula has unique effects on respiratory physiology that allow it to better match inspiratory demand during respiratory distress and thereby reduce the work of breathing.[9]

Nasal cannula is the most common low-flow device used. It is meant to be set between 1–6 L/minute, which corresponds to FiO_2 of 24%–40%. For reference, room air is composed of 21% FiO_2 and each liter of flow adds 3%–4% FiO_2. A simple face mask can be set from 5–10 L/minute and provides FiO_2 of 35%–55%. A non-rebreather mask is a low-flow device that can provide a high FiO_2. It uses a reservoir bag to deliver up to 100% FiO_2 using a one-way valve that prevents patients from inhaling expired air.[10] Intermediate-flow devices, like Venturi masks, provide a consistent FiO_2, up to 60% FiO_2 with a total flow up to 24 L/minute. High-flow nasal cannula can provide flows up to 60 L/minute at 100% FiO_2.[11] Low- and intermediate-flow devices can be provided outside of the hospital setting. High-flow nasal cannula requires inpatient care.

When these methods of oxygen supplementation are not sufficient to treat hypoxemia or resolve respiratory distress, providers can turn to positive pressure ventilation. Positive pressure ventilation can be either noninvasive, such as bilevel or continuous positive airway pressure (bilevel [commonly referred to by brand name BiPAP] or CPAP, respectively), or invasive (mechanical ventilation via an endotracheal tube or a tracheostomy). At this point, a pulmonologist, critical care physician, or anesthesiologist should be considered to provide assistance in determining the appropriate methods of ventilation and oxygenation.

Patients with new, or acute, hypoxia should be evaluated and managed in an inpatient setting to determine the underlying cause and provide appropriate oxygen supplementation. Once patients have stabilized, they may be discharged home with low- or intermediate-flow oxygen devices. There are a number of supplemental oxygen devices that can deliver up to 10 L/minute of oxygen flow for patients outside of the hospital setting. For patients that require higher oxygen supplementation either via high-flow or invasive mechanical ventilation, they must be treated in the hospital. In most hospitals, patients who require invasive mechanical ventilation via an endotracheal tube require monitoring in an intensive care unit. Some intubated patients progress to chronic hypoxemic respiratory failure and may proceed to invasive mechanical ventilation via a tracheostomy, which will allow transfer out of the hospital to a long-term care facility or home if special accommodations can be made within the home.

Medication Implications

- Nebulized medications may be given to patients receiving all types of oxygen supplementation, both invasive and noninvasive. They can be delivered in-line with the oxygen tubing of ventilators and noninvasive positive pressure machines. Nebulized medications are often easier to use for patients with respiratory difficulty because they are not dependent on inspiratory effort, unlike metered dose inhalers (MDIs) and dry powder inhalers (DPIs). MDIs and DPIs are best used in patients on low- or intermediate-flow oxygen supplementation who have a preserved inspiratory capacity.
- Oral medications can be given to patients with low-, intermediate-, and high-flow supplemental oxygen. However, in patients on bilevel or CPAP, oral intake may be restricted to minimize mask leak and allow for optimal ventilation. Oral medications can be given during breaks from noninvasive ventilation. Patients who are mechanically ventilated will require enteral access to provide oral medications either via a nasogastric or orogastric tube. See Chapter 42: Nasogastric Tubes for more details.
- Transportation is often not possible when patients are requiring high-flow supplemental oxygen, as these systems require continuous high-pressure oxygen attachments. Patients on high-flow must be switched to intermediate-flow non-rebreather masks. Patients who are invasively mechanically ventilated can be easily transported, as they have a stable airway, but they should be accompanied by a respiratory therapist or critical care provider who is solely dedicated to monitoring the airway.

References

1. Chu DK, Kim LH, Young PJ, et al. Mortality and morbidity in acutely ill adults treated with liberal versus conservative oxygen therapy (IOTA): a systematic review and meta-analysis. *Lancet*. 2018;391:1693–1705.

2. Kane B, Decalmer S, O'Driscoll R. Emergency oxygen therapy: from guideline to implementation. *Breathe*. 2013;9(4):246–253.

3. Dunn JO, Mythen MG, Grocott MP. Physiology of oxygen transport. *BJA Educ*. 2016;16(10):341–348.

4. Macintyre NR. Tissue hypoxia: implications for the respiratory clinician. *Respir Care*. 2014;59:1590–1596.

5. O'Driscoll BR, Howard LS, Earis J, et al. British Thoracic Society Guideline for oxygen use in adults in healthcare and emergency settings. *BMJ Open Resp Res*. 2017;4.

6. Siemieniuk RA, Chu DK, Kim LH, et al. Oxygen therapy for acutely ill medical patients: a clinical practice guideline. *BMJ*. 2018;363:k4169.

7. Parshall MB, Schwartzstein RM, Adams L, et al. An official American Thoracic Society statement: update on the mechanisms, assessment, and management of dyspnea. *Am J Respir Crit Care Med*. 2012;185(4):435–452.

8. Abernethy AP, McDonald CF, Frith PA, et al. Effect of palliative oxygen *versus* room air in relief of breathlessness in patients with refractory dyspnoea: a double-blind, randomised controlled trial. *Lancet*. 2010;376:784–793.

9. Drake MG. High-flow nasal cannula oxygen in adults: an evidence-based assessment. *Ann Am Thorac Soc*. 2018;15:145–155.

10. Korupolu R, Gifford JM, Needham DM. Early mobilization of critically ill patients: reducing neuromuscular complications after intensive care. *Contemp Crit Care*. 2009;6:1–12.

11. Hardavella G, Karampinis I, Frille A, et al. Oxygen devices and delivery systems. *Breathe*. 2019;15:e108–e116.

CHAPTER 45

Patient-Controlled Analgesia

Tran H. Tran, PharmD, BCPS

Background

Pain management through patient-controlled analgesia (PCA) allows patients to self-administer predetermined doses of analgesic medication, typically through a computerized pump, eliminating the need for administration by a nurse or healthcare practitioner. This facilitates delivery of analgesia at shorter intervals and in smaller doses and reduces burden on nursing staff.

How to Use It

A Cochrane review of 49 studies reported lower visual analog scale (VAS) pain intensity scores with PCA versus non-PCA over most time intervals.[1] Higher patient satisfaction and greater amounts of opioids consumed in the PCA group compared with controls was also found. Aside from more pruritus in the PCA group, similar adverse events and length of hospitalization were reported in both groups. An additional benefit to the PCA pump is that the number of times the button is pressed can inform the need to titrate the analgesic doses up, in response to inadequate pain relief, or down, in response to resolution of pain. Common indications for the use of PCA include acute, chronic, postoperative, sickle cell, and labor pain.

How It Is Done

PCA has been in use since the 1970s, and its use is limited to settings that have the equipment and an interprofessional team of providers, pharmacists, and nurses to ensure safe use. Thus, PCAs are typically used in the hospital where a provider can order the medication, the pharmacist can verify the appropriateness of the order and prepare the medication, the nurse can set up the equipment and monitor its use, and the patient can press the button. Orders for analgesic medication through a PCA include a basal (continuous infusion) rate, patient-controlled bolus (demand) dose, lockout period, and hour limit. These settings are entered into a computerized PCA pump that will deliver the medication to the patient through an intravenous (IV) line. Other routes of administration include epidural, peripheral nerve catheter, or, less commonly, transdermal.[2] The pump can be set to deliver a continuous infusion of medication set as a basal rate or without a basal rate. Patient-controlled bolus (demand) doses are intermittent doses that are given when a patient presses the PCA button, which is attached to the pump using a cord of sufficient length that it can rest on the patient's bed. Lockout times are safety settings that restrict how frequently the medication can be delivered (typically every 5–10 minutes) even if the button is pressed more frequently. Hour limits must also be set to indicate the maximum amount of medication a patient can receive within a specific time frame (typically over 1 or 4 hours). If the maximum dose within that time frame is reached, no additional medication will be administered even if the button is pressed.

- There are a variety of PCA dosing strategies, and it is advisable to refer to current literature when available for dosing recommendations based on pain indication. As a reference, one example is shown here.

- Add up all scheduled and as-needed (PRN) opioid doses used by the patient in the previous 24-hour period to determine a total daily dose.[3]
- Because all opioids are not equipotent, every opioid dose will need to be converted to morphine milligram equivalents (MME) in order to calculate a total daily dose. It is best to use one's institution's preferred equianalgesic conversion table for consistency; however, a number of equianalgesic conversion tables are available.[4,5]
- Convert the total daily dose in MME to the desired IV opioid dose for use in the PCA. Reduce the desired IV opioid dose by 25%–50% to adjust for incomplete cross-tolerance to obtain the new adjusted IV dose.
- Use the new adjusted IV dose to calculate an hourly (basal) dose by dividing it by 24 hours.
- Calculate the demand (PRN) dose as 10%–20% of new adjusted IV opioid dose to use PRN every hour.
- For opioid-naive patients, standard dosing parameters for loading and demand doses are usually established at most institutions, and a basal dose is usually not needed.[3,6]
  - A continuous (basal) dose can be added after 12–24 hours if frequent demand doses are used or if pain is uncontrolled.
  - One method to determine a basal dose is to calculate an average hourly dose and use 30%–50% as the basal dose.

Medication Implications

- Patient should be alert and demonstrate cognitive and physical ability to administer demand doses for pain.
- Opioids are more frequently administered through PCA; however, local anesthetics, dissociatives, or other analgesics may also be used.[7]
- The three most common opioids administered via a PCA pump are morphine, hydromorphone, and fentanyl, in no particular order. Of note, meperidine is less frequently used due to concerns of accumulation of its neurotoxic metabolite, normeperidine.[8]
- Morphine is the reference opioid to which all other opioids are equated, and equianalgesic comparisons are usually made in units of MME.
- PCA orders should take into account the patient's current opioid regimen, opioid tolerance, severity and etiology of the pain, side effects from opioids, baseline drowsiness, and need for opioid rotation.
- In opioid-naive patients, morphine may be used because it is less potent than hydromorphone or fentanyl.
  - Morphine has active metabolites that can accumulate in renal impairment.[9] Thus, hydromorphone may be preferable in patients with renal impairment because it is hepatically metabolized into an inactive metabolite that is then renally cleared.[10]
- IV fentanyl is approximately 80–100 times more potent than IV morphine and should be reserved for patients who are opioid tolerant.[11] Nearly 90% of fentanyl is renally cleared as its inactive metabolite, norfentanyl. Thus, it is reasonable to use fentanyl, albeit cautiously, in patients with renal impairment.
- Specialty consultation is recommended for PCA ordering if[3]:
  - There are concerns about cognitive failure or significant anxiety.
  - There are significant side effects, drowsiness, confusion, respiratory, or central nervous system concerns.
- Respiratory depression can occur with all opioids, and it is important to monitor sedation, respiratory rate, and oxygen saturation, especially during the first 24 hours in opioid-naive patients.

- If there is concern for respiratory depression, hold opioids and provide supplemental oxygen.
- If patient becomes minimally responsive or unresponsive and respiratory rate is ≤6 breaths/minute, consider administering naloxone.
  - Prepare naloxone 0.4 mg diluted in 9 mL normal saline for total volume of 10 mL. Give 1 mL (0.04 mg) via slow IV push every 2–3 minutes until patient becomes more awake and respiratory status improves.[12]
    - This dosing is for airway protection and adequate oxygenation and is lower than the recommended dose for an opioid overdose, which is intended to fully reverse the effects of an opioid
    - The half-life of naloxone is short (approximately 30 minutes when given IV), and repeat doses or an infusion of naloxone may be needed for long-acting opioids
    - Opioid withdrawal may be precipitated by naloxone in patients who have been on chronic opioids
  - If no improvement occurs with naloxone, rule out other causes for respiratory depression.
  - If patient is actively dying, has do-not-resuscitate orders, and is receiving comfort care, naloxone administration may not be appropriate.
- Common side effects of opioids include nausea and vomiting, which can be treated with antiemetics PRN.
  - Scheduling antiemetics around the clock (as opposed to PRN) can be considered for 5 days followed by PRN dosing if there is a high risk of nausea.[3]
  - Nausea can be dose related, so consider using adjuvant analgesic medications to decrease the required doses of opioids.
  - Consider alternate opioid if nausea remains refractory.
- All patients receiving opioids should be started on a laxative bowel regimen that may include stool softeners and osmotic, stimulant, and lubricant agents for constipation associated with opioids.[13]
  - Peripherally acting μ-opioid receptor antagonists (PAMORAs) such as naldemedine and naloxegol may be considered in those with opioid-induced constipation that is refractory to two or more laxatives. Methylnaltrexone has fewer consistent outcomes from clinical studies.[13]
  - All PAMORAs should be avoided in those with a known or suspected mechanical gastrointestinal obstruction due to the risk of perforation.
- PCA by proxy occurs when activation of the PCA pump is performed by anyone other than the patient, whether authorized or not, and is not recommended or endorsed by The Joint Commission (it was previously considered a "Sentinel event") or Institute for Safe Medication Practices.[14,15]
  - Having someone else activate the PCA button can increase the risk of oversedation and respiratory depression by overcoming the built-in safety mechanism of PCA, which is that patients will not be able to push the button if they are sedated.
  - Methods to reduce the risk of PCA by proxy include providing family members with written instructions not to administer PCA doses unless they are designated as an authorized agent, warning staff of the dangers of PCA by proxy, and placing warning tags on all PCA delivery devices stating that only the patient should press the button.[14,16]

References

1. McNicol ED, Ferguson MC, Hudcova J. Patient controlled opioid analgesia versus non-patient controlled opioid analgesia for postoperative pain. *Cochrane Database Syst Rev.* 2015;6:CD003348.
2. Viscusi ER, Reynolds L, Chung F, et al. Patient-controlled transdermal fentanyl hydrochloride vs intravenous morphine pump for postoperative pain: a randomized controlled trial. *JAMA.* 2004;291(11):1333–1341.

3. Post-operative Pain Management. 2019. The University of Texas MD Anderson Cancer Center. https://www.mdanderson.org/documents/for-physicians/algorithms/clinical-management/clin-management-post-op-pain-web-algorithm.pdf. Accessed 3/6/2020.
4. McPherson ML. *Demystifying opioid conversion calculations: A guide for effective dosing.* 2nd ed. Bethesda, MD: American Society of Health-System Pharmacists, c2018.
5. This Equianalgesic Opioid Dose Conversion chart is based on the Centers for Disease Control and Prevention (CDC) recommendations (https://www.cdc.gov/drugoverdose/resources/data.html).
6. Weber LM, Ghafoor VL, Phelps P. Implementation of standard order sets for patient-controlled analgesia. *Am J Health Syst Pharm.* 2008;65(12):1184–1191.
7. Takieddine SC, Droege CA, Ernst N, et al. Ketamine versus hydromorphone patient-controlled analgesia for acute pain in trauma patients. *J Surg Res.* 2018;225:6–14.
8. Gordon DB, Dahl JL, Miaskowski C, et al. American Pain Society recommendations for improving the quality of acute and cancer pain management. *Arch Intern Med.* 2005;165:1574–1580.
9. Morphine [package insert]. Lake Forest, IL: Hospira Inc; 2011.
10. Hydromorphone [package insert]. Lake Forest, IL: Hospira Inc; 2008.
11. Fentanyl citrate injection [package insert]. Lake Forest, IL: Akorn Inc; 2016.
12. Naloxone hydrochloride [package insert]. Lake Forest, IL: Hospira Inc; 2019.
13. Rao VL, Micic D, Davis AM. Medical management of opioid-induced constipation. *JAMA.* 2019;322(22):2241–2242.
14. Wuhrman E, Cooney MF, Dunwoody CJ, et al. Authorized and unauthorized (PCA by Proxy) dosing of analgesic infusion pumps: position statement with clinical practice recommendations. *Pain Manag Nurs.* 2007;8(1):4–11.
15. Joint Commission Sentinel Event Alert. Patient controlled analgesia by proxy. December 20, 2004. http://www.jointcommission.org/SentinelEvents/SentinelEventAlert.
16. Institute for Safe Medication Practices. Safety issues with patient controlled analgesia, Part 1. How errors occur. *ISMP Medication Safety Alert.* 2003. July 10. https://www.ismp.org/resources/safety-issues-pca-part-i-how-errors-occur.

CHAPTER 46

Percutaneous Coronary Intervention

Amit Alam, MD ■ Ali Seyar Rahyab, MD ■
Gregory J. Hughes, PharmD, BCPS, BCGP

Background

Percutaneous coronary intervention (PCI) is a mainstay of treatment for coronary artery disease (CAD). There are approximately 18 million Americans with CAD, and one American will have a myocardial infarction (MI) approximately every 40 seconds.[1] A patient will classically present to the emergency department with chest discomfort along with other signs/symptoms that are suggestive of MI, which will prompt an electrocardiogram (EKG). If the EKG demonstrates ST-segment elevations (STEMI), the patient will undergo emergent evaluation for PCI. If the EKG does not demonstrate ST-segment elevations, the patient will undergo further evaluation including possible stress testing and evaluation of biomarkers (cardiac enzymes). See Chapter 53: Stress Tests for more details about these tests. If the patient has high-risk clinical features or has abnormal stress testing, he/she will also undergo evaluation for PCI. PCI involves deploying a stent device within the lumen of the coronary artery to keep the vessel open, or patent. Stent, originally a name and therefore spelled with a capital "S," is now so common a term and can be used as a noun with a lowercase "s" ("the patient received a stent") or even as a verb ("he was stented last week").

How to Use It

PCI is performed only after a coronary catheterization and angiogram are done. The coronary catheterization and angiogram are the diagnostic portion in which iodinated contrast dye is injected directly into the coronary arteries to visualize the arteries under a live X-ray (fluoroscopy) to diagnose areas of stenosis. Contrast-induced nephropathy is a possible adverse event, and the amount of dye that is used is related to the complexity of the case and the amount of vessel that needs to be intervened upon. See Chapter 17: Computed Tomography Scan for more details about iodinated contrast media. Once CAD is confirmed by coronary angiography, the interventional cardiologist will proceed to perform PCI on the culprit lesion(s) that have been diagnosed. The decision to intervene on a lesion factors into account multiple considerations including the acuity of the lesion, degree of stenosis, and location of the stenosis. If there are multiple lesions, the interventional cardiologist will consider intervention on the additional nonculprit lesions either at that time or at a later date depending on the stability of the patient.[2]

How It Is Done

Cardiac catheterization with coronary angiography and PCI are performed by interventional cardiologists. The procedure is performed in a cardiac catheterization laboratory that contains fluoroscopy and other specialized equipment to diagnose and subsequently treat CAD and MI. The interventional cardiologist obtains access to the arterial system by introducing a catheter into a peripheral artery, typically the radial or femoral artery. The catheter is subsequently guided to the aorta and gently inserted into the opening of the right and left coronary arteries successively.

Iodinated contrast dye is injected into the arteries to provide visualization of the lumen of the arteries, and this allows the cardiologist to determine if there is stenosis (blockage) in the arteries. Once stenosis has been confirmed, the interventional cardiologist will determine if placing a stent is appropriate. For patients with extensive disease or certain individuals with diabetes, a coronary artery bypass graft (CABG) operation may be more appropriate, and consultation with cardiothoracic surgery should be obtained. If stents are warranted, the interventional cardiologist will perform PCI by using specialized catheters to position a stent at the location of the stenosis. The stent will be expanded from the inner lumen of the artery, thus eliminating or reducing the stenosis and leading to improved blood flow. Patients with acute MI typically feel immediate relief of symptoms. Once the PCI is complete, the patient is transferred to a monitored bed either in the cardiac care unit or a telemetry unit in the hospital for further observation and management.

Medication Implications

BEFORE THE PROCEDURE

- In an emergency setting, when a patient presents with a STEMI, the patient will proceed directly to PCI due to the life-threatening nature of an acute MI.
- For routine (elective) PCI, as of the date of this publication, there are no randomized controlled trials to inform recommendations on the timing and use of oral anticoagulation. The cardiologist will make recommendations based on the individual patient's risk of bleeding and risk for thrombosis. It is reasonable to require an international normalized ratio (INR) less than 3 (or sometimes preferably around 2.0) for patients taking warfarin and to continue other oral anticoagulants (i.e., direct oral anticoagulants). Antiplatelet agents are also continued. A high risk of bleeding or a high risk of thrombosis may cause the cardiologist to deviate from this. For example, a patient with a high risk for bleeding and a low risk for thrombosis (such as a low CHA_2DS_2-VASc score) may have the INR below 2 for an elective PCI. See Chapter 4: Anticoagulation Management in the Periprocedural Period for more details about balancing these risks.
- Other medications such as antihypertensive agents, including beta blockers, and statins should be continued uninterrupted.

DURING THE PROCEDURE

- Conscious sedation is typically achieved with benzodiazepines and opioids for the procedure. General anesthesia is not typically necessary unless a patient is also in respiratory distress requiring intubation.
- Most patients who require PCI will receive a drug-eluting stent (DES). DES includes coatings that slowly release immunosuppressant drugs to reduce inflammation within the walls of the artery and reduce stent restenosis. Examples include zotarolimus- or everolimus-eluting stents.
- Anticoagulation is maintained with a continuous heparin infusion throughout the procedure. Other options include low-molecular-weight heparin or direct thrombin inhibitors.[3]
- Similar to cases in the operating room, any hypotension may be treated with vasopressors such as vasopressin, phenylephrine, or norepinephrine.

AFTER THE PROCEDURE

- If a DES is placed, patients are continued on dual antiplatelet treatment (DAPT). Typically, this is aspirin plus either clopidogrel, prasugrel, or ticagrelor ($P2Y_{12}$ inhibitors). For patients who undergo routine/elective PCI (i.e., stable CAD) with stent placement, DAPT is continued for at least 6 months, and for patients with MI, it is continued for at least 12 months.[4] See Chapter 20: Coronary Artery Bypass Grafting for more details about the $P2Y_{12}$ inhibitors.

- The decision to prolong DAPT beyond the above recommendation must balance the trade-off between further reducing ischemic events and increasing bleeding complications. This is the rationale behind recommending lower-ischemic-risk patients (those undergoing elective PCI) a $P2Y_{12}$ inhibitor for a minimum 6 months, but higher-ischemic-risk patients (MI undergoing urgent PCI) are recommended a minimum of 12 months.
  - A rough estimate is that prolonging (18–36 additional months) DAPT:
    - Decreases late stent thrombosis and ischemic complications by 1%–2%
    - Increases bleeding complications by 1%
- Aspirin is the antiplatelet that should almost always be continued indefinitely (with the $P2Y_{12}$ inhibitor being the agent considered for discontinuation).
  - Aspirin 81 mg orally daily is recommended, as it has shown less bleeding complications and comparable ischemic protection compared with higher doses
- When deciding among $P2Y_{12}$ inhibitors, the 2016 ACC/AHA guidelines give the following IIa recommendations (moderate strength) for patients with acute coronary syndrome and stent implantation.
  - It is reasonable to use ticagrelor in preference over clopidogrel
  - It is reasonable to use prasugrel in preference over clopidogrel in patients who are not at a high bleeding risk and do not have a history of stroke or transient ischemic attack
- Newer DES (like those with zotarolimus or everolimus) have lower risk of stent thrombosis when compared to older-generation DES. This evolution of devices partially explains why the antiplatelet strategy recommended over the past two decades has changed and decreases the validity of trials that used older stents.

GUIDELINE-DIRECTED LIPID LOWERING[5]

- Patients who are diagnosed with new CAD, whether or not a stent was placed, will need effective lipid-lowering therapy. The current guidelines recommend a stepwise approach to lipid management.[5]
  - Reduce low-density lipoprotein (LDL) cholesterol with a high-intensity statin (atorvastatin 40–80 mg orally daily or rosuvastatin 20–40 mg orally daily) at maximally tolerated doses to reduce LDL cholesterol by at least 50%.[5]
  - If the LDL cholesterol remains above 70 mg/dL, in very high-risk patients, it is reasonable to add ezetimibe (intestinal inhibitor of cholesterol absorption).[5,6]
  - If the LDL cholesterol remains above 70 mg/dL despite maximum doses of a high-intensity statin and ezetimibe, in very high-risk patients, it would be reasonable to consider a proprotein convertase subtilisin kexin type 9 enzyme (PCSK9) inhibitor.[5]
    - Evolocumab and alirocumab are Food and Drug Administration–approved PCSK9 inhibitors.[7,8] These medications are monoclonal antibodies that inhibit the PCSK9 enzyme in the liver and are administered via subcutaneous injection once or twice a month. These medications very potently lower the LDL cholesterol by roughly 50% from baseline, even when used as add-on therapy to maximally tolerated statins.[7,8]
- Side effects include:
  - Evolocumab[7]: Rash, upper respiratory tract infection, influenza, back pain, injection site reactions, diabetes mellitus
  - Alirocumab[8]: Rash, hypersensitivity vasculitis/hypersensitivity reactions, nasopharyngitis, influenza, injection site reactions

References

1. Benjamin EJ, Muntner P, Alonso A, et al. Heart disease and stroke statistics—2019 update: a report from the American Heart Association. *Circulation.* 2019;139:e56–e528.
2. Levine GN, Bates ER, Blankenship JC, et al. 2015 ACC/AHA/SCAI focused update on primary percutaneous coronary intervention for patients with ST-elevation myocardial infarction: an update of the 2011 ACCF/AHA/SCAI guideline for percutaneous coronary intervention and the 2013 ACCF/AHA guideline for the management of ST-elevation myocardial infarction. *J Am Coll Cardiol.* 2016;67(10):1235–1250.
3. Rao SV, Ohman M. Anticoagulant therapy for percutaneous coronary intervention. *Circ Cardiovasc Interv.* 2010;3:80–88.
4. Levine GN, Bates ER, Bittl JA, et al. 2016 ACC/AHA guideline focused update on duration of dual antiplatelet therapy in patients with coronary artery disease: a report of the American College of Cardiology/American Heart Association task force on clinical practice guidelines. *J Thorac Cardiovasc Surg.* 2016;152(5):1243–1275.
5. Grundy SM, Stone NJ, Bailey A, et al. 2018 AHA/ACC/AACVPR/AAPA/ABC/ACPM/ADA/AGS/APhA/ASPC/NLA/PCNA guideline on the management of blood cholesterol: a report of the American College of Cardiology Foundation/American Heart Association task force on clinical practice guidelines. *Circulation.* 2019;139:e1082–e1143.
6. Ezetimibe [package insert]. North Wales, PA: Merck/Schering-Plough Pharmaceuticals; 2007.
7. Evolocumab [package insert]. Thousand Oaks, CA: Amgen Inc.; 2017.
8. Alirocumab [package insert]. Bridgewater, NJ: Sanofi-Aventis U.S. LLC; 2015.

CHAPTER 47

Percutaneous Endoscopic Gastrostomy Tubes

Judith L. Beizer, PharmD, BCGP, FASCP, AGSF   ■   Lev Ginzburg, MD

Background

Gastrostomy tube placement is used in patients who are unable to maintain adequate oral intake yet have an otherwise intact digestive system. This type of enteral tube is used for patients who will need long-term enteral feeding, generally defined as longer than 4 to 6 weeks. Multiple ways to obtain access to the digestive system exist, including radiologic, surgical, and endoscopic. The most commonly used method is percutaneous endoscopic gastrostomy (PEG). Gastrostomy tubes may also be referred to as G-tubes or PEG tubes. To clarify, the actual definition is: percutaneous (through the skin); endoscopic (pertaining to the examination of the interior of a canal or hollow organ); gastrostomy (establishment of a new opening into the stomach).

How to Use It

Enteral feeding via PEG tube is indicated for patients with dysphagia (difficulty swallowing), which is usually due to neurologic disorders such as Parkinson's disease, stroke, or multiple sclerosis. A PEG tube may also be placed for patients with oropharyngeal or esophageal malignancies who may have difficulty swallowing.

How It Is Done

PEG tube placement is generally performed in an inpatient setting and requires two operators. A variety of methods to place PEG tubes are available, with the "pull" method being the most common.[1] Preprocedure antibiotics covering skin flora are given to prevent wound infections, and the patient is placed in a supine position. After adequate sedation (or anesthesia, based on specific situation) is achieved, an endoscope is passed through the mouth into the stomach and proximal duodenum.

The mucosa is carefully inspected to ensure there are no anatomical restrictions to the planned procedure, and a proper site for the gastrostomy placement is identified. Typically, a combination of techniques is used—transillumination (visualizing the endoscope light inside the stomach through the abdominal wall) and finger palpation (a second operator presses on the abdominal wall and the endoscopist identifies a clear indentation of the gastric wall inside the stomach). The skin is then cleaned with betadine, and local anesthetic is infiltrated; next, a hollow introducer needle is passed into the stomach and visualized endoscopically. The endoscopist places a snare around the needle to secure it in place, and the second operator next passes a long soft blue wire through the needle into the stomach. The wire is then grasped with the snare and withdrawn retrograde through the esophagus and out of the mouth, thus creating a loop (one end of the wire enters the abdominal wall and the other exits the oral cavity). The oral end of the wire is next attached to a loop at the end of a PEG tube, and the entire assembly is "pulled" through the mouth into the stomach by the second operator applying traction to the wire end that exits the abdominal wall. Once the tapered end of the tube exits the abdominal wall, traction is applied until the internal bolster of the PEG tube rests along the gastric wall. An external bolster is then placed over the tube at the abdominal wall level and the tube is trimmed to a desired length. An access port is then attached to the external end of the tube (typically Y-shaped), and a repeat endoscopy is done to confirm adequate placement of the internal bolster inside the stomach. Standard outcome of the procedure is the creation of a patent tube to allow access to the patient's stomach for nutrition, hydration, and medication administration. After completion of the procedure, it is recommended to wait 2 hours to begin medication administration via the PEG tube. Feedings may be started 6–8 hours after the procedure.

Medication Implications

BEFORE THE PROCEDURE

- The patient should have nothing by mouth or nasogastric tube for a period of time before the procedure. See Chapter 6: Introduction to Anesthesia for specific recommendations for holding enteral nutrition.
- Antiplatelet agents should be held for 5 days before the procedure; warfarin should be held until the international normalized ratio (INR) is <1.5; direct oral anticoagulants (DOACs) such as rivaroxaban or apixaban should be held for 24–48 hours; intravenous heparin should be held for 6 hours; and low-molecular-weight heparins, such as enoxaparin, should have one dose held.

AFTER THE PROCEDURE

- Medications can be restarted and given via PEG tube 2 hours after the procedure, and feedings may be started 6–8 hours after the insertion of the tube.
  - Medications and feedings are typically administered by nurses in an inpatient or long-term care setting (e.g., nursing homes, rehabilitation facilities) but can safely be given at home by the patient's family or the patient him/herself if they are cognitively intact and have the physical capability to do so.

DOSE FORMULATION ISSUES

- Liquid preparations are preferred to prevent occlusion of the PEG tube. Elixirs and suspensions are preferred over syrups, which are generally more acidic (pH <4) and can therefore cause clumping by coagulating the proteins in the enteral feeding.[2]
- Adjustment in the dosing schedule may be necessary when converting from a sustained-release product to a liquid formulation or an immediate-release tablet or capsule.
- Many liquid medications are hyperosmotic and/or contain large amounts of sorbitol, which can cause diarrhea, particularly if the patient is taking more than one liquid preparation. Hyperosmotic liquids can be diluted with water before administration to decrease the incidence of diarrhea.[3]
- If an acidic syrup must be administered, it is recommended to stop the enteral feeding and flush the PEG tube with 30 mL of water before and after the dose of the syrup.[3]
- Most compressed tablets that are immediate-release can be crushed. A commercially available tablet crusher or a mortar and pestle should be used to crush tablets. The powder should be mixed with 15–30 mL before pouring down the PEG tube. To ensure that the whole dose is administered, the container of crushed medications should be rinsed with additional water as necessary.

- Powder-filled capsules can be opened and the powder mixed with 10–15 mL of water.
  - Capsules containing pellets or beads can be cautiously opened and the contents emptied into the feeding tube. Care should be taken to not crush the beads or pellets.[4]
- Ideally, if multiple medications are to be administered, they should be given separately and the PEG tube flushed with 5–10 mL of water between each medication. After all medications are given, the tube should be flushed with an additional 15–30 mL water.
- The following dosage formulations should NOT be given via PEG tube: enteric-coated tablets, liquid-filled gelatin capsules, buccal or sublingual tablets, and controlled-release tablets (usually indicated by the suffix ER, XL, XR, CR, CD, SR). Viscous liquids should be avoided unless they can be diluted.
- Crushing carcinogenic or teratogenic medications should be avoided due to the risk to administering personnel. If that is not possible, the person crushing the tablets should wear gloves and a mask to protect themselves from contact with the crushed tablet.
- When in doubt about whether a tablet can be crushed, refer to a reference such as the Institute for Safe Medication Practices' "Do Not Crush" list. http://ismp.org/recommendations/do-not-crush.

SPECIAL CONSIDERATIONS

- For medications that should be administered on an empty stomach, if a patient is receiving continuous feeding, ideally the enteral feeding should be held for 1 hour before and 2 hours after the dose. If that is not possible, then the feeding should be held for at least 30 minutes before and after the dose.[2]
- Phenytoin has been noted to bind to the proteins in many enteral products. Feedings should ideally be held for 2 hours before and after a dose, and serum phenytoin concentrations should be measured.[3]
- Cases of warfarin resistance have been reported in patients receiving enteral feeding. Patients taking warfarin should have their INR monitored closely, and some clinicians suggest holding the feeding for 1 hour before and after the warfarin dose.[5]
- Fluoroquinolones, such as ciprofloxacin and levofloxacin, may have impaired absorption when given with enteral feedings due to the presence of minerals such as calcium and iron in the enteral products.[3]

CLOGGED TUBES

- To prevent the occlusion or clogging of the PEG tube, care should be taken to flush the tube after feedings and medication administration, as described previously. Tablets should be thoroughly crushed before administration, and acidic solutions should be avoided.
- In clinical practice, there are a number of techniques to unclog tubes, though few have been shown to be more effective than warm water.[6] Various other liquids such as colas, cranberry juice, or a slurry of meat tenderizer have been used. The liquid is instilled down the PEG tube via a syringe, and then the administering person uses a gentle back-and-forth motion on a syringe to try to disperse the clog. It is important to note that colas and cranberry juice are acidic and could actually make the clog worse by causing coagulation of the proteins in the enteral feeding product.
- There are commercially available products for clearing clogged tubes. A study compared an enzyme treatment, Clog Zapper, and a mechanical occlusion clearing device, TubeClear. The latter product was found superior to the enzyme treatment and to warm water.[7]

References

1. ASGE Technology Committee. Enteral nutrition access devices. *Gastrointestinal Endoscopy.* 2010;72(2):236–248.
2. Magnuson BL, Clifford TM, Hoskins LA, et al. Enteral nutrition and drug administration, interactions, and complications. *Nutr Clin Pract.* 2005;20(6):618–624.

3. Williams NT. Medication administration through enteral feeding tubes. *Am J Health Syst Pharm.* 2008;65(24):2347–2357.
4. Beckwith MC, Feddema SS, Barton RG, et al. A guide to drug therapy in patients with enteral feeding tubes: dosage form selection and administration methods. *Hosp Pharm.* 2004;39(3):225–237.
5. Dickerson RN, Garmon WM, Kuhl DA, et al. Vitamin K-independent warfarin resistance after concurrent administration of warfarin and continuous enteral nutrition. *Pharmacotherapy.* 2008;28(3):308–313.
6. Dandeles LM, Lodoice AE. Efficacy of agents to prevent and treat enteral feeding tube clogs. *Ann Pharmacother.* 2011;45(5):676–680.
7. Garrison CM. Enteral feeding tube clogging: what are the causes and what are the answers? A bench top analysis. *Nutr Clin Pract.* 2018;33(1):147–150.

CHAPTER 48

Peritoneal Dialysis

Yuriy Khanin, MD

Background

Peritoneal dialysis (PD) is a modality of renal replacement therapy using a patient's peritoneal cavity and extensive capillary vasculature as a dialysis membrane. The concept is exactly the same as hemodialysis (HD); both involve the transport of solutes and water across a membrane that separates two fluid-containing compartments. In HD the dialyzer is the membrane, whereas in PD the peritoneal lining is the membrane. This form of dialysis consists of three processes that occur simultaneously—diffusion, ultrafiltration, and fluid absorption.[1] See Chapter 33: Hemodialysis for more details about that procedure.

How to Use It

PD is performed at home by patients with end-stage renal disease, providing convenience and independence that is lacking in patients receiving in-center HD. PD comes in two forms—continuous ambulatory peritoneal dialysis (CAPD) and automated peritoneal dialysis (APD) that uses hydraulic cyclers. The preferred mathematical method for measuring PD dose is similar to that for HD in that both are expressed as a Kt/V (where K is urea clearance, t is time, and V is volume of distribution of urea). However, the actual calculation requires the 24-hour drain volume (consists of the fluid instilled + ultrafiltrate removed) and knowledge of the individual's peritoneal transport capabilities.[1]

How It Is Done

As mentioned earlier, PD involves instilling a dialysis solution directly into a patient's peritoneal cavity. This is accomplished via a PD catheter that is inserted into the abdominal cavity using local anesthesia with sedation. The catheter can be inserted via open surgical technique, laparoscopically (preferred), or percutaneously by experienced surgeons or interventional radiologists/nephrologists to ensure appropriate position. The PD catheter consists of silicone rubber tubing with two polyester cuffs; the deep cuff is implanted into the rectus muscle to provide fixation, and the superficial cuff is positioned inside the subcutaneous tissue 2–4 cm from the exit site. PD solution (generally 2 L) is then instilled into the peritoneal cavity for a few hours before being removed and replaced with an additional "exchange" of 2 L of PD solution. This process is repeated several times throughout the day if a patient does manual exchanges or overnight for patients using a machine. The amount of dialysis achieved and the extent of fluid removal depend on the volume of dialysis solution infused (dwell volume), duration (dwell time), how often this dialysis solution is exchanged (number of exchanges), and the concentration of crystalloid osmotic or colloid oncotic agent present. The physiology of PD is complex and outside the scope of this chapter; for greater detail, refer to Chapter 59 in the *Primer on Kidney Diseases*.[3] PD, unlike HD, is performed daily at home, either throughout the day or at night depending on the individual's preferences. A PD prescription performed manually by the patient is referred to as CAPD, and when using a machine (a cycler) overnight as APD (or CCPD).[1–3]

Medication Implications

- Solute (including medication) movement in PD, like HD, is mainly by diffusion and is therefore based on the concentration gradient between the instilled dialysate fluid and the blood. PD is a less efficient modality of solute clearance, which is why it needs to be performed daily unlike HD.
  - In HD the proper timing of medications, in particular antibiotics, is essential due to the possible abrupt medication clearance that may occur with HD. This is not an issue with PD, as solute clearance is considerably slower.[4] See Chapter 33: Hemodialysis for more details.
  - Since volume and solute removal is slower and at times unpredictable, PD is not as safe and efficient as HD for the treatment of certain emergencies such as acute pulmonary edema, life-threatening hyperkalemia, toxin exposure, and medication overdoses.
- Ultrafiltration (fluid movement) is dependent on the concentration of an osmotically active agent. Dialysate fluid can be dextrose, icodextrin (brand name Extraneal), or amino acid–based (not available in the United States).
  - Dextrose is the most commonly used dialysate in PD; it is available in varying concentrations of 1.5%, 2.5%, and 4.5%. The higher percentage yields greater ultrafiltration.
    - The main advantage of dextrose is that it is cheap and readily available. The disadvantage of the solution is the generation of glucose degradation products (GDPs). The products damage the peritoneal membrane and eventually lead to ultrafiltration failure. It is difficult to predict exactly when this will occur; however, at 6 years, up to 50% of patients will experience ultrafiltration failure.[5]
    - In addition, during PD a proportion of the dextrose in the dialysate is absorbed systemically and leads to hyperglycemia, which is especially profound in patients with diabetes mellitus. Therefore, adjustments in insulin therapy may be required with increased frequency of glucose monitoring, particularly when initiating PD.
  - Icodextrin is a starch-derived glucose polymer, available in 7.5% solution, and uses oncotic pressure to accomplish ultrafiltration. It is generally reserved for patients who require more ultrafiltration than dextrose can provide, as it is absorbed slower than dextrose solutions. Benefits include improved glycemic control, decreased weight gain, and preservation of the peritoneal membrane. The main disadvantage is added cost.[1,6]
- During PD, proteins in the blood, primarily albumin, move down their concentration gradient and therefore are lost. This obligate protein loss and increased glucose absorption can lead to higher low-density lipoprotein cholesterol and triglyceride levels. Surprisingly, multiple randomized controlled trials failed to show a consistent mortality benefit with lipid-lowering agents, and they are therefore recommended to not be initiated in the Kidney Disease Improving Global Outcomes (KDIGO) guidelines.[7]
- PD in general causes minimal medication removal. Medications that have a low molecular weight and low volume of distribution are more likely to be removed. Medications that are highly protein bound are removed more with PD than with HD given the large protein losses experienced with PD. Generally, PD is never utilized for toxic ingestions due to the relatively slow rate of clearance compared with HD.[1]
- As much as 30% of patients on PD will develop hypokalemia requiring daily supplementation. This is explained by the greater potassium removal during dialysis (as PD solutions have no added potassium), transcellular shift (induced by insulin released in response to the obligatory glucose absorption), and renal losses with diuretics (PD patients have preserved kidney function).[1]
- Catheters that are not being used require irrigation weekly with 1 L of normal saline or dialysate fluid to maintain patency. Heparin (dosed at 1000 U/L) is administered via the

dialysate if there is visible fibrin in the drain bag, as it can lead to slow fills, drains, and ultimately ultrafiltration failure. If no improvement occurs with heparin, the next step would be fluoroscopic intervention with a guidewire.[1,2]

- Antiplatelet and anticoagulant medications generally do not need to be held, as PD access and use carry a low bleeding risk.
- PD complications usually revolve around the catheter and can be either mechanical or infectious in nature. The most important noninfectious complications in PD are abdominal wall hernias, dialysate leaks, and inflow/outflow obstruction.
  - Before inserting a PD catheter, all significant abdominal wall hernias must be corrected, as the presence of significant dialysate fluid in the peritoneal cavity can increase intra-abdominal pressures and worsen existing hernias. The most frequently occurring hernias are incisional, umbilical, and inguinal. PD generally can be continued postoperatively at the nephrologist's/surgeon's discretion using low-dwell volumes (1 L) and supine position to avoid increased intra-abdominal pressures.[1,2]
  - Leakage of peritoneal fluid is often a result of catheter implantation technique or trauma. The presentation depends on the location of the leak. Treatment involves stopping PD momentarily (2–4 weeks), switching over to HD, or performing low-volume PD in the supine position. The majority of these leaks seal spontaneously, and surgical repair is the last resort for refractory leaks.[1,2]
  - Infusion pain, drain pain, and drain failure can occur, especially during new start dialysis, and is usually a result of catheter malposition, fibrin clot in the catheter, or constipation. Radiologic studies such as abdominal X-ray can be used to confirm correct anatomical placement (catheter tip should always be located a few centimeters above the pubic symphysis). Patients are often placed on bowel regimens to maintain adequate bowel movements and prevent constipation from developing. Avoid routine nonsteroidal anti-inflammatory drug (NSAID) use if treating pain, as they are known to worsen kidney function.
  - Peritoneal catheter infections can occur at the exit site, the tunnel, or both simultaneously. The presentation can include erythema, purulent discharge, edema, or tenderness overlying the subcutaneous tunnel pathway. *Staphylococcus aureus* is the most common organism isolated. Hence all PD patients, regardless of *S. aureus* carrier status, must indefinitely apply mupirocin ointment daily to the exit site.[1,2]
  - Peritonitis is the major complication of PD. Empiric antibiotics must cover gram-positive and gram-negative organisms. An empiric regimen of vancomycin with cefepime or ceftazidime is appropriate. Intraperitoneal (IP) administration of antibiotics is preferred, though intravenous (IV) antibiotics should be used when there is also a systemic infection (i.e., bacteremia).[1]
    - *S. aureus* peritonitis with concurrent exit-site or tunnel infection is unlikely to respond to antibiotic therapy without catheter removal.[1]
    - With effective treatment, the patient should begin to improve clinically within 12–48 hours, and the total cell count and percentage of neutrophils in the peritoneal fluid should begin to decrease. Often, visual inspection of the drained fluid (effluent) will suffice, but if there is no improvement within 48 hours, repeat cell count and peritoneal fluid culture are necessary.[1]
    - With any case of peritonitis, it is imperative to refer to the International Society for Peritoneal Dialysis for the current recommendations regarding management and antibiotic regimens.[8]
  - Encapsulating peritoneal sclerosis (EPS) is a rare condition characterized by dense fibrosis, thickening of the peritoneum with bowel adhesions, and eventual encapsulation of the bowels. EPS incidence increases significantly with >5 years of PD; the exact

mechanisms are unclear, but GDPs and recurrent peritonitis episodes are risk factors. Clinically, it presents with progressive failure of ultrafiltration, ileus, and bowel obstruction. Computed tomography (CT) scan shows peritoneal calcifications; however, it is not diagnostic of EPS, and the disease remains a clinical diagnosis. Laparotomy or laparoscopy are the only confirmatory tests; however, they are rarely performed due to the high-risk nature and invasiveness. Immediate discontinuation of PD is the mainstay of treatment, and surgical intervention is reserved for patients with an established abdominal encapsulation or recurrent bowel obstructions.[1,2]

- Several case series primarily from Japan provide evidence for corticosteroids as a possible treatment for EPS. No standardized dosage exists, though prednisolone 0.5–1 mg/kg/day is the most utilized regimen with a slow taper over a year. In addition, tamoxifen has been studied as a potential antifibrotic therapy, but once again no established dosing regimen exists. The majority of the studies utilized tamoxifen 10–40 mg once daily for one year and tapered off.[9]

- PD compared with HD in the first few years is characterized by a lower mortality rate, but afterward the survival between PD and HD is comparable. One possible explanation is that there is better preservation of residual renal function in PD, which is a major determinant of survival while on dialysis.[10] Therefore, patients should be on angiotensin-converting enzyme inhibitors (ACE-I) or angiotensin II receptor blockers (ARB) (especially if they have hypertension). Nephrotoxic medications such as NSAIDs, aminoglycosides, and iodinated contrast should be avoided.

References

1. Daugirdas JT, Blake PG, Ing TS. *Handbook of Dialysis*. 5th ed.; 2015.
2. Khanna R. Solute and water transport in peritoneal dialysis: a case-based primer. *Am J Kidney Dis*. 2017;69:461.
3. Gilbert S, Weiner D. *National Kidney Foundation Primer of Kidney Disease*. 7th ed.: Elsevier; 2017.
4. Floege J, Johnson RJ, Feehally J. *Comprehensive clinical nephrology*. 4th ed. St Louis, MI: Elsevier; 2010.
5. Heimburger O, Wang T, Lindholm B. Alterations in water and solute transport with time on peritoneal dialysis. *Perit Dial Int*. 1999;19:S83–S90.
6. Cho Y, Johnson DW, Badve S, et al. Impact of icodextrin on clinical outcomes in peritoneal dialysis: a systematic review of randomized controlled trials. *Nephrol Dial Transplant*. 2013;28:1899–1907.
7. Willis K, Cheung M, Slifer S. Kidney Disease: Improving Global Outcomes (KDIGO) lipid work group. KDIGO clinical practice guideline for lipid management in chronic kidney disease. *Kidney Int Suppl*. 2013;3:259–305.
8. International Society of Peritoneal Dialysis. https://ispd.org/ispd-guidelines/.
9. Danford CJ, Lin SC, Smith MP, et al. Encapsulating peritoneal sclerosis. *World J Gastroenterol*. 2018;24:3101–3111.
10. Moist LM, Port FK, Orzol SM, et al. Predictors of loss of residual renal function among new dialysis patients. *J Am Soc Nephrol*. 2000;11:556–564.

CHAPTER 49

Positron Emission Tomography

Chung-Shien Lee, PharmD, BCPS, BCOP ■ Nagashree Seetharamu, MD, MBBS

Background

Positron emission tomography (PET) is a nuclear medicine test that provides a measurement of the metabolic activity of the cells in body tissues. Positron comes from the combination of English words "positive" and "electron." The test is commonly called a "PET scan."[1-4] The first large-scale PET scanner was developed in the 1950s.[5,6] Currently, the test is usually performed along with a computed tomography (CT) scan, which involves the digital capture of images produced by combining data from several X-rays. See Chapter 17: Computed Tomography Scan for more details.

How to Use It

PET is a useful tool in getting information about biochemical changes, such as metabolism, taking place in the body in patients with cancer or certain conditions of the heart or brain. This information can be used in detecting biochemical changes in an organ, tissue, or tumor and, when combined with a CT, can provide information about anatomical or structural changes related to a disease. In particular, PET is most commonly used to diagnose and evaluate cancers but can also be useful in evaluating epilepsy, coronary artery disease, and Alzheimer's disease.[1-4]

How It Is Done

A PET can be done in an inpatient or outpatient setting. Prior to the scan, a radioactive material, usually fluorine-18 fluorodeoxyglucose (18F-FDG), which is a glucose analog, is injected intravenously. These tracers are then circulated throughout the body. Other examples of tracers include N-13, O-15, C-11, and Rb82. After about 1 hour, the patient is placed in the supine position while the overhead PET scanner slowly moves over the areas of the body of interest. As the radioactive material can be taken up by any metabolically active area in the body, it is important that the patient lies still during this portion of the test, since body movements can not only blur images but also cause 18F-FDG to be taken up by the muscles, which are active during any movement. For the same reason, a rigorous diet is recommended prior to the test. While instructions for dietary restrictions prior to the procedure may vary among imaging centers, a typical diet involves absolute fasting for 4–6 hours prior to the scan. This means no consumption of any food including chewing gum, mints, candy, or vitamins for 4–6 hours prior to the scan. Plain water is the only beverage allowed for the 24 hours leading up to the procedure. In addition, a high-protein and low-carbohydrate diet is recommended for the 6 to 24 hours prior to the PET scan. The purpose of this rigorous dietary recommendation is to minimize the effect of glucose derived from food and drink on the accuracy of the test. Elevated blood glucose raises the insulin concentration, which in turn enables intake of glucose into the muscles instead of the areas of interest. For the same reason, strenuous physical activity should be avoided the day prior to the scan.[1-4]

Despite taking all these precautions, false negatives can occur when tumors or lesions are slow growing and have low metabolic activity, or if they are very small (generally less than

1 cm in size). False positives can be seen in pneumonia or granulomatous disease where the 18F-FDG uptake is related to the inflammation. Additional examples of each are listed in the following section.

Medication Implications

- 18F-FDG is similar to glucose; therefore, the balance between blood glucose concentrations and insulin concentrations can have an effect on the quality of the PET images, and patients should be normoglycemic when undergoing PET imaging. Increased glucose concentrations will lead to decreased uptake of 18F-FDG in the brain and tumors due to competition with glucose at binding sites but increased uptake in insulin-sensitive tissues such as skeletal muscle.
    - Medications that work directly on altering blood glucose concentrations in patients with diabetes should be held 6 hours before the PET scan.[1,7]
        - Metformin should be held 48 hours before the PET scan[8–12]
        - Peroxisome proliferator-activated receptor–gamma agonists (e.g., pioglitazone, rosiglitazone) have shown not to interfere with 18F-FDG uptake and do not need to be held before the PET scan
        - Short-acting insulins should be held 4–6 hours before the PET scan. One option is to have patients eat breakfast and use their short-acting insulin and undergo the PET scan 6 hours later in the afternoon
    - Patients using insulin pumps or continuous insulin should be scheduled early in the morning before breakfast, after an overnight fast. If a basal insulin is normally given in the morning, this may need to be adjusted to the evening before the PET scan.[7]
        - Patients using insulin pumps for a continuous infusion of insulin may continue the insulin at the basal rate before, during, and after the PET scan[7]
    - Patients with diabetes should have their blood glucose measured prior to the PET scan. If their blood glucose is ≥200 mg/dL, the PET scan may need to be rescheduled.[1,13]
- All prescription medications should be taken as directed unless instructed otherwise. Some medications that could potentially alter glucose concentrations include glucocorticoids, phenothiazines, lithium, tricyclic antidepressants, phenytoin, thiazide diuretics, isoniazid, rifampin, and ephedrine.[7,14,15]
    - Glucocorticoid use may result in hyperglycemia, which in turn can affect the accuracy of PET results. Temporary management of steroid-induced hyperglycemia with basal/bolus insulin may be necessary in cancer patients undergoing PET imaging.[7,16,17] Standardized uptake value (SUV) is reliable in patients undergoing corticosteroid treatment as long as the glucose concentration prior to the test is optimal. One retrospective study demonstrated that prednisone may statistically significantly increase glucose concentrations depending on the body part.[18]
- Benzodiazepines can be used for patients with claustrophobia, anxiety, or a need to relax skeletal muscles.[7]
- Brown adipose tissue (BAT) has prominent 18F-FDG uptake and can potentially mimic or mask malignant lesions. Beta blockers and benzodiazepines can be used to reduce BAT interference, although recommendations are conflicting.[7,19–22]
    - Beta blockers: Propranolol regimens of 80 mg orally 2 hours before, 20 mg orally 1 hour before, or 40 mg orally 1 hour before the PET have been shown to be effective in reducing BAT interference.[23–25]
    - Benzodiazepines: Any agent can be given 30–60 minutes prior to PET scan. Alprazolam 0.5 mg orally has been suggested by one group.[7,21]

- Sometimes PET can lead to false-positive findings. Some common causes of this include[20]:
  - Physiologic uptake in the salivary glands and lymphoid tissues in the head and neck, thyroid, BAT, thymus (more so in pediatric patients), lactating breast, areola, skeletal and smooth muscles (e.g., neck or paravertebral; hyperinsulinemia), gastrointestinal (e.g., esophagus, stomach, or bowel), urinary tract structures (containing excreted 18F-FDG), female genital tract (e.g., uterus during menses or corpus luteum cyst)
  - Inflammatory processes, such as postsurgical inflammation, infection, hematoma, biopsy site, amputation site, radiation pneumonitis, post chemotherapy, local inflammatory disease (especially granulomatous processes like sarcoidosis, fungal disease, or mycobacterial disease), ostomy site and drainage tubes, injection site, thyroiditis, esophagitis, gastritis, inflammatory bowel disease, acute and occasionally chronic pancreatitis, acute cholangitis and cholecystitis, osteomyelitis, recent fracture sites, joint prostheses, lymphadenitis
  - Benign neoplasms, such as pituitary adenoma, adrenal adenoma, thyroid follicular adenoma, salivary gland tumors (e.g., Warthin's tumor or pleomorphic adenoma), colonic adenomatous polyps and villous adenoma, ovarian thecoma and cystadenoma, giant cell tumor, aneurysmal bone cyst, leiomyoma
  - Hyperplasia or dysplasia, such as Graves' disease, Cushing's disease, bone marrow hyperplasia (e.g., anemia or cytokine therapy), thymic rebound hyperplasia, fibrous dysplasia, Paget's disease
  - Ischemia, such as hibernating myocardium
  - Misalignment between PET and CT data
- Sometimes PET scans can lead to false-negative findings. Some common causes of this include[20]:
  - Small size (<2 times the resolution of the system), tumor necrosis, recent chemotherapy or radiotherapy, recent high-dose steroid therapy, hyperglycemia and hyperinsulinemia, some low-grade tumors (e.g., sarcoma, lymphoma, or brain tumor), tumors with large mucinous components, some well-differentiated tumors, some bronchioloalveolar carcinomas, some lobular carcinomas of the breast, some skeletal metastases, especially osteoblastic or sclerotic tumors, some osteosarcomas
- Side effects of 18F-FDG include hypotension, hypoglycemia, hyperglycemia, and increase in alkaline phosphatase.[26,27]
  - The 18F-FDG exposure or dose in pregnant women is low and PET has been shown to be safe in pregnant women. Potential risks to the fetus should be considered and PET should not be administered to a pregnant woman unless the potential benefit justifies the risk.[26–28]
- Findings of a PET should be followed closely and discussed with the specialist who orders the test (i.e., oncologist). Treatment options may be altered based on test results. For many types of cancers, it may help decide if the intent of treatment is curative or palliative. It may also help ascertain modalities of treatment that might be necessary for a particular cancer. In addition, PET/CT scans may help target specific sites for biopsy.

References

1. Fitzgerald PA. Thyroid Cancer. In: Papadakis MA, McPhee SJ, Rabow MW, eds. *Current Medical Diagnosis and Treatment*. New York, NY: McGraw-Hill; 2020. http://accessmedicine.mhmedical.com/content.aspx?bookid=2683&sectionid=22513422. Accessed March 16, 2020.
2. Hutton BF, Segerman D, Miles KA, et al. Radionuclide and hybrid imaging. In: Adam A, Dixon AK, Gillard JH et al, eds. *Grainger & Allison's Diagnostic Radiology*. 6th ed. New York, NY: Elsevier Churchill Livingstone; 2015 Chap 6.
3. Meyer PT, Rijintjes M, Hellwig S, et al. Functional neuroimaging: functional magnetic resonance imaging, positron emission tomography, and single-photon emission computed tomography. In: Daroff RB,

Jankovic J, Mazziotta JC et al., eds. *Bradley's Neurology in Clinical Practice*. 7th ed. Philadelphia, PA: Elsevier; 2016 Chap 41.

4. Khuri FR. Lung cancer and other pulmonary neoplasms. In: Goldman L, Schafer AI, eds. *Goldman-Cecil Medicine*. 25th ed. Philadelphia, PA: Elsevier Saunders; 2016 Chap 191.

5. Rich DA. A brief history of positron emission tomography. *J Nucl Med Technol*. 1997;25(1):4–11.

6. Portnow LH, Vaillancourt DE, Okun MS. The history of cerebral PET scanning: from physiology to cutting-edge technology. *Neurology*. 2013;80(10):952–956. doi:10.1212/WNL.0b013e318285c135.

7. Surasi DS, Bhambhvani P, Baldwin JA, et al. ^{18}F-FDG PET and PET/CT patient preparation: a review of the literature. *J Nucl Med Technol*. 2014;42(1):5–13.

8. Hamidizadeh R, Eftekhari A, Wiley EA, et al. Metformin discontinuation prior to FDG PET/CT: a randomized controlled study to compare 24- and 48-hour bowel activity. *Radiology*. 2018;289:418–425.

9. Oh JR, Song HC, Chong A, et al. Impact of medication discontinuation on increased intestinal FDG accumulation in diabetic patients treated with metformin. *AJR Am J Roentgenol*. 2010;195(6):1404–1410.

10. Ozülker T, Ozülker F, Mert M, et al. Clearance of the high intestinal (18) F-FDG uptake associated with metformin after stopping the drug. *Eur J Nucl Med Mol Imaging*. 2010;37(5):1011–1017.

11. Lee SH, Jin S, Lee HS, et al. Metformin discontinuation less than 72 h is suboptimal for F-18 FDG PET/CT interpretation of the bowel. *Ann Nucl Med*. 2016;30(9):629–636.

12. Morris M, Saboury B, Chen W, et al. Finding the sweet spot for metformin in 18F-FDG-PET. *Nucl Med Commun*. 2017;38(10):875–880.

13. Boellaard R, O'Doherty MJ, Weber WA, et al. FDG PET and PET/CT: EANM procedure guidelines for tumour PET imaging: version 1.0. *Eur J Nucl Med Mol Imaging*. 2010;37(1):181–200.

14. Shreve P, Townsend DW, eds. *Clinical PET/CT in Radiology: Integrated Imaging in Oncology*. New York, NY: Springer; 2011.

15. Cohade C. Altered biodistribution on FDG-PET with emphasis on brown fat and insulin effect. *Semin Nucl Med*. 2010;40(4):283–293.

16. Gosmanov AR, Goorha S, Stelts S, et al. Management of hyperglycemia in diabetic patients with hematologic malignancies during dexamethasone therapy. *Endocr Pract*. 2013;19(2):231–235.

17. Baldwin D, Apel J. Management of hyperglycemia in hospitalized patients with renal insufficiency or steroid-induced diabetes. *Curr Diab Rep*. 2013;13(1):114–120.

18. Raplinger K, Chandler K, Hunt C, et al. Effect of steroid use during chemotherapy on SUV levels in PET/CT. *J Nucl Med*. 2012;53(no. supplement 1):2718.

19. Jacene HA, Cohade CC, Zhang Z, et al. The relationship between patients' serum glucose levels and metabolically active brown adipose tissue detected by PET/CT. *Mol Imaging Biol*. 2011;13(6):1278–1283.

20. Delbeke D, Coleman RE, Guiberteau MJ, et al. Procedure guideline for tumor imaging with 18F-FDG PET/CT 1.0. *J Nucl Med*. 2006;47(5):885–895.

21. Shankar LK, Hoffman JM, Bacharach S, et al. Consensus recommendations for the use of 18F-FDG PET as an indicator of therapeutic response in patients in National Cancer Institute Trials. *J Nucl Med*. 2006;47(6):1059–1066.

22. ACR–SPR Practice Guideline for performing FDG-PET/CT in Oncology. American College of Radiology Web site. https://www.acr.org/-/media/ACR/Files/Practice-Parameters/FDG-PET-CT.pdf. Published 2007. Amended 2009. Revised 2016. Accessed April 16, 2020.

23. Söderlund V, Larsson SA, Jacobsson H. Reduction of FDG uptake in brown adipose tissue in clinical patients by a single dose of propranolol. *Eur J Nucl Med Mol Imaging*. 2007;34(7):1018–1022.

24. Parysow O, Mollerach AM, Jager V, et al. Low-dose oral propranolol could reduce brown adipose tissue F-18 FDG uptake in patients undergoing PET scans. *Clin Nucl Med*. 2007;32(5):351–357.

25. Agrawal A, Nair N, Baghel NS. A novel approach for reduction of brown fat uptake on FDG PET. *Br J Radiol*. 2009;82(980):626–631.

26. FLUDEOXYGLUCOSE F-18- fludeoxyglucos e f-18 injection package insert. Grand Forks, ND: University of North Dakota; 2015 February.

27. FLUDEOXYGLUCOSE F-18- fludeoxyglucos e f-18 injection package insert. Bismarck, ND: Northland Nuclear Medicine; 2018 October.

28. Takalkar AM, Khandelwal A, Lokitz S, et al. 18F-FDG PET in Pregnancy and Fetal Radiation Dose Estimates. *J Nucl Med*. 2011;52:1035–1040.

CHAPTER 50

Renal Ultrasound

Devora Lichtman, MD, RDMS, RDCS, RVT

Background

Renal ultrasound is a noninvasive diagnostic test that uses high-frequency sound waves to create real-time images of the kidneys. The images are two-dimensional pictures of the kidneys that evaluate their size, shape, architecture, and location. It can also be used to evaluate the blood flow to and from the kidneys. The underlying complex architecture of the kidneys is represented by the variety of echotextures seen within the kidney parenchyma. The array of echotextures are a direct representation of the density of the tissues present within the kidneys. For example, the renal pyramids are darker than the renal cortex. A change in the renal architecture may represent a congenital deformity or a disease process.[1] Fig. 50.1 is an example of a renal ultrasound of a depth in the body and distance from the ultrasound probe. The more superficial structures are displayed toward the top of the screen, whereas the deeper structures are displayed near the bottom of the screen.

How to Use It

Renal ultrasound is a useful tool in evaluating the kidneys. The visual representation of the anatomy is also a representation of the physiology. The renal architecture has multiple tissue subtypes that are represented by degradations of grayscale on the ultrasound image. The information gleaned from the images is used to diagnose renal pathology, including renal cysts, hydronephrosis, diffuse renal cortical disease, pyelonephritis, neoplasms, nephrolithiasis, arterial stenosis, or venous thrombosis.[2] As renal ultrasound can identify this wide array of abnormalities, it is commonly performed when working up acute kidney injury, evaluating a patient for unexplained hypertension, and evaluating patients with chronic kidney disease. Renal cysts are displayed as anechoic or black circular lesions with a thin wall. Solid neoplasms are made up of varying echodensities and may or may not have blood flow within them when they are interrogated with color Doppler. Nephrolithiasis is seen as a bright white echogenic focus with shadowing behind it.[1]

How It Is Done

The patient is positioned in the supine position to start the exam and then repositioned to the right and left lateral decubitus positions as needed to better visualize the kidneys. A sonographer or other allied health care professional uses an ultrasound probe of 2–5 MHz to image the kidneys. There is no required preparation for renal ultrasound, and the patient does not need to fast. No medications are given during the procedure, and neither sedation nor analgesia is used. The test takes approximately 20 minutes to complete. A small amount of ultrasound gel is applied to the ultrasound probe, and the probe is placed on the abdomen. The images are obtained in the sagittal/long axis and in the transverse/short axis. Pulsed high-frequency sound waves are emitted from an ultrasound probe, and the echoes from those pulsed sound waves are sent back to the probe. The kidneys and the renal arteries are interrogated with color Doppler and pulsed wave Doppler, which evaluates the kidneys for renal stenosis and renal vein thrombosis. A normal renal

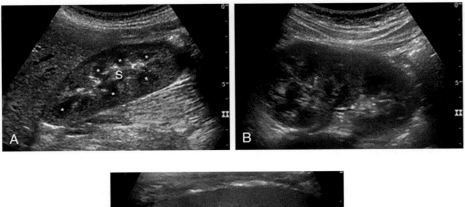

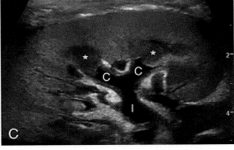

Fig. 50.1 (A–C) This is an ultrasound image of a normal kidney in the sagittal/longitudinal view. (A) The renal sinus (S) is echogenic (bright) and the renal pyramids (*) are hypoechoic (dark). (C) The renal calices (C) are clearly seen draining into the infundibulum (I) which is all part of the normal renal urinary drainage.[1]

ultrasound typically states the size of the kidneys, which are approximately 10–13 cm in length, 3–5 cm in width, and 3 cm in anterior-posterior thickness and that there is no hydronephrosis present. The renal ultrasound is used in both outpatient and inpatient settings including the emergency, radiology, and intensive care units.[1]

Medication Implications

■ Renal ultrasound is noninvasive, and no medications are given prior to or during the exam.
■ If renal ultrasound reveals hydronephrosis, it usually indicates that there is a downstream obstruction that needs to be alleviated. Many times this means that the patient will need a urinary catheter or nephrostomy tube placed to alleviate the obstruction. See Chapter 59: Urinary Catheters and Chapter 43: Nephrostomy Tubes for more details.
■ If the renal ultrasound reveals increased echogenicity in the cortex, there is concern for chronic kidney disease, which can be correlated with increased serum blood urea nitrogen (BUN) and creatinine. When a patient is diagnosed with chronic kidney disease, it is extremely important to preserve the remaining renal function. In an effort to preserve renal function, it is important to avoid nephrotoxic medications. See the following list of nephrotoxic agents, though note that this is not an all-inclusive list[3]:
  ■ Vasoconstriction/hemodynamic alterations: due to decreased blood flow to the glomerulus—nonsteroidal anti-inflammatory drugs (NSAIDs), angiotensin-converting enzyme (ACE) inhibitors, angiotensin II receptor blockers (ARBs), calcineurin inhibitors

- Note ACE inhibitors and ARBs are nephroprotective with chronic use in certain populations[4]
- Direct tubular toxicity: aminoglycosides, amphotericin, cisplatin, ifosfamide, calcineurin inhibitors, methotrexate, cocaine
- Interstitial nephritis: hypersensitivity reaction—NSAIDs, sulfonamides, ciprofloxacin, diuretics, anticonvulsants
- Crystal formation: medications that are poorly soluble in urine can form crystals and the crystals accumulate in the urinary space and can cause acute tubular necrosis—methotrexate, acyclovir, sulfonamides
- Thrombotic microangiopathy: caused by the creation of platelet-rich thrombi in the microvasculature, can be caused by the following medications—cyclosporine, quinine, tacrolimus, interferon, clopidogrel, cocaine
- Glomerular injury/podocytopathy: lithium, sirolimus, NSAIDs
- If renal ultrasound reveals nephrolithiasis, then an alpha blocker such as tamsulosin 0.4 mg orally once daily for up to 4 weeks can help with stone passage.[5] This is known as medical expulsive therapy (MET) in the literature.
  - A 2018 Cochrane systematic review and meta-analysis found that alpha blockers significantly improved ureteral stone clearance, reduced stone expulsion time, reduced pain episodes, and reduced hospitalizations. Important subgroup analyses found that stone size was an important factor. Stones 5 mm or smaller did not benefit from alpha blockers in terms of stone clearance or expulsion time, but stones larger than 5 mm did benefit from alpha blockers for the same outcomes.[6]
- Specific medications can also be used to prevent recurrence of nephrolithiasis, the choice of which is based on the composition of the stone.
  - If the stone is composed of calcium oxalate, thiazide diuretics can be used to decrease urinary calcium.[7]
  - If the stone is composed of uric acid, then treatment can include potassium citrate (to alkalinize the urine) and the xanthine oxidase inhibitor allopurinol (to decrease uric acid formation).[8,9]

References

1. Hertzberg BS, Middleton WD. Chapter 5: Kidney. In: *Ultrasound: The Requisites,* 3e. Elsevier; 2016.
2. O'Neill WC, Bardelli M, Yevzlin AS. Imaging for renovascular disease. *Semin Nephrol.* 2011;31(3):272–282.
3. Perazella MA. Pharmacology behind common drug nephrotoxicities. *Clin J Am Soc Nephrol.* 2018; 13(12):1897–1908.
4. Kidney Disease: Improving Global Outcomes (KDIGO) Blood Pressure Work Group. KDIGO Clinical Practice Guideline for the Management of Blood Pressure in Chronic Kidney Disease. *Kidney Int Suppl.* 2012;2:337–414.
5. Hollingsworth JM, Rogers MA, Kaufman SR, et al. Medical therapy to facilitate urinary stone passage: a meta-analysis. *Lancet.* 2006;368(9542):1171–1179.
6. Campschroer T, Zhu X, Vernooij RWM, et al. Alpha-blockers as medical expulsive therapy for ureteral stones. *Cochrane Database Syst Rev.* 2018;4.
7. Fink HA, Wilt TJ, Eidman KE, et al. Medical management to prevent recurrent nephrolithiasis in adults: a systematic review for an American College of Physicians Clinical Guideline. *Ann Intern Med.* 2013;158(7):535–543.
8. Trinchieri A, Esposito N, Castelnuovo C. Dissolution of radiolucent renal stones by oral alkalinization with potassium citrate/potassium bicarbonate. *Arch Ital Urol Androl.* 2009;81(3):188–191.
9. Kenny JE, Goldfarb DS. Update on the pathophysiology and management of uric acid renal stones. *Curr Rheumatol Rep.* 2010;12(2):125–129.

CHAPTER 51

Sleep Study

Annamaria Iakovou, MD

Backgound

There are multiple diagnostic tests to evaluate sleep disorders. Common tests include polysomnograph (PSG), home sleep apnea test (HSAT), multiple sleep latency test (MSLT), oximetry, and actigraphy.[1] PSG, also known as an "in-lab sleep study or sleep test," is derived from the Greek roots "poly," meaning many, "somno," meaning sleep, and "graphy," meaning to write, and refers to testing performed on patients while they sleep. HSAT, often referred to as "home sleep test" (HST), is an unattended study that is not performed in a sleep center and typically done at home. PSG with MSLT consists of a PSG followed by a daytime nap study performed in a sleep testing center. Overnight oximetry is a measure of continuous pulse oximetry that is worn when asleep. Oximetry is derived from the Greek roots, "oxys," from "sharp, acid" and is a shortened form of the word oxygen, and "metry," to measure. Actigraphy is a measure of movement and is derived from Latin "activus," "a doing," and "graphy," from the Greek for writing or recording.

Therapeutic testing modalities are also performed for the treatment of sleep disorders known as "titration studies." They evaluate different therapies for effectiveness. Continuous positive airway pressure (CPAP), bilevel positive airway pressure (PAP), adaptive servoventilation (ASV), and volume-assured pressure support (AVAPS/iVAPS) are examples of such modalities.

Diagnostic and therapeutic PSG, known as a "split study," is an attended test during which the first portion is a diagnostic PSG. If the findings fulfill criteria for sleep-disordered breathing, the remainder of the test is a titration study. Home testing including automatic PAP titration is an option for evaluating PAP therapy.

How to Use It

Sleep testing is used when there is a complaint about sleep quality or abnormal behaviors. Oftentimes there is an effect on daytime function, including excessive daytime sleepiness, cognitive disturbance, and headaches. It can be part of evaluation of comorbid conditions such as cardiac arrhythmias, uncontrolled hypertension, and seizures.

PSG is used to diagnose many disorders, including sleep-disordered breathing, abnormal behaviors either during non-rapid eye movement (NREM) sleep (known as parasomnias) or during rapid eye movement (REM) sleep (known as REM behavior disorders), periodic limb movements (PLMs), and nocturnal seizures. Sleep-disordered breathing includes obstructive sleep apnea (OSA), nocturnal hypoxemia or hypoventilation, central sleep apnea (CSA), and Hunter-Cheyne-Stokes respiration (HCSR).

HSTs may also be used to diagnose sleep-disordered breathing, including OSA, CSA/HCSR, and nocturnal hypoxemia; however, they are limited to patients that do not have significant cardiopulmonary or neuromuscular disease in which additional monitoring is required.

PSG with MSLT consists of an overnight PSG followed by a daytime nap study to evaluate for the presence of central disorders of hypersomnia, including type 1 and 2 narcolepsy and idiopathic hypersomnia.

Oximetry is a measure of continuous pulse oximetry that is worn when asleep. This is done to determine the presence of nocturnal hypoxemia related to pulmonary disease. Actigraphy is a measure of movement and position. It is worn continuously over 7–14 days and evaluates sleep-wake patterns for the diagnosis of insufficient sleep syndrome and circadian rhythm disorders.

How It Is Done

PSG is an attended study that is performed by sleep technicians in a sleep laboratory. Monitoring includes electroencephalography (EEG), electromyelography (EMG), electrocardiography (EKG), inspiratory flow, thermistor, pulse oximetry, body plethysmography, and carbon dioxide (CO_2) monitoring.[2] See Chapter 27: Electroencephalography, Chapter 26: Electrocardiography, and Chapter 44: Oxygen Supplementation for more details about these tests. PSG findings include EEG architecture (time to sleep onset, time to REM onset, percentages of NREM and REM sleep, wake time after sleep onset [WASO]), respiratory parameters (obstructive apneas, hypopneas, central apneas, and inspiratory flow limitation), and increased muscle tone and movements. There is also video monitoring for abnormal behaviors. PSG is typically a one-night study. Patients do not need to fast or alter their medications other than to avoid stimulants in the afternoon such as caffeine and prescribed stimulants. Other medications that may interfere with sleep architecture and quality should also be addressed prior to the study, and their effects are discussed below. A normal study would show evidence of normal sleep architecture and quality and a normal apnea-hypopnea index (AHI) of <5 per hour and normal pulse oximetry of >90%.[3]

HST is an unattended study performed at home. Monitoring consists of pulse oximetry, inspiratory flow, and body plethysmography. A normal HST will show evidence of AHI <5 per hour and normal pulse oximetry.

PSG with MSLT consists of an overnight PSG followed by a daytime nap study. This is performed in the sleep laboratory by sleep technicians. MSLT includes four to five nap opportunities examining average sleep-onset latency (SOL) as well as the presence or absence of REM during the naps. An abnormal or positive finding on MSLT includes a mean SOL of ≤ 8 minutes as well as two or greater REM periods during the naps.

Actigraphy is a measure of movement and position over a 24-hour period and involves a sensor that is worn on the wrist continuously over a 7- to 14-day course. The data provides typical sleep-wake patterns for the patient according to the time of day.

Oximetry consists of a finger probe with a wrist monitor that is worn when sleeping at home. A normal oximetry shows oxygen saturation levels >90% when asleep.

Medication Implications

Medications can affect multiple aspects of the PSG and influence diagnosis.[1] EEG can be affected with resultant changes in sleep architecture and sleep quality as well as respiratory monitoring for thoraco-abdominal effort, pulse oximetry, and CO_2.

- Benzodiazepines: diazepam, clonazepam, lorazepam
  - Treat anxiety and insomnia
  - Reduce SOL
  - Decrease the amount of N1 sleep, and increase spindle activity in N2 sleep and the amount of N2 sleep. Can decrease REM sleep when used at high doses
- Nonbenzodiazepine receptor agonists: zolpidem, zaleplon, and eszopiclone (sometimes referred to as the "Z-drugs")
  - Treat insomnia, sleep onset, and maintenance
  - Reduce SOL
- Antidepressants:
  - Tricyclic agents (TCAs): amitriptyline, doxepin

- Monoamine oxidase inhibitors (MAOIs): selegiline
- Selective serotonin reuptake inhibitors (SSRIs): sertraline, fluoxetine, escitalopram
- Prolong REM onset, suppress REM sleep
- Stimulants: modafinil, amphetamines, methylphenidate, solriamfetol, pitolisant
  - Prolong SOL
- Opioids: methadone, oxycodone
  - Chronic opioid use: increase WASO, decrease total sleep time. Sleep quality not affected in naive users
  - Decrease N3 sleep, higher doses decrease REM
  - Cause CSA with pauses to breathing, hypoxemia, and arousals
- Atypical antipsychotics: quetiapine, olanzapine, and clozapine
  - Psychiatric indications, often used as hypnotics
  - Reduce SOL and WASO, increased total sleep time
  - Suppress REM
- Beta blockers: metoprolol, propranolol
  - Lipophilic and cross the blood-brain barrier
    - Causes sleep disturbances and insomnia, increase WASO and number of awakenings
    - Suppress REM
    - Can cause nightmares and hallucinations
  - Other beta blockers such as atenolol and labetalol are hydrophilic and do not cross the blood-brain barrier as easily, and therefore do not have the same effects on sleep
- Centrally acting alpha adrenergic agonist: clonidine
  - Inconsistent data on sleep quality
  - Suppresses REM

MEDICATION CONSIDERATIONS PRIOR TO SLEEP TESTING

- REM suppressants
  - These agents limit the diagnostic accuracy of PSG in patients being evaluated for sleep-disordered breathing, REM behavior disorder, and central disorders of hypersomnia.
  - Rapid withdrawal of SSRI/serotonin norepinephrine reuptake inhibitors (SNRIs) can lead to REM rebound and can increase the percentage of REM sleep.
  - Patients should have these agents weaned and discontinued prior to sleep testing, as they can affect the presence of REM and REM latency (time to first REM episode).
- How to wean and discontinue any specific medication depends on several factors such as the medication half-life, the potential for rebound or withdrawal effects, and the acute need of the medication.
- Stimulants
  - Patients should wean off of these agents if able or hold dosing the day of the study, including abstaining from caffeine at least 8 hours prior to the study.
- Sedative hypnotics
  - Patients should have these agents weaned and discontinued prior to sleep testing, as they can affect SOL from either their direct effects of promoting sleep or due to withdrawal with rebound insomnia.

THERAPY FOR SLEEP DISORDERS

- OSA
  - CPAP or automatic PAP therapy, oral mandibular advancement device, weight loss, hypoglossal nerve stimulator (e.g., brand name Inspire)

- Difficulty maintaining sleep secondary to PAP therapy
  - Eszopiclone
- Residual daytime sleepiness despite adherence with PAP therapy
  - Modafinil, armodafinil
- CSA
  - Treat the underlying causes, as CSA is typically related to congestive heart failure, stroke, opioid use, end-stage renal disease
  - CPAP therapy; however, patients are often poor responders and require bilevel S/T ("spontaneous/timed"—a certain type of PAP) or ASV
  - Phrenic nerve stimulator (e.g., brand name Remede) for those intolerant or not benefiting from noninvasive therapy
- Insomnia
  - Sleep hygiene and behaviors related to sleep
  - Nonbenzodiazepine receptor agonists ("Z-drugs" mentioned above), benzodiazepines, suvorexant
- Narcolepsy
  - Sleep hygiene, scheduled naps
  - Sodium oxybate (brand name Xyrem) for consolidating sleep, venlafaxine to suppress cataplexy
  - Stimulants: modafinil/armodafinil, amphetamines, pitolisant
- Hypoventilation syndromes
  - Treat underlying causes, including congenital, obesity, neuromuscular, pulmonary disease
  - Trial of CPAP, may require bilevel PAP
  - Respiratory stimulants such as theophylline have not been shown to be effective
- Restless legs syndrome (RLS)
  - Diagnosis: clinical history, does not require PSG for diagnosis
  - Evaluation: ferritin deficiency, identification of medications that can trigger (i.e., SSRIs), and identification of underlying diseases that can predispose, such as advanced kidney dysfunction
  - Treatment
    - Treat underlying causes
    - Medications
      - Dopamine agonists: pramipexole, ropinirole
      - GABA analogs: gabapentin and gabapentin enacarbil
      - Opioids
- PLMs
  - Diagnosis: clinical history, PSG
  - Treatment similar to RLS
- Circadian rhythm disorders (including advanced sleep-wake disorder, delayed sleep-wake disorder, jet lag sleep-wake disorder, shift work sleep-wake disorder, non-24-hour sleep-wake disorder)
  - Evaluation: actigraphy, sleep logs
  - Treatment: behavioral techniques, melatonin, and ramelteon

References

1. Kryger M, Roth T, Dement WC. *Principles and Practice of Sleep Medicine*. 7th ed.: Saunders; 2015.
2. Berry RB, Brooks R, Gamaldo CE, et al. *The AASM Manual for Scoring of Sleep and Associated Events: Rules, Terminology, and Technical Specifications*. Version 2.2. *American Academy of Sleep Medicine*; 2015.
3. Sateia MJ. *International Classification of Sleep Disorders*. 3rd ed.: American Academy of Sleep Medicine; 2014.

CHAPTER 52

Speech-Language and Swallow Evaluations

Kara E. Bain, MA, CCC-SLP

Background

As a whole, speech-language pathology assessments are conducted for the examination of speech, language, cognitive abilities, and swallowing safety and function. Within the medical setting, there are a number of types of evaluations performed by speech-language pathologists (SLPs) that provide valuable information to guide medical management of patients. These assessments include clinical swallowing evaluations and instrumental swallowing exams such as modified barium swallow (MBS) study and the fiberoptic endoscopic evaluation of swallowing (FEES). Other assessments are of communication, including assessment of speech, language, voice, cognition, and the need for supportive devices to facilitate communication.[1-3]

Medications may affect many aspects of the skills involved in speech, language, cognition, and swallowing, including alertness, awareness, motor functioning, lubrication of the oropharyngeal mucosa, and esophageal health and functioning. Many medications may affect a patient's ability to swallow safely. This can occur potentially both in the short term during performance of an exam and with chronic medications used over time by affecting overall presentation of the oropharyngeal swallow mechanism. Many of these medications may also affect a patient's performance on assessments of speech, language, and cognitive functioning if they affect parameters such as alertness, awareness, cognitive levels, and muscular integrity for articulatory precision and speech production.[1,3,4]

How to Use It

In the medical setting, particular emphasis is placed upon evaluation of swallowing function and safety to identify and reduce the risk of aspiration. Reducing the risk of aspiration limits morbidity due to aspiration pneumonia and resultant respiratory compromise. The purpose of the swallowing assessment is to examine whether oral feeding is safe and appropriate at the time of exam, and, if so, to determine the least restrictive dietary consistencies and appropriate swallow strategies to maximize safety for oral intake. Swallowing assessments also provide guidance for rehabilitation of swallow function in dysphagia therapy if clinically indicated based upon etiology, prognosis, and ability to participate.[1-3]

Assessment of speech, language, and cognition serves to identify impairments in varied aspects of communication, and to identify need for assistive communication devices. Working closely with physicians, SLPs play an important role in assisting with differential medical diagnoses for neurologic and communication disorders based upon types of motor speech impairments or language impairments. These collaborations also assist in providing access to communication for those with respiratory compromise requiring a tracheostomy tube, or for patients with head and neck cancer requiring laryngectomy. These evaluations ascertain needs for rehabilitative services, needs for assistive communication devices, and the findings provide goals for therapeutic interventions to facilitate improvement in effectiveness of communication.[1,4]

How It Is Done

SWALLOWING ASSESSMENTS

CLINICAL SWALLOW EVALUATION

A clinical swallow evaluation is an assessment by the SLP to determine candidacy for oral feeding, most appropriate oral diet textures, and/or need for instrumental assessment of swallowing. It begins with collection of medical history, notably any history of dysphagia, to determine potential aspiration risks based upon known diagnoses. It then proceeds with a clinical assessment of alertness, orientation, and respiratory status to determine candidacy for participation in food and drink trials. It includes an oral mechanism exam to assess cranial nerve functioning, strength, range of motion, and coordination of the oral structures. If appropriate to proceed, it involves food and drink trials of different textures (various liquid consistencies, purees, and chewable solid foods). Recommendations for oral or non-oral feeding are made based upon clinical observations, including respiratory status, level of alertness and overall cognitive status, orientation to feeding task, patient complaints, observation of coordination of oral mechanism for feeding, and signs and symptoms of aspiration during oral trials. It may be determined that an instrumental exam (MBS or FEES) is indicated to obtain more objective information.[1,3]

MODIFIED BARIUM SWALLOW/VIDEOFLUOROSCOPIC SWALLOW STUDY

An MBS/videofluoroscopic swallow study (VFSS) is an instrumental exam conducted in a radiology suite, under fluoroscopy (or video X-ray), by an SLP with collaboration of a radiologist. The patient is positioned in lateral, and potentially anteroposterior views, so that oral and pharyngeal structures and the upper esophagus can be seen during oral trials of foods and drinks containing barium. The patient is administered trials of various consistencies of liquids, puree, and chewable solids to assess strength, coordination, and safety for oral intake of the provided consistencies. It is within the scope of practice of SLPs to perform esophageal sweeps during MBS/VFSS exams, given that esophageal motility and/or retrograde flow can have pressure effects on the pharyngeal swallow and can lead to aspiration risk. While SLPs are not the clinicians directly treating esophageal findings, they frequently receive referrals for generalized complaints of dysphagia, some of which require referrals for gastroenterology workup.[1,3,5]

FIBEROPTIC ENDOSCOPIC EVALUATION OF SWALLOWING

FEES is an instrumental exam by the SLP using a transnasal flexible scope to examine the anatomy and physiology of the pharynx and larynx before and after swallowing from approximately the level of the velum, at the level of the uvula, or just below. The patient is administered trials of various consistencies of liquids, puree, and chewable solids, typically colored with blue or green food dye for contrast. Structures are observed prior to and during food trials, and observations are made regarding flow of food and drink, including details that might be representative of pharyngeal dysphagia and laryngeal penetration and/or aspiration. These observations include timeliness of swallow initiation, degree of pharyngeal retention, and entry/residual of any material in the laryngeal vestibule and/or below the vocal folds within the trachea. Observations allow for inference of strength and coordination, and may allow visualization of retrograde flow of material into the pharynx from the esophagus, which could indicate potential esophageal dysfunction.[1,3,6]

SPEECH-LANGUAGE EVALUATION

A speech-language evaluation is performed by an SLP to assess functional communication, oral motor functions, speech production skills, comprehension and production of spoken and written language, and cognitive aspects of communication. These assessments identify language disorders, including the various types of aphasias (e.g., Broca's [expressive], Wernicke's). They may identify disorders of speech production, including voice disorders, motor speech disorders (e.g., acquired apraxia of speech), and the various types of dysarthria. Cognitive-linguistic impairments may also be identified, including behavioral changes, memory and attention deficits, executive function deficits, and impairments of problem solving and reasoning. These deficits may be due to acute-onset conditions such as stroke or traumatic brain injury, or else due to progressive medical conditions, commonly neurologic in nature. These evaluations may also determine the need and appropriateness for supportive communication devices, including speaking valves for patients requiring tracheostomy tubes for respiratory support, assistive speech devices for patients post laryngectomy, such as electrolarynx or tracheo-esophageal prosthesis, and alternative/augmentative communication devices for those unable to communicate via speech, such as low-tech picture communication boards or high-tech computerized speech-generating devices.[1,4]

Medication Implications

PREMEDICATION CONSIDERATIONS THAT MAY PROVIDE BENEFIT PRIOR TO THE EXAMS DESCRIBED PREVIOUSLY

Patients may benefit from premedication prior to the performance of the above evaluations, in order to enhance participation or performance, if it is determined that the benefits outweigh possible detrimental effects on swallow function during the exam.

- **Pain management:** Nonsteroidal anti-inflammatory drugs (NSAIDs), acetaminophen, or opioids in dosages that do not significantly affect alertness may be considered if they will improve patient comfort to maximize the ability to participate in the assessment in the optimal upright posture.
- **Antiemetics:** These agents may be considered if they will improve tolerance of oral intake to allow patients to participate in swallowing exams, as well as to enhance tolerance to meet nutrition/hydration needs.
- **Anxiolytic medications:** For patients who are significantly anxious or confused, careful use of anxiolytics may improve the ability to cooperate with testing instructions that require full participation and direction-following. However, too high a dose may have detrimental effects on test performance if it contributes to impaired alertness or slowed motor function.
- **Parkinson's disease medications** (e.g., carbidopa/levodopa): In patients with Parkinson's disease, there is mixed evidence regarding Parkinson's disease medication benefit to oropharyngeal dysphagia, with literature reviews suggesting a general lack of clear evidence to support it.[7-9] However, some studies have suggested that administration of these medications prior to oral intake may benefit oral management and timing of oral anterior-posterior transport of bolus, timing of pharyngeal swallow trigger, and timing of pharyngeal transit. Additionally, Parkinson's disease medications may improve rigidity and posture for enhanced participation in all exams, and particularly in assessment of speech-language and cognition.[7,8,10]

POTENTIALLY BENEFICIAL MEDICATIONS FOR DYSPHAGIA, WHICH MAY AFFECT OVERALL PRESENTATION

- **Beta blockers** (e.g., atenolol, metoprolol): These medications have been shown to potentially have protective effects against dysphagia related to preservation of the pharyngeal musculature and production of less thick secretions.[7]
- **Calcium channel blockers** (e.g., nimodipine): These agents have been shown to be useful in treatment of achalasia and esophageal spasms associated with dysphagia.[7]

- **Botulinum toxin:** This toxin may be beneficial for patients with hypertonicity of the upper esophageal sphincter, achalasia, or hypersalivation.[7]

IMPORTANT SIDE EFFECTS/COMPLICATIONS OF THERAPEUTIC ACTIONS OF MEDICATIONS THAT MAY NEGATIVELY AFFECT SWALLOWING PERFORMANCE ON THE PREVIOUS ASSESSMENTS

NEUROMUSCULAR BLOCKING AGENTS

This class of medications (including succinylcholine and vecuronium) has a direct effect on striated muscle, which may contribute to impaired muscular strength and coordination for both motor speech and swallowing performance. Effects are temporary and resolve fully as medication effects wear off, so it is important to wait for resolution of effects prior to performance of any assessment of speech and/or swallowing.[11]

DRUGS THAT CAUSE SEDATION OR CONFUSION

Many medications affect performance on cognitive-linguistic tasks, may affect motor speech ability, and may impair performance and safety for swallowing assessments due to reduced alertness, awareness, and impaired motor function. These may need to be held, if possible, to improve accuracy of assessment.[2,7,12,13]

- Antiemetics (e.g., droperidol, diphenhydramine)
- Antiepileptic drugs (e.g., phenytoin, levetiracetam)
- Antipsychotics (e.g., haloperidol, quetiapine)
- Barbiturates (e.g., phenobarbital)
- Benzodiazepines (e.g., clonazepam, alprazolam)
- Opioids (e.g., codeine, hydromorphone, oxycodone)
- Skeletal muscle relaxants (e.g., baclofen, cyclobenzaprine)

DRUGS THAT CAUSE XEROSTOMIA

Dry mouth affects the ability to manipulate and transport foods effectively, impairing safety particularly with solid foods requiring mastication. Additionally, significant xerostomia may affect performance on motor speech tasks, resulting in imprecise articulation due to poor lubrication. Hydration and use of saliva substitutes may improve symptoms and performance for these tasks.[2,7,12–15]

- Angiotensin-converting enzyme (ACE) inhibitors (e.g., lisinopril, enalapril)
- Antiarrhythmics (e.g., procainamide, disopyramide)
- Antibiotics (e.g., penicillin)
- Antiemetics (e.g., metoclopramide, ondansetron)
- Antiepileptics (e.g., phenytoin)
- Antihistamines and decongestants (e.g., diphenhydramine, pseudoephedrine)
- Atypical antipsychotics (e.g., risperidone, quetiapine)
- Diuretics (e.g., furosemide, torsemide)
- Selective serotonin reuptake inhibitors (SSRIs) (e.g., fluoxetine, sertraline)
- Tricyclic depressants (TCAs) (e.g., amitriptyline)

LOCAL ANESTHETICS

These medications may be used for nasal endoscopy, nasogastric tube insertion, or dental procedures (e.g., lidocaine, benzocaine). These medications cause reduced sensation and impaired motor function. Sensorimotor effects resolve as effects of medications wear off, so it is advisable to wait for resolution prior to performance of any assessment of speech and/or swallowing.[14]

While topical anesthetics may be used for nasal endoscopy performed by an otolaryngologist (or ear, nose, and throat physician) for pharyngeal and laryngeal exam, it is not generally advised to use them during a FEES exam due to the negative effects on sensation and motor function for swallowing.[16]

DRUGS THAT CAUSE DYSKINESIAS AND/OR OTHER EXTRAPYRAMIDAL SYMPTOMS

Use of antipsychotic medications is associated with extrapyramidal symptoms that may start out as a Parkinsonian presentation with tremor, rigidity, and bradykinesia, which may lead to oropharyngeal dysphagia. These symptoms may progress to tardive dyskinesia, or involuntary, repetitive body movements that may affect swallowing coordination and coordination of motor speech, and contribute to risk for choking episodes and aspiration pneumonia. Generally, these are long-term effects (i.e., years) that may or may not be reversible with discontinuation of the relevant medication depending on duration of use and other factors. Both presentations are more frequent in typical than atypical antipsychotics. Use of these medications has been noted to have significantly more frequent and more severe adverse effects in older patients.[2,12,13,17,18]

- Antipsychotics/neuroleptics (e.g., chlorpromazine, haloperidol).
- Atypical antipsychotics (e.g., risperdone, quetiapine) may have lower risk for tardive dyskinesias, but may cause sedation, orthostatic hypotension, and xerostomia.
- Chronic use of Parkinson's disease medications (e.g., levodopa) is frequently associated with the development of motor fluctuations including dyskinesias (or uncontrollable motor movements) that occur more frequently in younger patients in the presence of higher doses of levodopa, alternating with end-of-dose wearing-off, when patients may present with worsening of their Parkinsonian symptoms including rigidity, tremor, and bradykinesia. These fluctuations can contribute to fluctuations in dysphagia presentation, severity, and type of dysarthria (hyperkinetic versus hypokinetic presentations).[19]

DRUGS THAT CAUSE ESOPHAGITIS, ESOPHAGEAL INJURY, OR GASTROESOPHAGEAL REFLUX DISEASE

Drug-induced esophagitis typically presents with complaints of dysphagia, odynophagia, or retrosternal pain. Typical treatment is use of proton pump inhibitors (PPIs) and discontinuation of the causative medication, if possible.[7,12–15,20]

- Antibiotics (e.g., penicillin, tetracycline, erythromycin)
- ACE inhibitors (e.g., ramipril)
- Anticholinergics (e.g., diphenhydramine, ipratropium)
- Antianginals (e.g., nitroglycerin, isosorbide mononitrate)
- Anxiolytic/benzodiazepines (e.g., alprazolam)
- Bisphosphonates (e.g., alendronate)
- Bronchodilators (e.g., fluticasone/salmeterol)
- Calcium channel blockers (antihypertensives) (e.g., nifedipine, diltiazem)
- Warfarin
- NSAIDs (e.g., ibuprofen, aspirin)
- Antiarrhythmic (quinidine)
- Steroids (e.g., prednisone, dexamethasone)
- Minerals/vitamins (e.g., potassium chloride, ascorbic acid, ferrous sulfate, or ferrous succinate)

DRUGS THAT MAY AFFECT ESOPHAGEAL MUSCLE TONE

- Steroids (e.g., prednisone, dexamethasone): When used in high dosages, can cause muscle wasting of the skeletal muscles of the esophagus, which is typically chronic and not reversible.[11]

Decrease Lower Esophageal Tone

These medications contribute to reflux of stomach contents into the esophagus, which may be viewed on esophageal sweep.[12–14]

- Alpha blockers (e.g., doxazosin, tamsulosin)
- Anticholinergics (e.g., diphenhydramine, ipratropium, scopolamine)
- Antidepressants – SSRIs/TCAs (e.g., trazodone, citalopram)
- Antipsychotics (e.g., clozapine, quetiapine)
- Barbiturates (e.g., phenobarbital)
- Benzodiazepines (e.g., clonazepam, alprazolam)
- Beta agonists (e.g., albuterol)
- Calcium channel blockers (e.g., nifedipine, diltiazem)
- Dopaminergic drugs (e.g., levodopa)
- Estrogen replacement medications (e.g., estradiol)
- Muscle relaxants (e.g., baclofen)
- Nitrates (e.g., nitroglycerin)

Increase Lower Esophageal Tone

These agents can contribute to impaired peristalsis or achalasia, which is associated with reduced lower esophageal sphincter relaxation.[12]

- Antacids (e.g., calcium carbonate)
- Antiemetics (e.g., metoclopramide, ondansetron)
- Beta blockers (e.g., propranolol)
- Cholinergic agonists (e.g., bethanechol, pilocarpine)

DRUGS THAT MAY CAUSE DIFFUSE MUCOSAL INJURY[7,11–14]

Chemotherapeutic agents may lead to direct injury of the oropharyngeal and esophageal mucosa as a result of the cytotoxic effects of the medications, leading to mucositis, which may present with painful oral, pharyngeal, and esophageal phases of swallow, and dysphagia.[11] As a complication of therapeutic action, antineoplastic agents may also cause immunosuppression that can lead to opportunistic infections such as oropharyngeal and/or esophageal candidiasis or viral esophagitis, which may present with dysphagia, odynophagia, and retrosternal pain.[11,14]

MEDICATION ADMINISTRATION CONCERNS

As a result of the findings of any of the above swallow exams, it may be recommended that patients take medications crushed in pureed foods, in liquid form, or with other suggested modifications for safety, rather than as a whole with a liquid wash. It may be determined that for safety, it would be best to administer medications non-orally (e.g., intravenously or via gastrostomy tube). See Chapter 37: Intravenous Access, Chapter 42: Nasogastric Tubes, and Chapter 47: Percutaneous Endoscopic Gastrostomy Tubes for more details. These recommendations all have significant implications for effectiveness and safety of the medications administered and ease of administration to patients with oropharyngeal dysphagia and increased aspiration risk.[21,22]

References

1. American Speech-Language-Hearing Association. *Scope of practice in speech-language pathology [Scope of practice]*; 2016. Available from www.asha.org/policy/.
2. Gallagher L, Naidoo P. Prescription drugs and their effects on swallowing. *Dysphagia*. 2009;24:159–166.
3. Logemann JA. *Evaluation and Treatment of Swallowing Disorders*. 2nd ed. Austin, TX: Pro-Ed, Inc; 1998.

4. Rampello L, Rampello L, Patti F, et al. When the word doesn't come out: a synthetic overview of dysarthria. *J Neurol Sci.* 2016;369:354–360.
5. American Speech-Language-Hearing Association. (2004). Knowledge and skills needed by speech-language pathologist performing videofluoroscopic swallowing studies. Available from www.asha.org/policy.
6. American Speech-Language-Hearing Association. *The role of the speech-language pathologist in the performance and interpretation of endoscopic evaluation of swallowing: position statement*, 2005. Available from www.asha.org/policy.
7. Alonso JSE, Garcia IZ. Drugs and dysphagia. In: Desuter G, ed. *Oropharyngeal Dysphagia* Springer: Cham; 2019.
8. Baijens LWJ, Speyer R. Effects of therapy for dysphagia in Parkinson's disease: systematic review. *Dysphagia.* 2009;24:91–102.
9. Melo A, Monteiro L. Swallowing improvement after levodopa treatment in idiopathic Parkinson's disease: lack of evidence. *Parkinsonism Relat Disord.* 2013;19(3):279–281.
10. Fonda D, Schwarz J, Clinnick S. Parkinsonian medication one hour before meals improves symptomatic swallowing: a case study. *Dysphagia.* 1995;10(3):165–166.
11. Balzer KM. Drug-induced dysphagia. *Int J MS Care.* 2000;2(1):40–50.
12. Brandt N. Medications and dysphagia: how do they impact each other? *Nutr Clin Pract.* 1999;14:S27–S30.
13. Carl L, Johnson P. Drugs and dysphagia: perspectives on swallowing and swallowing disorders. *Dysphagia.* 2008;17(4):143–148.
14. Al-Shehri AM. Drug-induced dysphagia. *Ann Saudi Med.* 2003;23(5):249–253.
15. Gallagher L. The impact of prescribed medication on swallowing: an overview: perspectives on swallowing and swallowing disorders. *Dysphagia.* 2010;19(4):98–102.
16. Lester S, Langmore SE, Lintzenich CR, et al. The effects of topical anesthetic on swallowing during nasoendoscopy. *Laryngoscope.* 2013;123:1704–1708.
17. Aldridge KJ, Taylor NF. Dysphagia is a common and serious problem for adults with mental illness: a systematic review. *Dysphagia.* 2012;27:124–137.
18. Miarons Font M, Rofes Salsench L. Antipsychotic medication and oropharyngeal dysphagia: systematic review. *Eur J Gastroenterol Hepatol.* 2017;29(12):1332–1339.
19. Stocchi F, Tagliati M, Olanow CW. Treatment of levodopa-induced motor complications. *Mov Disord.* 2008;23:S599–S612.
20. Kim SH, Jeong JB, Kim JW, et al. Clinical and endoscopic characteristics of drug-induced esophagitis. *World J Gastroenterol.* 2014;20(31):10994–10999.
21. Fusco S, Cariati D, Schepisi R, et al. Management of oral drug therapy in elderly patients with dysphagia. *J Gerontol Geriatr.* 2016;64:9–20.
22. Stegemann S, Gosch M, Breitkreutz J. Swallowing dysfunction and dysphagia is an unrecognized challenge for oral drug therapy. *Int J Pharm.* 2012;430(1–2):197–206.

CHAPTER 53

Stress Tests

Amit Alam, MD   ▓   Ali Seyar Rahyab, MD   ▓
Gregory J. Hughes, PharmD, BCPS, BCGP

Background

Cardiac stress tests are common procedures that are performed to evaluate patients for evidence of coronary artery disease (CAD). The gold standard for the diagnosis of CAD is cardiac catheterization and angiography; however, this is an invasive procedure that is not indicated for all patients. Therefore, many patients with a low to intermediate risk for CAD will undergo stress testing first to ascertain whether a subsequent cardiac catheterization is needed.[1] There are two components to a stress test. The first is the method in which the patient's heart will be stressed. The options are exercise (on a treadmill or stationary bike) or pharmacologic (several agents are available), as tolerated, typically to achieve at least 85% of the age-adjusted maximum predicted heart rate (220 beats per minute – the patient's age = maximum predicted heart rate). The second component is the method by which the heart is assessed for evidence of ischemia to the coronary arteries. The typical options are electrocardiogram (EKG) monitoring, nuclear imaging to evaluate coronary blood flow, or echocardiography to evaluate left ventricular systolic function. Which components are optimal for a given individual is based on multiple variables. For example, a patient with severe arthritis who cannot exercise on a treadmill will typically undergo a pharmacologic stress test.

The most common stress tests (in no particular order) are treadmill exercise EKG stress test, treadmill exercise or pharmacologic nuclear stress test, and exercise (treadmill or stationary bike) or pharmacologic (e.g., dobutamine) stress echocardiography.[1]

How to Use It

A stress test is performed to evaluate a patient for evidence of CAD. Typically, a patient will report chest discomfort or symptoms with exertion that are suggestive of heart disease, prompting the test. A stress test may also be performed in patients with established CAD to evaluate the progression of disease. A patient with a positive stress test will undergo further testing, usually with cardiac catheterization. A patient with a negative stress test will typically be reassured that his or her symptoms are not from CAD. Stress testing may have false-negative results; however, if a patient continues to have symptoms concerning for CAD, he or she may still undergo cardiac catheterization.[2,3] Any of the stress tests can be performed in the inpatient or outpatient settings.

An exercise EKG stress test will evaluate a patient for evidence of EKG changes while undergoing exercise. A test is considered abnormal (positive) if characteristic ST-segment depressions or ST-segment elevations (suggesting ischemia) are noted on the EKG during the test.[4] See Chapter 26: Electrocardiography for more information about the EKG.

A nuclear stress test may be done with either exercise on a treadmill or by administering a pharmacologic agent. A cardiologist will compare the rest and stress nuclear images, and a study will be deemed abnormal (positive) if there is worse flow on the stress images.[4,5] Patients who are actively wheezing should not undergo a pharmacologic nuclear stress test.

Stress echocardiography can also be done with exercise or by administering a pharmacologic agent. The cardiologist will compare the function of the left ventricle at rest compared with stress.

If there are parts of the ventricle that are not contracting properly, the test will be considered abnormal (positive).[6] See Chapter 25: Echocardiography for more information about this test.

How It Is Done

EXERCISE EKG STRESS TEST[4]

- EKG leads will be placed on the patient and will remain in place during exercise (treadmill or stationary bike).
- EKG is continuously obtained and reviewed for evidence of characteristic changes suggestive of underlying coronary ischemia.
- The Bruce protocol is commonly used to standardize the amount of exercise that is performed. It comprises specified stages of exercise. Each subsequent stage increases the incline and speed of the treadmill.[6]
- The test may be terminated if the patient is unable to continue, if a hemodynamically unstable arrhythmia or heart block occurs, or if symptoms occur such as fatigue, chest discomfort, shortness of breath, or a reduction in blood pressure.
- A positive stress test may lead to cardiac catheterization or an imaging study such as a nuclear stress test or a stress echocardiogram.

NUCLEAR STRESS TEST[5]

- A radioactive imaging tracer is injected into the patient.
- A set of resting images will be obtained using a form of computed tomography (CT) known as single-photon emission computed tomography (SPECT), and the result will be an image that demonstrates blood flow to the heart that is proportional to the amount of radioactive tracer uptake. An area of the heart that has abnormal blood flow will demonstrate a lack of color on the SPECT image owing to less tracer uptake.
- The patient will then undergo stress either by exercising on a treadmill or by receiving an intravenous vasodilator or dobutamine. A vasodilator is the preferred agent. It causes coronary artery vasodilation that leads to increased blood flow with increased tracer uptake (which is visualized on the SPECT image) in areas with normal coronary arteries. However, if there is an area of the heart with occluded coronary arteries, this area will not demonstrate increased blood flow, since the vasodilator will not lead to further dilation of an occluded artery. These areas will subsequently not demonstrate increased tracer uptake and will demonstrate less activity on the SPECT image.
- The cardiologist will compare the resting images to the stress images to determine if there is evidence of reduced blood flow and, if so, in which coronary artery territory.

STRESS ECHOCARDIOGRAPHY[6]

- See Chapter 25: Echocardiography for more information about this test.

Medication Implications

BEFORE THE PROCEDURE

- Patients are instructed to abstain from eating or drinking anything with caffeine and should fast (aside from water) for at least 3 hours prior to the test.
- Beta blockers and calcium channel blockers are stopped 1–2 days prior to the test in many patients (patients who cannot tolerate being off these medications may undergo stress testing without stopping beta blockers or calcium channel blockers).

- Medications used to cause vasodilation work through stimulating adenosine receptors so other medications that interact with this pathway can interfere with a stress test.
  - Examples of these interacting medications include caffeine and theophylline. Patient use of caffeine-containing drugs or ingestion of caffeine-containing foods has been shown to decrease the vasodilating effects of some of these agents, invalidating the results of the test. Patients may only be queried about their use of these agents when about to undergo the stress test, and the test must then be cancelled and rescheduled for another day. This can result in important delays in getting information about cardiovascular health and cost additional resources in the form of hospital length of stay (for inpatients) or lost productivity (for outpatients).
    - Caffeine can be found not only in many foods, drinks, and candy but also in prescription medications (e.g., Fioricet) and over-the-counter medication (e.g., Excedrin, Midol, weight loss supplements), which patients may forget to list as medications.
  - Another interacting medication is the chronic use of oral dipyridamole, which is one of the medications also used as a vasodilator for the stress test itself. If a patient has recently taken oral dipyridamole and has a stress test performed in which adenosine is administered, this drug interaction can exaggerate the hemodynamic effects of adenosine resulting in a potentially fatal arrhythmia.
    - Dipyridamole is taken daily as part of a combination product with aspirin for stroke prevention (brand name Aggrenox) and as a single-agent antiplatelet.
- For these reasons, patients should be screened several days in advance of a stress test for the use of any caffeine-, theophylline-, or dipyridamole-containing products with special attention given to over-the-counter medications and diet. If identified, these medications, supplements, or foods should be held prior to the procedure (>12 hours for caffeine and >48 hours for dipyridamole).

DURING THE PROCEDURE

- Exercise EKG stress testing: no pharmacologic agents are routinely administered.
- Nuclear stress testing[5]:
  - All patients will receive the radioactive imaging isotope. Examples include technetium-99m sestamibi and technetium-99m tetrofosmin which have similar pharmacologic characteristics. The uptake of these compounds in the heart is proportional to blood flow through the heart.[7] Possible side effects include seizure, transient arthritis, angioedema, arrhythmia, dizziness, syncope, abdominal pain, vomiting, or hypersensitivity reactions.[8]
  - For patients who will not exercise, the common vasodilator options are regadenoson, adenosine, or dipyridamole. Regadenoson is preferred due to having fewer side effects. Contraindications are second- or third-degree heart block or sinus node dysfunction (unless the patient has a functioning permanent pacemaker). For regadenoson and adenosine, warnings include:
    - Risk for myocardial ischemia and use should be avoided in patients with unstable symptoms
    - Bronchospasm, shortness of breath, or respiratory distress may occur in patients with chronic obstructive pulmonary disease (COPD) or asthma
    - Risk of seizures
    - Risk of stroke
    - The most common side effects are shortness of breath, headache, flushing, chest discomfort, dizziness, and nausea. A low level of walking during regadenoson infusion can help ameliorate side effects.[9]

- Aminophylline may be given for the relief of side effects from regadenoson, though it also reverses its intended pharmacologic effects. It is important to note that aminophylline has many noted drug interactions, as it is a substrate of cytochrome P450 1A2.[10]
- Stress echocardiography[6]
  - No pharmacologic agents are routinely administered for patients who will exercise.
  - For patients who will not exercise, the pharmacologic agent commonly utilized is dobutamine. See Chapter 25: Echocardiography for more details.

AFTER THE PROCEDURE[1,3]

- Negative stress test results:
  - If the patient has resolution of symptoms and/or has atypical or low-risk symptoms, the patient is reassured and no further testing is indicated.
  - If the patient has persistent symptoms and/or has concerning typical or high-risk symptoms, the patient is considered for cardiac catheterization and angiography.
- Positive stress test results:
  - In a patient with no prior diagnosis of CAD, cardiac catheterization and angiography are typically performed with the timing determined based on the results of the test. Patients with more severe findings may undergo urgent or even emergent cardiac catheterization, whereas individuals with less significant findings will schedule the procedure for the future.
    - Antianginal medications including beta blockers, nitrates, and calcium channel blockers may be started along with a statin and antiplatelet agents prior to cardiac catheterization.
  - In a patient with known CAD, medical management with antiplatelet agents, statins, beta blockers, and antianginal medications may be indicated without further invasive workup.
- Equivocal stress results (i.e., normal imaging results with abnormal EKG results or inconclusive results on imaging):
  - Further testing will be considered based on clinical judgment.
    - Patients with low-risk clinical features may not undergo further testing
    - Patients with high-risk clinical features will proceed to coronary catheterization
  - Patients who had inconclusive results with one stress test modality may undergo another modality rather than proceeding with coronary catheterization.

References

1. Multimodality Writing Group for Stable Ischemic Heart DiseaseWolk MJ, Bailey SR, et al. ACCF/ AHA/ASE/ASNC/HFSA/HRS/SCAI/SCCT/SCMR/STS 2013 multimodality appropriate use criteria for the detection and risk assessment of stable ischemic heart disease: a report of the American College of Cardiology Foundation Appropriate Use Criteria Task Force, American Heart Association, American Society of Echocardiography, American Society of Nuclear Cardiology, Heart Failure Society of America, Heart Rhythm Society, Society for Cardiovascular Angiography and Interventions, Society of Cardiovascular Computed Tomography, Society for Cardiovascular Magnetic Resonance, and Society of Thoracic Surgeons. *J Card Fail*. 2014;20(2):65–90. doi:10.1016/j.cardfail.2013.12.002.
2. Fihn SD, Gardin JM, Abrams J. 2012 ACCF/AHA/ACP/AATS/PCNA/SCAI/STS Guideline for the diagnosis and management of patients with stable ischemic heart disease: a report of the American College of Cardiology Foundation/American Heart Association Task Force on Practice Guidelines, and the American College of Physicians, American Association for Thoracic Surgery, Preventive Cardiovascular Nurses Association, Society for Cardiovascular Angiography and Interventions, and Society of Thoracic Surgeons. *J Am Coll Cardiol*. 2012;60(24):e44–e164. doi:10.1016/j.jacc.2012.07.013.
3. Fihn SD, Blankenship JC, Alexander KP. 2014 ACC/AHA/AATS/PCNA/SCAI/STS focused update of the guideline for the diagnosis and management of patients with stable ischemic heart disease: a report

of the American College of Cardiology/American Heart Association Task Force on Practice Guidelines, and the American Association for Thoracic Surgery, Preventive Cardiovascular Nurses Association, Society for Cardiovascular Angiography and Interventions, and Society of Thoracic Surgeons. *J Thorac Cardiovasc Surg*. 2015;149(3):e5–23. doi:10.1016/j.jtcvs.2014.11.002.

4. Henzlova MJ, Cerqueira MD, Mahmarian JJ, et al. Stress protocols and tracers. *J Nucl Cardiol*. 2006;13(6).
5. Dorbala S, Ananthasubramaniam K, Armstrong IS, et al. Single photon emission computed tomography (SPECT) myocardial perfusion imaging guidelines: instrumentation, acquisition, processing, and interpretation. *J Nucl Cardiol*. 2018;25:1784–1846. https://doi.org/10.1007/s12350-018-1283-y.
6. Pellikka PA, Arruda-Olson A, Chaudhry FA, et al. Guidelines for performance, interpretation, and application of stress echocardiography in ischemic heart disease: from the American Society of Echocardiography. *J Am Soc Echocardiogr*. 2020;33(1):1–41. e48. https://doi.org/10.1016/j.echo.2019.07.001.
7. Okada RD, Glover D, Gaffney T, et al. Myocardial kinetics of technetium-99m-hexakis-2-methoxy-2-methylpropyl-isonitrile. *Circulation*. 1988;77(2):491.
8. Technetium Tc 99m Sestamibi [package insert]. N. Billerica, MA: Lantheus Medical Imaging; 2007.
9. Regadenoson [package insert]. Northbrook, IL: Astellas Pharma US, Inc.; 2018.
10. Aminophylline [package insert]. Lake Forest, IL: Hospira, Inc.; 2017.

CHAPTER 54

Thyroid Ablation

Jamie M. Pitlick, PharmD, BCPS, BC-ADM

Background

Thyroid ablation is a procedure where the thyroid tissue is destroyed via radioactive iodine (RAI), percutaneous ethanol injection, radiofrequency, or laser ablation.[1] The most common form of thyroid ablation used in the United States is RAI, in the form of ^{131}I.[2]

How to Use It

Thyroid ablation is done in certain patients after the diagnosis of thyroid-stimulating hormone (TSH)-induced hyperthyroidism (i.e., Graves' disease), toxic adenomas (TA), or toxic multinodular goiters (TMNG).[1] It is considered the best treatment option for toxic or hot nodules, which show increased iodine uptake during a thyroid uptake and scan.[1] See Chapter 55: Thyroid Uptake and Scan for more details about this test. It is also used as adjunctive therapy in some intermediate- and high-risk patients with thyroid cancer post surgical removal of the cancer, to kill remnant cancer cells.[3] Other treatment options for these disease states include surgery or use of thionamides (e.g., methimazole, propylthiouracil).[1] The treatment choice is individualized based on several factors including type and severity of hyperthyroidism, age, sex, comorbidities, and response to previous therapy.[1]

RAI cannot be performed during pregnancy or breastfeeding, since this would lead to exposure and subsequent destruction of fetal/infant thyroid tissue, and pregnancy should be deferred for 6 to 12 months postablation.[2] All women of childbearing age should have a negative pregnancy test within 48 hours prior to RAI administration.[1,3] Breastfeeding women should not have RAI for at least 6 weeks after lactation stops, as RAI will accumulate in the breast milk and breast tissue. Furthermore, breastfeeding should not be resumed after therapy.[1] RAI is also contraindicated in patients with moderate to severe orbitopathy associated with Graves' disease, as the orbital antigen is released with RAI treatment, and this could worsen the eye disease.[1,2]

How It Is Done

RAI is administered orally, in an outpatient environment, as ^{131}I, a colorless, tasteless liquid available as an oral solution or in a carrier capsule, that is well absorbed with a half-life of 8 days and a radiation time of 56 days (99% expended).[2,4] Acutely, it works by being incorporated into thyroid hormones and thyroid globulin and disrupting normal hormone synthesis.[2,4] During this time, serum thyroid hormone will transiently increase, exacerbating hyperthyroid symptoms due to release of preformed thyroid hormone.[2] After a few weeks, because of exposure to beta and gamma radiation from RAI, the follicles that take up RAI and surrounding follicles develop cellular necrosis and start to break down.[2] There is little to no damage to other parts of the thyroid gland.[4] Hypothyroidism occurs months to years following RAI.[2] Other side effects that can occur immediately after RAI include mild thyroidal tenderness and dysphagia.[2] Patients should be monitored monthly after RAI until they reach a euthyroid state.[1,2] Dietary recommendations to follow prior to the treatment are reviewed in the "Medication Implications" section.

For patients with Graves' disease, sufficient radiation should be administered in a single fixed dose of 10–15 millicuries (mCi) or 150 microcuries per gram of tissue corrected for 24-hour RAI uptake to render the patient hypothyroid.[1] With this dose, 60% of patients will be euthyroid by 6 months or less.[2] There is currently no consensus on how to determine the optimal dose of RAI (i.e., fixed dose or calculation based on uptake); however, in thyroid glands that are estimated to weigh more than 80 g, larger doses are usually required.[1] For patients with TMNG and TA, sufficient radiation should be administered in a single dose to alleviate hyperthyroidism.[1] Doses required are generally higher than those needed to treat Graves' disease, ranging from 150 to 200 microcuries per gram of tissue corrected for 24-hour RAI uptake for TMNG and TA or a fixed dose of 10–20 mCi for TA.[1] RAI for remnant thyroid cancer ablation will use doses of 30–150 mCi.[3] A second dose may be given for all indications at 6 months if the patient remains hyperthyroid, and some patients with minimal response can be considered for a second dose in as soon as 3 months.[1]

Medication Implications

- Elderly patients and those with high-risk comorbidities (e.g., atrial fibrillation, heart failure, pulmonary hypertension, renal failure, infection, trauma, poorly controlled diabetes, cerebrovascular or pulmonary disease) should be treated for a minimum of 2 months with thionamides prior to RAI to decrease thyroid hormone to normal levels.[1,2,5] This decreases the risk of a cardiac event if the patient would have an elevation in thyroid levels postablation.[5] Methimazole is preferred, as propylthiouracil may result in a higher rate of treatment failure and has a higher risk of hepatotoxicity.[2] These should be stopped 2–3 days prior to RAI treatment and may be resumed 3–7 days after therapy.[1] Use of thionamides in the week before or after RAI may result in a higher rate of treatment failure (e.g., post-treatment recurrence).[1,2] However, higher doses of RAI may offset this reduced effectiveness.[1]
  - Common adverse reactions to thionamides include transient leukopenia, pruritic maculopapular rashes, arthralgias, and fevers.[2] More severe reactions include agranulocytosis (including fever, malaise, gingivitis, oropharyngeal infection, granulocyte count <250/mm³), and hepatotoxicity (boxed warning for propylthiouracil).[2]
  - Propylthiouracil is preferred in the first trimester of pregnancy due to increased risk of birth defects with methimazole.[6] However, due to higher risk of adverse hepatotoxicity, methimazole is preferred thereafter. Both should be used at the least effective dose.
  - Although a small amount is transferred into the breast milk, studies have shown that both are safe to use in breastfeeding women at low to moderate doses (propylthiouracil <450 mg daily; methimazole <20 mg daily).[6]
- Beta blockers, which are given to decrease the symptoms of hyperthyroidism, may be given any time without affecting RAI therapy.[2] It is especially important to give beta blockers to patients at increased risk for complications due to worsening hyperthyroidism (i.e., elderly patients and those with comorbidities), even when asymptomatic, as RAI can acutely worsen hyperthyroidism.[1]
  - Propranolol has the most evidence for use and may block the conversion of levothyroxine (T4) to triiodothyronine (T3) at high doses.[1] In addition, it is preferred for pregnant and nursing mothers. Other beta blockers that have evidence for use include atenolol, metoprolol, and nadolol.[1] Esmolol can also be used intravenously in the setting of thyroid storm.[1]
- Saturated solution potassium iodide (SSKI), 38 mg per drop, may be used starting at 3–10 drops daily as an adjunct for 3–7 days after RAI treatment.[2] This blocks the release of thyroid hormone and helps concentrate RAI in the thyroid.[2]

- If iodides, like SSKI, are given prior to RAI, they prevent the uptake of RAI in the thyroid gland.[2] It takes weeks for the effects of the iodide to stop working on the gland.[4] In patients exposed to high doses of iodides, a 24-hour radioiodine measurement should be performed prior to RAI to ensure there is adequate uptake to accomplish the desired ablation.[4]
- A special diet is not required before RAI for patients with Graves' disease, but the patient should be counseled to avoid nutritional supplements that may contain excess iodine and seaweed.[1] A patient undergoing RAI to ablate remnant cancerous cells should be instructed to have a low-iodine diet (<50 mcg/day) for 1–2 weeks prior to RAI treatment, as retrospective studies show that the uptake of RAI into the thyroid was improved by following a low-iodine diet.[3] Foods highest in iodine include iodized salt, milk and other dairy products, seafood, and egg yolks. Additional information about low-iodine diets can be found at www.thyroid.org/low-iodine-diet.[7]
- Amiodarone contains 37% iodine by weight, which translates to 6 mg/day of iodine for a patient taking 200 mg of amiodarone.[2] This is over the recommended daily amount of 150 mcg of iodine per day, resulting in iodine-exacerbated thyroid dysfunction in patients with preexisting thyroid disease.[2] The thyroid dysfunction can manifest as hyperthyroidism with increased synthesis of thyroid hormone (type I) or destructive thyroiditis with leakage of thyroid globulin and thyroid hormone (type II).[1] RAI is not effective as a treatment for either of these types of thyroid dysfunction.[1]
- Lithium may be used as an adjunctive therapy to RAI, as it increases RAI retention in the thyroid and inhibits thyroid hormone release from the gland.[2] Use is associated with increased cure rate, shortening time to cure, and preventing post-therapy increase in thyroid hormone levels.[8]
- Patients on levothyroxine therapy prior to RAI should be taken off the hormone therapy for 3–4 weeks prior to RAI.[3] In addition, liothyronine should be withdrawn for at least 2 weeks prior to RAI.[3] Patients with hyperthyroidism could potentially be on these agents in combination with thionamides as part of their hyperthyroidism treatment prior to RAI.
- Levothyroxine replacement therapy is used if the patient develops hypothyroidism after a thyroid ablation with the goal of maintaining TSH and free T_4 within the normal range.[2]
- Ethanol can be considered in patients to treat TA and TMNG when the preferred therapy options are inappropriate or refused. It is percutaneously injected into the TA or autonomous area of a TMNG. Although it can produce a functional cure in 78%–93% of patients, use has been limited due to adverse reactions of pain associated with extravasation, transient thyrotoxicosis, permanent ipsilateral facial dysesthesia, paramodular fibrosis, and toxic necrosis of the larynx and adjacent skin.[9,10]

References

1. Ross DS, Burch HB, Cooper DS, et al. 2016 American Thyroid Association Guidelines for diagnosis and management of hyperthyroidism and other causes of thyrotoxicosis. *Thyroid*. 2016;26:1343–1421. doi:10.1089/thy.2016.0229.
2. Kane MP, Bakst G, et al. Thyroid Disorders. In: DiPiro JT, Yee GC, Posey L et al, eds. *Pharmacotherapy: A Pathophysiologic Approach*. 11th ed. New York, NY: McGraw-Hill. http://accesspharmacy.mhmedical.com/content.aspx?bookid=2577&sectionid=223397495. Accessed March 23, 2020.
3. Haugen BR, Alexander EK, Bible KC, et al. 2015 American Thyroid Association Management Guidelines for adult patients with thyroid nodules and differentiated thyroid cancer. *Thyroid*. 2016;26:1–133. doi:10.1089/thy.2015.0020.
4. Brent GA, Koenig RJ. Thyroid and Antithyroid Drugs. In: Brunton LL, Hilal-Dandan R, Knollmann BC, eds. *Goodman & Gilman's: The Pharmacological Basis of Therapeutics*. 13th ed. New York, NY: McGraw-Hill. http://accesspharmacy.mhmedical.com/content.aspx?bookid=2189&sectionid=172481901 5. Accessed March 23, 2020.

5. Burch HB, Solomon BL, Cooper DS, et al. The effects of antithyroid drug pretreatment on acute changes in thyroid hormone levels after (131)I ablation for Graves' disease. *J Clin Endocrinol Metab.* 2001;86:3016–3021. doi:10.1210/jcem.86.7.7639.

6. Alexander EK, Pearce EN, Brent GA, et al. 2017 guidelines of the American Thyroid Association for the diagnosis and management of thyroid disease during pregnancy and the postpartum. *Thyroid.* 2017;27(3):315–389. doi:10.1089/thy.2016.0457.

7. Low Iodine Diet. American Thyroid Association. https://www.thyroid.org/low-iodine-diet. Accessed February 24, 2020.

8. Bogazzi F, Giovannetti C, Fessehatsion R, et al. Impact of lithium on efficacy of radioactive iodine therapy for Graves' disease: a cohort study on cure rate, time to cure, and frequency of increase serum thyroxine after antithyroid drug withdrawal. *J Clin Endocrinol Metab.* 2010;95:201–208. doi:10.1210/jc.2009-1655.

9. Tarantino L, Francica G, Sordelli I, et al. Percutaneous ethanol injection of hyperfunctioning thyroid nodules: long-term follow-up in 125 patients. *Am J Roentgenol.* 2008;190:800–808. doi:10.2214/AJR.07.2668.

10. Monzani F, Caraccio N, Goletti O, et al. Five-year follow-up of percutaneous ethanol injection for the treatment of hyperfunctioning thyroid nodules: a study of 117 patients. *Clin Endocrinol (Oxf).* 1997;46:9–15. doi:10.1046/j.1365-2265.1997.d01-1752.x.

CHAPTER 55

Thyroid Uptake and Scan

Kwan Cheng, MD ■ Lubaina S. Presswala, DO

Background

Radioactive iodine (RAI) uptake and scan is a direct, noninvasive test used to assess the function of the thyroid gland. RAI uptake and scan is frequently interchangeable with "RAI scan" or "RAI uptake" in clinical practice. However, the RAI test involves two separate phases including the uptake and the scan. Thus, to be clear, RAI uptake and scan will be the term used in this section. Physiologically, the thyroid gland actively transports and traps iodine inside the cell to synthesize thyroid hormones. The test uses a radioactive isotope of iodine (^{123}I) as a tag for the body's stable form of iodine (nonradioactive ^{127}I) to measure the fractional uptake by the thyroid gland.[1] The goal of a RAI uptake and scan is to determine the percent of the radiopharmaceutical that becomes trapped in the thyroid gland.[2] The scan (or scintigraphy) provides an image, allowing for assessment of homogeneity or heterogeneity of the radiotracer distribution within the thyroid gland.

How to Use It

There are several factors that influence the 24-hour thyroid iodide uptake as listed in Box 55.1.[1,3,4] RAI uptake and scan is commonly performed to determine the etiology of thyrotoxicosis when the diagnosis is not clear, usually in the case of a patient with nodular thyroid disease. The etiology of thyrotoxicosis includes Graves' disease, toxic multinodular goiter (MNG), toxic adenoma, thyroiditis, intrathoracic mass, ectopic thyroid tissue, and human chorionic gonadotropin (hCG)-mediated hyperthyroidism. When ^{123}I is administered to a patient with a normal thyroid gland, the tracer activity will be fairly homogeneous throughout the gland, as shown in Fig. 55.1. In Graves' disease, the tracer activity is also homogenous but more intense throughout the gland, as shown in Fig. 55.2. In cases of MNG (Fig. 55.3), there can be thyroid areas with lower than normal uptake of ^{123}I that correspond to hypofunctioning thyroid nodules (also called cold nodules), areas with supranormal uptake suggestive of hyperfunctioning thyroid nodules (also called hot nodules), and areas of homogeneous uptake that correspond to thyroid tissue without nodules. A toxic nodule has significant uptake, whereas the remainder of the thyroid uptake is low to absent. On the contrary, in cases of thyroiditis (Fig. 55.4), the tracer activity in the gland will be minimal to absent, reflecting the reduced function of the inflamed thyroid gland. A low thyroid uptake will also be noted in cases of iatrogenic hyperthyroidism, iodine-induced hyperthyroidism, amiodarone-induced thyroiditis, and, rarely, in cases of struma ovarii.

How It Is Done

RAI uptake and scan is typically performed in the outpatient setting while the patient is awake. ^{123}I is administered orally or intravenously by the nuclear medicine technician supervised by the nuclear medicine radiologist. Patients are advised not to eat or drink for at least 4 hours before taking the oral ^{123}I to aid absorption. RAI uptake is measured at 6 hours and 24 hours after oral ^{123}I

BOX 55.1 ■ Factors That Influence 24-Hour Thyroid Iodide Uptake

FACTORS THAT INCREASE UPTAKE

- Hyperthyroidism (Graves' disease, toxic MNG, toxic adenoma, intrathoracic functional mass, ectopic thyroid tissue)
- hCG-mediated (pregnancy, hydatidiform mole, choriocarcinoma)
- Excessive hormone losses (nephrotic syndrome, chronic diarrhea, excessive soybean ingestion)
- Amiodarone-induced thyroiditis type 1

FACTORS THAT DECREASE UPTAKE

- Primary or secondary hypothyroidism
- Exogenous thyroid hormone ingestion
- Thyroiditis (infectious, inflammatory, or drug toxicity such as amiodarone-induced thyroiditis type 2)
- Diet or drugs (excessive ingestion of kelp-containing substances or supplements)
- Antithyroid medications
- Iodinated contrast media

hCG, human chorionic gonadotropin; *MNG*, multinodular goiter.

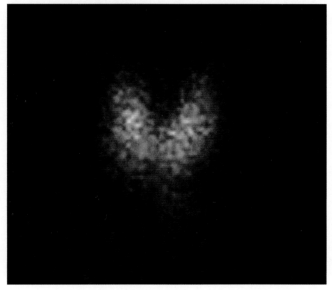

Fig. 55.1 This is a radioactive iodine (^{123}I) uptake and scan image for a normal thyroid gland. There is a 13% uptake diffusely noted in all lobes. Normal uptake ranges from 5% to 25%.

administration with a stationary probe.[5] Thyroid scintigraphy is performed on a gamma camera at the 24-hour period with a pinhole collimator for ^{123}I. Images are obtained in anterior and bilateral oblique positions and in the supine position with the neck hyperextended.

Radioactive isotope ^{123}I has a half-life of 0.55 days and is an ideal agent used for diagnosing thyroid conditions.[1,4] The low gamma radiation dose emitted by ^{123}I permits external detection and quantitation within the thyroid gland, which can then be compared with normalized values for the local imaging center. Iodine uptake can vary by geographical location and is usually dependent

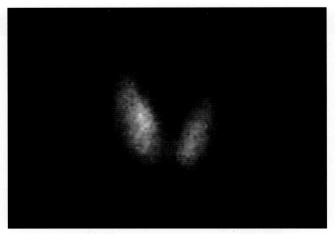

Fig. 55.2   This is a radioactive iodine (^{123}I) uptake and scan image for a patient with Graves' disease. There is intensely increased radioactive iodine uptake of 60% diffusely in all lobes.

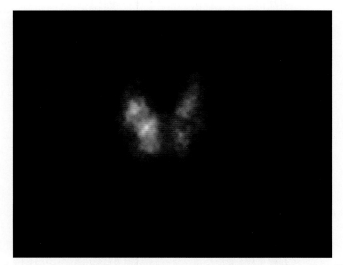

Fig. 55.3   This is a radioactive iodine (^{123}I) uptake and scan image for a patient with toxic multinodular goiter. There is increased radioactive iodine uptake of 34% in right mid-lower lobe with a focus of a cold nodule in left lower lobe and decreased uptake in the rest of the gland.

on iodine-deficient or iodine-replete areas.[6] It can range from 5% to 35% at 24 hours.[2] These characteristics contrast with ^{131}I, which has a longer half-life of 8.1 days and a higher radiation dose, making it a suitable agent to treat (or ablate) hyperthyroidism.[1,4] See Chapter 54: Thyroid Ablation for more details about treating hyperthyroidism and ^{131}I. Technetium-99m (Tc-99m) pertechnetate can also be used to image the thyroid, as pertechnetate is trapped in the thyroid, but organification does not occur, leading to rapid washout.[2] Due to a lower radiation dose to the thyroid, Tc-99m pertechnetate is preferentially used in children and will not be of focus in this section.

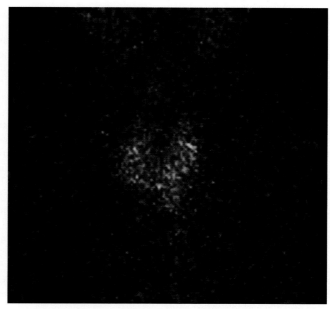

Fig. 55.4 This is a radioactive iodine (^{123}I) uptake and scan image for a patient with thyroiditis. There is decreased radioactive iodine uptake (only 3%) diffusely noted in all lobes.

TABLE 55.1 ■ Medications That May Affect Iodine Uptake and Recommended Withdrawal Time[7]

Medication	Recommended Time to Stop in Advance
Amiodarone	4–6 months
Methimazole, PTU	3–7 days
Levothyroxine, liothyronine	4 weeks
Intravenous contrast agents	1–2 months
Corticosteroids	1 week
Kelp supplement	2–3 weeks
Iodine solution (e.g., Lugol's, SSKI®)	2–3 weeks

PTU, propylthiouracil; *SSKI,* saturated solution of potassium iodide.

Medication Implications

There are several medications and agents that can interfere with RAI uptake and scan. Table 55.1 includes a list of these agents and the suggested timeline for holding them prior to attempting a thyroid uptake and scan.

- Methimazole and propylthiouracil (PTU) can decrease iodine uptake in the thyroid gland and are usually held for 3–7 days prior for optimal results. Thionamides should not be held in patients with severe hyperthyroidism preparing for thyroid ablation, as it can exacerbate thyrotoxicosis and potentially lead to thyroid storm in rare cases.[4]
- Increased iodine load from dietary sources or medications (e.g., amiodarone, intravenous contrast agents, kelp supplements, iodine solutions) can increase iodide in the blood and

compete with radioiodine, which may significantly reduce the uptake. Patients are not recommended to change their dietary salt intake prior to RAI uptake and scan, as reference ranges for this test accommodate for the geographic salt intake of the population.

- Amiodarone contains a large dose of free iodine and is stored in adipose tissues with a half-life of 100 days; therefore, it is recommended to stop amiodarone for 4–6 months before RAI uptake and scan.[8]
- Corticosteroids can decrease RAI uptake and potentially decrease the effectiveness of ablative therapy, though the exact pathophysiology is unclear.[9]
- For Graves' disease, the recommended treatment includes thionamide oral agents (e.g., methimazole, PTU) in addition to a beta blocker. The most dangerous side effect of methimazole is agranulocytosis manifesting with fevers and infection.[4] Hepatitis, vasculitis, and lupus-like syndrome are rare but recognized complications.[4] Milder side effects include pruritus, rash, transient granulocytopenia, fever, arthralgia, and gastric symptoms.[4] See Chapter 54: Thyroid Ablation for more details about treating hyperthyroidism.
- For toxic adenomas or MNG, treatment for hot nodules would be ablative therapy targeted to the nodule with ^{131}I or partial or total thyroidectomy.[10]
- In cases of acute thyroiditis, treatment is usually conservative with supportive management (such as anti-inflammatory agents and analgesics). Follow-up treatments may include glucocorticoids with or without thionamides.
- For drug toxicity–related cases (such as amiodarone), treatment can include stopping the offending medication if feasible or treating the hyperthyroid state with thionamides, beta blockers, and possibly with glucocorticoids.
- In cases of thyrotoxicosis-related hyperthyroidism, treatment is for the underlying etiology in addition to acute management with thionamides, beta blockers, possibly glucocorticoids, iodine solution, and anxiolytics.
- Iodinated contrast media exposes patients to an acute iodine load that can be several hundred thousand times the normal daily intake of iodine. The iodine load decreases RAI uptake and can potentially lead to hyperthyroidism (Jod-Basedow effect) or hypothyroidism (Wolff-Chaikoff effect).[11]
- ^{123}I
  - Allergy
    - RAI is safe to use in patients with a history of allergy to seafood or contrast. Iodine is essential as part of thyroid physiology and is added to salt in the United States. The allergic reaction is to compounds containing iodine rather than iodine itself.[12]
  - Fertility/pregnancy
    - A long-term study has revealed that radioiodine in doses used to treat hyperthyroidism does not increase the risk of infertility. The radiation doses in RAI uptake and scan are smaller and unlikely to cause infertility.[13]
    - RAIs are absolutely contraindicated in pregnancy. A pregnancy test should be obtained before RAI is administered. Fetal thyroid begins to uptake iodine by week 12–13 of gestation, and an accidental ^{131}I exposure can potentially lead to fetal hypothyroidism. There is no study specifically examining whether ^{123}I has adverse fetal outcomes, but it is contraindicated because of placental transport of radioactive isotope. RAI can also be excreted into the breast milk. Breastfeeding can resume after pumping and dumping for 3–4 days after administration of ^{123}I.[14]
      - Data on the optimal time to conceive after a RAI uptake and scan are limited, but there is evidence that conception 6 months or more after ^{131}I is not associated with adverse pregnancy outcomes. ^{123}I has 100 times less radiation than ^{131}I and a much shorter half-life. There is currently no recommendation to delay pregnancy after RAI uptake and scan; however, it should be considered if ablation is considered as a treatment option.[15]

References

1. Salvatore D, Davies T, Schlumberger M, et al. Thyroid Physiology and Diagnostic Evaluation of Patients with Thyroid Disorders. In: Melmed S, Polonsky K, Larsen P, et al., eds. *Williams Textbook of Endocrinology*. 13th ed. Philadelphia, PA: Elsevier; 2016:351–364.
2. Brandon D, Thomas A, Ravizzini G. Introduction to Nuclear Medicine. In: Elsayes K, Oldham S, eds. *Introduction to Diagnostic Radiology*. China: McGraw Hill; 2014.
3. Pantalone K, Nasr C. Approach to a patient with low TSH: patience is a virtue. *Clevel Clin J Med*. 2010;77(11):803–811.
4. Oszukowska L, Knapska-Kucharska M, Lewinski A. Effects of drugs on the efficacy of radioiodine (^{131}I) therapy in hyperthyroid patients. *Arch Med Sci*. 2010;6(1):4–10.
5. Intenzo CM, Dam HQ, Manzone TA, et al. Imaging of the thyroid in benign and malignant disease. *Semin Nucl Med*. 2012;42:49–61.
6. Al-Muqbel K, Tahtoush R. Patterns of thyroid radioiodine uptake: Jordanian experience. *J Nucl Med Technol*. 2010;38(1):32–36.
7. Mettler FA, Guiberteau MJ. Thyroid, parathyroid, and salivary glands. *Essentials of Nuclear Medicine and Molecular Imaging*. 2019:85–115.
8. Basaria S, Cooper DS. Amiodarone and the thyroid. *Am J Med*. 2005;118(7):706–714.
9. Halstenberg J, Kranert WT, Korkusuz H, et al. Influence of glucocorticoid therapy on intratherapeutic biodistribution of ^{131}I radioiodine therapy in Graves' disease. *Nuklearmedizin*. 2018;57:43–49.
10. Ross DS, Burch HB, Cooper DS, et al. 2016 American Thyroid Association guidelines for diagnosis and management of hyperthyroidism and other causes of thyrotoxicosis. *Thyroid*. 2016;26(10):1343–1421.
11. Rhee CM, Bhan I, Alexander EK, et al. Association between iodinated contrast media exposure and incident hyperthyroidism and hypothyroidism. *Arch Intern Med*. 2012;172(2):153–159.
12. Coakley FV, Panicek DM. Iodine allergy: an oyster without a pearl. *Am J Roentgenol*. 1997;169:951–952.
13. Read CH, Tansey MJ, Menda Y. A 36-year retrospective analysis of the efficacy and safety of radioactive iodine in treating young Graves' patients. *J Clin Endocrinol Metab*. 2004;89(9):4229–4233.
14. Alexander EK, Pearce EN, Brent GA, et al. 2017 guidelines of the American Thyroid Association for the diagnosis and management of thyroid disease during pregnancy and the postpartum. *Thyroid*. 2017;27(3):315–389.
15. Kim HO, Lee K, Lee SM, et al. Association between pregnancy outcomes and radioactive iodine treatment after thyroidectomy among women with thyroid cancer. *JAMA Intern Med*. 2020;180:54–61.

CHAPTER 56

Transcatheter Aortic Valve Replacement

Amit Alam, MD ■ Ali Seyar Rahyab, MD

Background

The most common valvular disease of the heart in adults is aortic stenosis (AS) with a noted increased incidence with aging.[1,2] Patients typically experience a slow decline in the aortic valve area over many years. The tipping point is the development of symptoms, after which there is increased mortality if the AS is left untreated.[1,2] Patients may experience shortness of breath, chest discomfort, syncope, or may present with heart failure. Surgical aortic valve replacement (SAVR) has been known to improve survival and leads to a resolution of symptoms. However, mortality and risk of complications from operative repair increases with age, and many patients are therefore unable to undergo SAVR.[2] Transcatheter aortic valve replacement (TAVR or transcatheter aortic valve implantation [TAVI]) is the minimally invasive insertion of a bioprosthetic valve, and it is approved by the Food and Drug Administration for patients who are at high, intermediate, or low risk for SAVR. Clinical trials have demonstrated similar outcomes overall for patients following TAVR versus SAVR, with TAVR generally demonstrating fewer adverse events and the procedure is typically well tolerated.[3,4]

How to Use It

The diagnosis of severe AS is made with echocardiography. See Chapter 25: Echocardiography for more details about this test. Patients may have a characteristic systolic murmur on examination or symptoms such as shortness of breath, chest discomfort, or syncope that prompts the test. The indications for TAVR include patients with severe symptomatic AS.[5] The decision regarding SAVR or TAVR is typically made in conjunction with the heart team (which includes interventional cardiology and cardiothoracic surgery) and will factor in the patient's surgical risk and anatomy. Once the decision has been made to proceed to TAVR, the patient will undergo computed tomography imaging of the chest to evaluate the patient's anatomy and determine the proper valve that will be utilized for the procedure. The patient will also undergo cardiac catheterization to evaluate for the presence of coronary artery disease.[2] See Chapter 17: Computed Tomography Scan and Chapter 46: Percutaneous Coronary Intervention for more details about these tests.

How It Is Done

TAVR may be performed by an interventional cardiologist or a cardiothoracic surgeon independently, or they may perform the procedure together. The procedure may be performed in the cardiac catheterization laboratory or in a hybrid operating room. It may be done via a transfemoral approach through the femoral vein and artery. The catheters and valve are all inserted via the minimally invasive peripheral access. A transapical approach may also be considered, and this requires a small lateral thoracotomy, and the valve is inserted through the left ventricular apex. A little over half of the TAVR patients will be discharged within 3 days, with a longer length of stay (past 72 hours) associated with worse outcomes.[6]

Medication Implications

BEFORE THE PROCEDURE[2]

- Anticoagulation is stopped prior to the procedure (both vitamin K antagonists and direct oral anticoagulants [DOACs]).
- Patients are treated with antimicrobial and antithrombotic prophylaxis.
  - Intravenous antibiotics generally include cefazolin (or vancomycin in certain circumstances) and are given just before the procedure (within 60 minutes for cefazolin or 120 minutes prior for vancomycin) and continued for 48 hours. Dosing regimens for these or other antibiotics used are consistent with those used for general surgical site infection prophylaxis.[7]
  - Aspirin (160–325 mg) and clopidogrel (300 mg) are given orally at least 24 hours prior to the procedure.

DURING THE PROCEDURE

- Conscious sedation or general anesthesia may be utilized. However, if transesophageal echocardiography is being performed during the procedure, then general anesthesia is preferred.
- Heparin is administered via continuous intravenous infusion throughout the procedure for anticoagulation.

AFTER THE PROCEDURE

- The ideal use of antiplatelet agent(s) and/or anticoagulation is an area of active research. Given that TAVR utilizes bioprosthetic valves, they do not require indefinite anticoagulation as with mechanical valves, and randomized controlled trials are attempting to answer the question of the ideal agent(s) and duration of therapy. In addition, technologic advances and improvement in procedural techniques have led to improved safety, potentially making earlier trial data less applicable to modern-day patients. Given the lack of conclusive data, the recommendations from various guidelines are not in agreement.[8]
  - The American College of Cardiology/American Heart Association 2017 update recommendations are[5]:
    - Aspirin 75–100 mg orally daily is continued indefinitely, and clopidogrel 75 mg orally daily may be reasonable for the first 6 months.
    - In patients without a preexisting indication for anticoagulation, an alternative approach is anticoagulation with a vitamin K antagonist alone (target international normalized ratio [INR] 2.5) for at least 3 months in patients at low risk of bleeding. The guidelines do not make a specific recommendation for patients with a preexisting indication for anticoagulation, such as atrial fibrillation.
  - Given the lack of uniform evidence-based recommendations, actual clinical practice varies and may include shorter duration of dual antiplatelet agents, single antiplatelet agent strategies, or use of DOACs.
  - According to expert opinion, in patients with new-onset atrial fibrillation or subclinical valve leaflet thrombosis (while on antiplatelet agents), anticoagulation should be started.[9]
  - Ongoing studies are evaluating the ideal anticoagulation agent including the use of DOACs.[8,9]

- Patients are followed up closely for routine monitoring including assessment for postprocedure complications, which include[2]:
  - Heart block: Approximately 4%–9% of patients ultimately require a permanent pacemaker, with a higher percentage observed in individuals with prior conduction disease.
  - Renal dysfunction: Acute kidney injury is associated with increased mortality, and it occurs less frequently in TAVR than in SAVR.
  - Severe aortic regurgitation: It is rare, and great care is undertaken to ensure proper sizing of the valve prior to the procedure and proper position of the valve during the procedure to limit this complication.
  - Embolization of the valve from the aortic position or aortic root dissection: Emergent surgical intervention is required to address these major complications.
  - Vascular complications: Occur in approximately 6% of cases. Vascular complications are more common in the transfemoral approach but are more fatal in the transapical approach.
  - Obstruction of the coronary arteries: Occurs rarely in about 0.6% of cases and is not relevant if there are coronary artery bypass grafts that are not occluded. If the patient does not have grafts, coronary artery bypass grafting would be performed on an emergent basis.

References

1. Bonow RO, Greenland P. Population-wide trends in aortic stenosis incidence and outcomes. *Circulation.* 2015;131(11):969–971.
2. Topol E, Teirstein P. Balloon-expandable trans-catheter aortic valve replacement systems. In *Textbook of Interventional Cardiology*, 8th ed. Elsevier; 2019:838–855.
3. Mack MJ, Leon MB, Thourani VH, et al. Transcatheter aortic-valve replacement with a balloon-expandable valve in low-risk patients. *N Engl J Med.* 2019;380(18):1695–1705.
4. Popma JJ, Deeb GM, Yakubov SJ, et al. Transcatheter aortic-valve replacement with a self-expanding valve in low-risk patients. *N Engl J Med.* 2019;380(18):1706–1715.
5. Nishimura RA, Otto CM, Bonow RO, et al. 2017 AHA/ACC Focused Update of the 2014 AHA/ACC Guideline for the management of patients with valvular heart disease: a report of the American College of Cardiology/American Heart Association Task Force on Clinical Practice Guidelines. *J Am Coll Cardiol.* 2017;70(2):252–289.
6. Wayangankar SA, Elgendy IY, Xiang Q, et al. Length of stay after transfemoral transcatheter aortic valve replacement: an analysis of the Society of Thoracic Surgeons/American College of Cardiology Transcatheter Valve Therapy Registry. *JACC Cardiovasc Interv.* 2019;12(5):422–430.
7. Bratzler DW, Dellinger EP, Olsen KM, et al. Clinical practice guidelines for antimicrobial prophylaxis in surgery. *Surg Infect (Larchmt).* 2013;14(1):73–156.
8. Lugo LM, Romaguera R, Gomez-Hospital JA, et al. Antithrombotic therapy after transcatheter aortic valve implantation. *Eur Cardiol.* 2020;15:e09.
9. Saito Y, Nazif T, Baumbach A, et al. Adjunctive antithrombotic therapy for patients with aortic stenosis undergoing transcatheter aortic valve replacement. *JAMA Cardiol.* 2020;5(1):92–101.

CHAPTER 57

Transjugular Intrahepatic Portosystemic Shunt

Michelle T. Martin, PharmD, FCCP, BCPS, BCACP ▪ Wadih Chacra, MD

Background

Transjugular intrahepatic portosystemic shunt (TIPS), introduced in the 1980s, is a procedure that is performed with imaging to connect the portal vein to the hepatic vein through the liver. Sequelae of advanced liver disease and cirrhosis include portal hypertension, which is defined by increased pressure in the portal circulation due to high resistance to blood flow through the cirrhotic liver; a TIPS will decrease this pressure gradient between the portal and hepatic veins.

How to Use It

TIPS is performed for secondary prevention of variceal hemorrhage or refractory ascites to minimize the complications of portal hypertension.[1] A specific description of refractory ascites can be found in the "Medication Implications" section. TIPS is not recommended for primary prevention of variceal hemorrhage due to increased risk of hepatic encephalopathy (HE) and mortality.[2] The indication for TIPS procedure can impact survival; one study found >60 months of survival with variceal hemorrhage versus >29 months of survival with refractory ascites ($P = .009$).[3] It is contraindicated in patients with severe HE, right-sided heart failure, and pulmonary hypertension. The model for end-stage liver disease (MELD) score, currently used in a modified format of the MELD-Na for allocation of organs for liver transplant recipients, was initially developed to predict mortality following elective TIPS placement.[4] The MELD and MELD-Na scores reflect the severity of liver disease. They are calculated using the international normalized ratio (INR), total bilirubin, and serum creatinine with the addition of the serum sodium concentration for the MELD-Na. A MELD or MELD-Na >18 is generally considered a contraindication for TIPS placement.

How It Is Done

The TIPS procedure requires anesthesia and imaging and can be performed as an elective procedure in an outpatient setting followed by observation, or as an emergent or planned procedure in an inpatient setting. It is typically performed by interventional radiologists with ultrasound or X-ray imaging guidance and takes about 60–90 minutes. Success rates are over 90%.[5]

The vessel of entry is the jugular vein, as indicated in the name of the procedure. A catheter is inserted and a balloon and metal stent are guided into one of the hepatic veins. Contrast dye is injected into the vein to aid placement of the stent. The stent is placed between the portal (hypertensive) and hepatic (normotensive) veins to facilitate blood flow from the splanchnic circulation to the hepatic vein. Hence, the TIPS bypasses the cirrhotic liver (the cause of the high resistance to blood flow) and reduces portal venous pressure. The goal portosystemic gradient post-TIPS is <12 mmHg to reduce the risk of variceal bleeding and development of ascites.[2] The preferred stent is coated with polytetrafluoroethylene ("Teflon"), which has been shown to

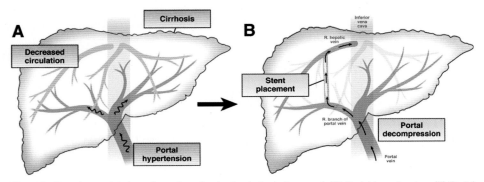

Fig. 57.1 Transjugular intrahepatic portosystemic shunt stent placement. (A) Portal hypertension. (B) Portal decompression. (From Bhogal HK, Sanyal AJ. Using transjugular intrahepatic portosystemic shunts for complications of cirrhosis. *Clin Gastroenterol Hepatol* 2011;9:936–46.)

decrease rebleeding rates compared with bare metal stents (10% versus 29%, $P < 0.001$).[6] See Fig. 57.1 for an illustration of TIPS.

Recovery includes monitoring the patient's vital signs and monitoring for bleeding. Patency of the TIPS should be assessed by Doppler ultrasound 5 days after the procedure and every 6 months thereafter.[2]

Post-TIPS, the diversion of blood flow past the liver into the hepatic veins reduces the ability of the liver to remove toxins. Ammonia concentrations may increase, which causes HE. The risk of developing HE can be over 10%–50% following TIPS.[5–7] Hence, the presence of preexisting HE is a contraindication for TIPS given the risk of it worsening. A reduction in the shunt diameter can reverse HE but may exacerbate the condition that necessitated TIPS in the first place.

Medication Implications

- Prior to TIPS procedures, patients with portal hypertension and medium to large varices that have not yet bled are medically managed.[2]
  - Nonselective beta blocker (NSBB)
    - NSBB are avoided in patients with ascites.
    - Nadolol Starting at 20–40 mg once daily; can adjust the doses every 2–3 days. The maximum dose is 160 mg/day. Monitor heart rate and blood pressure for nadolol dose optimization. The target heart rate is 55–60 beats/minute and the systolic blood pressure should not be <90 mmHg.[2]
    - Propranolol Starting at 20–40 mg twice daily; can adjust the doses every 2–3 days up to 160 mg/day if well tolerated. Monitor heart rate and blood pressure for propranolol dose optimization. The target heart rate is 55–60 beats/minute and the systolic blood pressure should not be <90 mmHg.[2]
    - Carvedilol (NSBB with anti-α1 adrenergic activity) Starting at 3.125 mg twice daily, increase to 6.25 mg twice daily after 3 days. The maximum dose is 12.5 mg/day (due to the decrease in arterial pressure that is not recommended in patients with refractory ascites). The systolic blood pressure should remain >90 mmHg.[2]
- Endoscopic variceal band ligation is used in patients who bleed or cannot tolerate NSBB to eradicate esophageal varices and reduce the risk of rebleeding.
  - If patients have recurrent bleeding despite band ligation and do not tolerate NSBB therapy (or have ascites or other complication), TIPS is recommended.
    - After TIPS, as long as the stent is patent, portal hypertension should be reduced, and therefore there is no need for NSBB, endoscopic surveillance, or treatment of varices.[2]

- Acute variceal hemorrhage
  - Octreotide, a long-acting somatostatin analog (or other vasoactive medication such as terlipressin, if outside the United States), is administered immediately after variceal hemorrhage is suspected. It controls the hemorrhage by splanchnic vasoconstriction, which decreases portal pressure. The dosing is 50 mcg intravenous (IV) bolus, repeated in 1 hour if continued bleeding, and continuation of 50 mcg/hour IV infusion for up to 5 days after variceal band ligation.[2]
  - Antibiotic prophylaxis should be started to decrease the risk of infection, recurrent bleed, and death in patients with cirrhosis and gastrointestinal hemorrhage whether or not TIPS is planned.[2]
    - The preferred agent is ceftriaxone 1g IV every 24 hours for up to 7 days.[2,8]
- If the TIPS procedure is planned, providers should hold warfarin, direct oral anticoagulants (DOACs), and some providers may elect to hold aspirin prior to the procedure. Clinicians should consider thrombocytopenia instead of elevated INR as a predictive factor for bleeding risk in cirrhotic patients; INR elevation in patients with liver disease is not limited to disruption in vitamin-K-dependent clotting factors as with warfarin's mechanism of action.[9] A MELD or MELD-Na score, which includes the INR, should be assessed, but an INR greater than 5 is also a relative contraindication to TIPS.[1] The number of days (1–4) for holding a DOAC will depend on the agent, the patient's renal function, and its indication for use.
  - Anticoagulation is used after TIPS in cases such as superior mesenteric vein thrombus or preexisting occlusive portal vein thrombus.
- Iodine-based contrast is administered to allow for fluoroscopic visualization during TIPS procedure. Assess patients for iodine allergy prior to administration and for contrast-induced nephropathy following the procedure. See Chapter 17: Computed Tomography Scan for more details.
- Refractory ascites is defined as persistent ascites despite the use of high-dose diuretics (spironolactone up to 400 mg/day and furosemide up to 160 mg/day) and dietary sodium restriction (2000 mg [88 mmoles] sodium per day), or ascites that recurs rapidly after large volume paracentesis. It can also be defined as failure of diuretic therapy manifesting as worsening kidney function, hyponatremia, and hyperkalemia.[10]
  - In patients who receive TIPS for refractory ascites, diuretics may be slowly tapered to lower doses after the procedure over several months based on clinical response.[11]
- Routine HE prophylaxis is not recommended after TIPS.[7]
  - In patients who experience HE after TIPS, treatment includes:
    - Lactulose, a nonabsorbable disaccharide and inexpensive oral liquid, is initially dosed every 1–2 hours until at least two loose stools are produced daily, then titrated to 30–45 mL (20–30 g) 2–4 times/day to achieve two to three soft bowel movements daily. The medication has a sweet taste that can be diluted with other liquids to help mask the taste, yet patients must ensure that the dilution is a volume that is able to be consumed. Lactulose can cause electrolyte abnormalities, which is particularly problematic as these, combined with dehydration, can precipitate HE. Reported adverse drug reactions include flatulence, belching, diarrhea, abdominal cramping, and nausea.
    - Ammonia concentrations are not useful for the diagnosis, prognosis, or staging of HE patients and should not be trended.[7] Response to treatment of HE is assessed clinically and does not correlate with ammonia levels.
    - Rifaximin, a nonaminoglycoside semi-synthetic nonsystemic antibiotic derivative of rifamycin, is an add-on to lactulose, dosed at 550 mg orally twice daily. The cost of rifaximin is approximately one hundred times the cost of lactulose and often requires prior authorization from third-party payers. Copay assistance may be available from

the manufacturer and, depending on the payer, 90-day supplies may decrease out-of-pocket costs for patients. Reported adverse drug reactions from clinical trials include peripheral edema, nausea, dizziness, fatigue, and ascites.[12]

■ Several other agents are available for treating HE, many of which have limited or conflicting data (e.g., neomycin, metronidazole, L-ornithine-L-aspartate, probiotics, branched-chain amino acids, polyethylene glycol, zinc).[7]

References

1. Boyer TD, Haskal ZJ. The role of transjugular intrahepatic portosystemic shunt (TIPS) in the management of portal hypertension. *Hepatology*. 2005;41:386–400.

2. Garcia-Tsao G, Abraldes JG, Berzigotti A, et al. Portal hypertensive bleeding in cirrhosis: risk stratification, diagnosis, and management: 2016 practice guidance by the American Association for the Study of Liver Diseases *Hepatology*. 2017;65:310–335.

3. Heinzow HS, Lenz P, Köhler M, et al. Clinical outcome and predictors of survival after TIPS insertion in patients with liver cirrhosis. *World J Gastroenterol*. 2012;18:5211–5218.

4. Kamath PS, Wiesner RH, Malinchoc M, et al. A model to predict survival in patients with end-stage liver disease. *Hepatology*. 2001;33:464–470.

5. Casadaban LC, Parvinian A, Minocha J, et al. Clearing the confusion over hepatic encephalopathy after TIPS creation: incidence, prognostic factors, and clinical outcomes. *Dig Dis Sci*. 2015;60:1059–1066.

6. Bucsics T, Schoder M, Diermayr M, et al. Transjugular intrahepatic portosystemic shunts (TIPS) for the prevention of variceal re-bleeding – a two decades experience. *PLoS One*. 2018;13:e0189414.

7. Vilstrup H, Amodio P, Bajaj J, et al. Hepatic encephalopathy in chronic liver disease: 2014 practice guideline by the American Association for the Study of Liver Diseases and the European Association for the Study of the Liver. *Hepatology*. 2014;60:715–735.

8. Fernandez J, dA Ruiz, Gomez C, et al. Norfloxacin vs ceftriaxone in the prophylaxis of infections in patients with advanced cirrhosis and hemorrhage. *Gastroenterology*. 2006;131:1049–1056.

9. Valla DC, Rautou PE. The coagulation system in patients with end-stage liver disease. *Liver Int*. 2015;35:139–144.

10. Runyon BA. Introduction to the revised American Association for the Study of Liver Diseases Practice Guideline management of adult patients with ascites due to cirrhosis 2012. *Hepatology*. 2013;57:1651–1653.

11. Garcia-Tsao G. Transjugular intrahepatic portosystemic shunt in the management of refractory ascites. *Semin Intervent Radiol*. 2005;22:278–286.

12. Xifaxin [package insert]. Bridgewater, NJ: Salix Pharmaceuticals; 2019.

CHAPTER 58

Urinalysis

Michael Kaplan, MD ▪ Bruce E. Hirsch, MD

Background

The concept that ordinary bodily fluids could yield insight into physiology emerged from the examination of urine. In fact, laboratory medicine began 6,000 years ago when Sumerian and Babylonian physicians recorded onto clay tablets their reflections on urine, thus introducing the objective study of human urine (a feat that would be called *uroscopy*, now called *urinalysis* [UA]).[1]

UA is a simple, cheap, noninvasive test that can be helpful in diagnosing and monitoring a range of diseases. From a small sample of urine, a correctly performed and interpreted UA allows clinicians to quickly learn a great deal about a patient. Many medications can change the nature of the urine, from its color to its performance on UA; therefore, it is important to be mindful of a patient's medication when reviewing their UA.

How to Use It

UA includes microscopic and macroscopic examination of the urine, as well as chemical analysis.[2] Clues to a patient's illness begin with macroscopic examination of their urine: What is the color? Is it clear or cloudy? Color indicates anything from dehydration (the most common cause of darker urine) to a drug effect (see "Medication Implications" section), while cloudy appearance predicts the presence of white cells (pyuria) or crystals (crystalluria). Likewise, a frothy or bubbly appearance implies the presence of protein, suggesting a range of diseases from fever to glomerulonephritis. Foul odor may indicate anything from dehydration to the ingestion of asparagus.[2]

Microscopic analysis can demonstrate white cells, red cells (hematuria), or clumps of protein and/or cells called *casts*. Casts help to diagnose the etiology of an acute kidney injury: muddy brown casts diagnose acute tubular necrosis (ATN), and red blood cell casts indicate glomerulonephritis. White blood cell casts suggest infection or acute interstitial nephritis.

Chemical examination is done most often with reagent strip testing (commonly referred to as a "dipstick"). Chemical analysis can indicate quite a bit, from the likelihood of infection (*leukocyte esterase* is a product of white blood cells, while *nitrites* are a product of gram-negative bacilli and rare gram-positive bacteria) to the likelihood of acute and chronic disease through various surrogate markers; these include pH (important in evaluating systemic acidosis), urine osmolality (important in disorders of sodium and water retention), specific gravity (helpful in evaluating hydration), protein, glucose, and ketones (relevant in starvation, stress, alcohol). A separate order for urine electrolytes can be helpful, as they can also indicate various disorders of the kidney and the body's ability to maintain equilibrium.

An important caveat is that urine tests in and of themselves are not sufficient to diagnose urinary tract infections (UTIs). Asymptomatic bacteriuria and pyuria are rarely indications for antibiotic therapy in the absence of signs and symptoms of infection. (And, interestingly, what exactly constitutes symptoms of a UTI is a controversial issue in itself.[3]) See Chapter 23: Culture - Urine for details about UTIs.

Clearly, there is a tremendous amount of information that can be gleaned from UA, so the authors recommend avoiding the use of terms like "dirty," "clean," "positive," or "negative" to describe the results of UA. These descriptors are vague and ripe for miscommunication.

How It Is Done

Several milliliters of urine are obtained from the patient. This is achieved by urinating in a cup ("clean catch"), introducing a catheter if the patient is incontinent ("straight cath"), or by sampling from an indwelling catheter. If attempting a clean catch, a midstream sample is ideal and the external genitalia should be cleaned first. Urine is then examined macroscopically, spun down in a centrifuge, and then the sediment at the bottom is microscopically examined. It is also sent to a laboratory for further chemical analysis. If there is delay in analysis, the sample must be refrigerated.

The prototypical UA of a well-hydrated healthy person is clear to light yellow in color, has a pH of 6 (range, 4.5–8), and lacks blood, protein, casts, leukocyte esterase, and nitrites.

Medication Implications[2,4,5–8]

- No drugs need to be held prior to the procedure, though several drugs can influence results.
- There are many different techniques used to analyze urine and, depending on the specific methods used, the nuance and details of drug interference may vary.
  - Exercise extra caution if attributing a finding secondary to a drug as a serious disease could be missed.
- Ascorbic acid (vitamin C) can cause false-negative results of the dipstick.[4]
  - Ascorbic acid is present in high quantities in many fruits and vegetables (citrus fruits, berries, broccoli), as well as most multivitamins.
    - Ascorbic acid is a strong reducing agent that can make oxidation reactions on the UA strip falsely negative, as the strip is coated with reagents that become oxidized by the presence of different analytes[4]
    - Ascorbic acid can, therefore, be associated with false-negative dipstick results, including urine blood and glucose, as well as leukocytes, nitrites, and bilirubin[4]
  - One small study looked at the potential for interference of ascorbic acid on the dipstick's detection of several analytes. Overall, the proportion of ascorbic acid–induced discrepancy was small, though present for blood, glucose, nitrites, and bilirubin. The effect was a function of the specific commercial dipstick used, as well as the urinary concentration of ascorbic acid and the concentration of analyte present.[4]
- Bilirubin/urobilinogen
  - There may be false-negative results with ascorbic acid use.
  - There may be false-positive results with phenothiazines (some antipsychotics).
  - Antibiotics kill gut flora, which decreases conversion of bilirubin to urobilinogen in the gut. This lowers systemic and thus urinary urobilinogen.
- Drug- and food-induced color change[2,5,6]
  - This is a nonexhaustive list. Also, some drugs are associated with a spectrum of colored urine.
    - Orange (rifampin, riboflavin, phenazopyridine, sulfasalazine, warfarin, excessive carrot consumption)
    - Red (beets, blackberries, rifampin, phenazopyridine)
    - Blue or green (amitriptyline, indomethacin, cimetidine, methylene blue, excessive black licorice)
    - Brown (fava beans, metronidazole, nitrofurantoin, chloroquine)
    - Black (L-dopa, senna, alpha-methyldopa)

- Glucosuria
  Sodium-glucose cotransporter-2 (SGLT2) inhibitors (e.g., empagliflozin, dapagliflozin, canagliflozin) will increase urine glucose. This is because of the medication's mechanism of action and is not an unintended side effect.
  - There may be false-negative results with ascorbic acid use.
- Hematuria
  - Consider a urinary catheter itself as introducing trauma to the urethra to explain hematuria. See Chapter 59: Urinary Catheters for more details.
  - If an asymptomatic patient is found to have a positive dipstick but no red blood cells on microscopy, then they have "dipstick pseudohematuria," usually a clinically insignificant finding.
    - One may find false-positive screening for blood on the dipstick because of menstrual blood, vigorous exercise, hemoglobinuria, or myoglobinuria.[7]
  - If there is macroscopic hematuria, assess if the patient is taking anticoagulants, antiplatelet medications, nonsteroidal anti-inflammatory drugs, or other medications or supplements that increase bleeding risk.
  - There may be false-negative results with ascorbic acid or captopril use.
  - Cyclophosphamide can cause hemorrhagic cystitis.
    - Cyclophosphamide is an alkylating agent used in the treatment of cancer and rheumatologic disease. Renal excretion of a urotoxic metabolite, acrolein, is thought to be the culprit of cyclophosphamide-induced hemorrhagic cystitis.
    - Hemorrhagic cystitis is prevented through administration of mesna, a medication that conjugates acrolein in the urine.
    - Severe refractory cyclophosphamide-associated hemorrhagic cystitis can be treated with a number of advanced measures, including intravesicular sodium hyaluronate and hyperbaric oxygenation.[8]
- Ketones
  - Mesna and metabolites of L-dopa can cause false-positive results.
- Nitrite/leukocyte esterase
  - False-negative results can be seen after a patient takes antibiotics.
    - Oxidizing antibiotics like cephalexin and nitrofurantoin in particular can cause false negatives
  - There may be false-negative results with ascorbic acid use.
  - There may be false-positive nitrites with exposure to air.
  - There may be false-positive leukocyte esterase with low specific gravity (increased cell lysis) or a false-negative result with high specific gravity.
  - There may be false-positive results for both leukocyte esterase and nitrite with phenazopyridine.
- pH
  - Acetazolamide will cause urine to be more basic. This is an expected outcome as a result of its mechanism as a carbonic anhydrase inhibitor. Inhibiting carbonic anhydrase reduces hydrogen secretion into the renal tubule.
  - Cranberries, in capsules with high quantities, make the urine more acidic.
    - This is one mechanism to explain the thought that cranberries could treat or prevent UTIs. Unfortunately, a clinical trial in which 185 elderly women were randomized to receive high-dose cranberry capsules or placebo failed to demonstrate any protective effect of cranberries[9]
- Proteinuria
  - Angiotensin-converting enzyme inhibitors and angiotensin II receptor blockers will decrease the amount of protein in the urine. This is not a false negative, as it is the intended therapeutic effect.

- Specific gravity[2]
  - Iodinated contrast can increase the urine specific gravity.
  - Alkaline urine (e.g., from acetazolamide) can lower specific gravity.
- Urine electrolytes
  - Urine electrolyte interpretation is obfuscated if the patient is taking diuretics (including medications such as loop diuretics [e.g., furosemide, bumetanide] and thiazide diuretics [e.g., hydrochlorothiazide, chlorthalidone]).
    - In these cases, urine electrolytes reflect not pathophysiology, but the medication's mechanism of action

References

1. Armstrong JA. Urinalysis in Western culture: a brief history. *Kidney Int.* 2007;71(5):384–387.
2. Simerville JA, Maxted WC, Pahira JJ. Urinalysis: a comprehensive review. *Am Fam Physician.* 2005;71(6):1153–1162.
3. McKenzie R, Stewart MT, Bellantoni MF, et al. Bacteriuria in individuals who become delirious. *Am J Med.* 2013;127(4):255–257.
4. Ko DH, Jeong TD, Kim S, et al. Influence of vitamin C on urine dipstick test results. *Ann Clin Lab Sci.* 2015;45(4):391–395.
5. Mayo Clinic. Urine Color. 2017. Available at: https://www.mayoclinic.org/diseases-conditions/urine-color/symptoms-causes/syc-20367333. Accessed 1/17/2020.
6. Gill B. Discoloration, discoloration, urine. *Medscape.* 2014. Available at: https://emedicine.medscape.com/article/2172371-overview. Accessed 1/17/2020.
7. Rao PK, Jones JS. How to evaluate 'dipstick hematuria:' what to do before you refer. *Cleve Clin J Med.* 2008;75(3):227–233.
8. Tsai CJ, Wang SS, Ou YC. Cyclophosphamide-induced intractable hemorrhagic cystitis treated with hyperbaric oxygenation and intravesical sodium hyaluronate. *Urol Sci.* 2014;25(4):155–157.
9. Juthani-Mehta M, Van Ness PH, Bianco L, et al. Effect of cranberry capsules on bacteriuria plus pyuria among older women in nursing homes: a randomized clinical trial. *JAMA.* 2016;316(18):1879–1887.

CHAPTER 59

Urinary Catheters

Kimberly Means, PharmD, BCCCP

Background

Urinary catheters are used in the inpatient and outpatient settings to assist in draining the bladder of urine. Indwelling catheters are placed in about 25% of hospitalized patients during their hospital stay.[1] Indwelling catheters (commonly called "Foley catheters") have been in use since the 1930s.[2] The origin of the word "catheter" comes from ancient Greek word *kathiénai*, meaning "to thrust into" or "to send down."[2] There are several forms of catheters including external devices (e.g., condom catheters), catheters used intermittently (e.g., "straight cath"), or catheters that remain in the bladder (e.g., indwelling urethral catheters or suprapubic catheters). There are two forms of indwelling catheters: 1) Foley catheters that are typically inserted through the urethra into the bladder and 2) suprapubic catheters that are surgically placed through the abdomen into the bladder.

How to Use It

Urinary catheters are used for a variety of indications and based on the indication, used for varying lengths of time. About 70% to 80% of hospital-acquired urinary tract infections (UTIs) are catheter-associated UTIs.[1] To prevent potential complications and catheter-associated infections, catheters should only be placed in the appropriate patients and should be removed as soon as medically feasible. A Foley catheter should be inserted as aseptically as possible to prevent potential infectious complications. Long-term catheter use is classified as being in place more than 30 days.[2]

Catheters historically have been made from latex, but are more recently being made with silicone due to adverse effects from latex.[2] Foley catheters are typically approximately 400 mm in length and have two channels, one for drainage of urine and another to allow the balloon at the end of the catheter to be inflated to keep the catheter anchored within the bladder.[2] Some catheters have a third channel that can be used for continuous bladder irrigation.[3] Coudé or biCoudé catheters are curved and designed to decrease risk of urethral trauma during insertion.[2] The curved tip of the catheter has holes in the end to allow urine to flow through the catheter.[2] The catheter can be connected to tubing that can then be attached to a collection device so that urine can be measured or collected.

Urinary catheters can be external, as with a condom catheters, or more invasive, as with catheters used intermittently or indwelling and suprapubic catheters. There are advantages and disadvantages to each type of catheter.

CONDOM CATHETERS

The least invasive urinary catheter for males is the condom catheter, which can be used for short- or long-term use.[2] Tubing connects the end of the sheath to a bag to collect urine.[2] Disadvantages to this method include skin breakdown, displaced sheath and subsequent urine leaking, and potential for UTI.[2]

INTERMITTENT CATHETERIZATION

Intermittent catheterization can be performed by patients at home in the outpatient setting, or it can be performed by healthcare providers in the inpatient setting. Intermittent catheterization can be used to collect urine samples (e.g., urinalysis or urine cultures) or to drain the bladder of urine without the catheter needing to remain in place. This method of catheterization can be used periodically, at specific time intervals (e.g., at certain times of day or every few hours), or when a patient is unable to void spontaneously.

INDWELLING CATHETERS

Indwelling catheters that remain in the bladder can be used to continually drain urine in patients who are comatose, terminally ill, or unable to void spontaneously due to altered mental status.[2] Indwelling catheters can also be used to irrigate the bladder or administer chemotherapy and other medications.[2] Patients who will undergo certain types of surgery or other medical procedures (e.g., childbirth, urologic, gynecologic) will also require an indwelling catheter.[2] Critically ill patients often require indwelling urinary catheters to closely monitor urinary output or pressure measurements during urodynamic studies.[2]

Another possible indication for indwelling catheters is to prevent urine from damaging skin, precipitating pressure injuries or wounds.[2] There are a few relative contraindications for inserting an indwelling urinary catheter, including previous urethral surgery or suspected or known urethral trauma.[3] Indwelling urinary catheters serve as potential entryway for microorganisms to reach the bladder.[4] In addition to microorganisms entering the bladder via a catheter, biofilms can also form on the catheter leading to potential infection. Biofilms consist of microbial organisms surrounded by a polysaccharide extracellular matrix.[4]

SUPRAPUBIC CATHETERIZATION

Suprapubic catheterization may be indicated when urethral catheterization is not possible for various reasons. These catheters are inserted above the pubic symphysis into the urinary bladder.[5] Suprapubic catheterization may be used for severe benign prostatic hyperplasia, false urethral passages, morbid obesity, urethral strictures, bladder neck contracture, genital malignancies, urogenital trauma, and long-term diversion with neurogenic bladder.[5] Foley catheters (those with a balloon, typically placed through the urethra) are also typically the catheter used for suprapubic placement and is most commonly inserted by a physician or surgeon specializing in the genitourinary system.[5] There are several potential complications associated with suprapubic catheter placement including injury to the bowel or surrounding structures, bleeding, vascular injury, and infection.[5]

How It Is Done

The smallest size catheter is preferably used when possible. Catheters are classified in French (Fr) gauge where the gauge size is three times the diameter.[2] For short-term catheterization in adults, catheters of 14–18 Fr are typically sufficient.[3] Some men with prostatic hypertrophy may require a larger-size catheter such as 20–22 Fr.[3] During routine use, patients are awake for this procedure and usually do not require medication for placement of a catheter. Patients may receive local or general anesthesia for placement of suprapubic catheters.[5]

Urethral catheter insertion techniques differ between males and females due to anatomic differences. Catheters should be inserted as aseptically as possible, and providers should begin each procedure by performing proper hand hygiene. Before inserting a catheter into a male, the urethral meatus and glans penis should be sterilely prepared with an antiseptic solution.[6] A lubricated catheter should then be inserted into the urethral meatus and advanced toward the hub of the catheter until there is spontaneous return of urine.[6] Once there is return of urine and the catheter is confirmed to be in the bladder, the catheter balloon is then inflated with sterile water or saline depending on the manufacturer of the catheter.[6] The catheter can then be secured in place using various methods.

To insert a urethral catheter into a female, the perineum and urethral meatus should be prepared with an antiseptic solution.[6] A lubricated catheter is then inserted into the urethral meatus and advanced toward the hub of the catheter until there is spontaneous return of urine and placement within the bladder is confirmed.[6] The catheter balloon is then inflated with sterile water or saline depending on the manufacturer of the catheter.[6]

Medication Implications

- The Infectious Diseases Society of America (IDSA) has published guidelines regarding practices associated with urinary catheters.
  - Prophylactic antibiotics are not routinely recommended for short-term or long-term catheter use.[7]
  - Guidelines make no recommendation regarding prophylactic antibiotics upon catheter removal as there is a knowledge gap in the literature.[8]
  - Guidelines recommend against screening for or treating asymptomatic bacteriuria in patients with short- or long-term indwelling urethral catheters.[8]
  - Guidelines make no recommendation on whether to use antimicrobial catheters for short- or long-term catheterization to prevent catheter-associated UTIs.[7]
    - Catheter-associated UTI is defined as an infection in a person who is currently catheterized or who was catheterized within the preceding 48 hours.[7]
  - Irrigation of the catheter with antimicrobial agents should not be routinely used to reduce infection in patients with indwelling catheters.[7]
  - Antimicrobial agents should not be routinely added to urinary drainage bags of catheterized patients to reduce risk of infection.[7]
  - Patients with catheter-associated UTIs with quick resolution of symptoms can be treated with 7 days of antibiotics.[7] Duration of antibiotics may depend on the antimicrobial agent chosen.
    - Patients who are not severely ill can consider a 5-day course of levofloxacin.[7]
    - Women aged ≤65 years without upper urinary tract symptoms can consider a 3-day antimicrobial regimen if the indwelling catheter is removed.[7]
  - Patients with catheter-associated UTIs with a delayed resolution of symptoms may be treated with 10–14 days of antibiotics.[7]
  - See Chapter 23: Culture - Urine for more details about treating UTIs.
- Medications can be administered through a catheter directly into the bladder.[9] This method of delivery allows for higher local concentrations of medication within the bladder and less systemic exposure.[9]
  - Disease states that may be treated this way include interstitial cystitis flares (e.g., treated with dimethyl sulfoxide) or non-muscle-invasive bladder cancer (e.g., treated with Bacillus Calmette-Guérin or mitomycin).[10]
  - Foley catheters may have an additional channel that can be used for infusing saline or other fluid for irrigation of the bladder if clots are present in the bladder.[2]

References

1. Clarke K, Hall CL, Wiley Z, et al. Catheter-associated urinary tract infections in adults: diagnosis, treatment, and prevention. *J Hosp Med.* 2019;14:E1–E5.
2. Feneley RCL, Hopley IB, Wells PNT. Urinary catheters: history, current status, adverse events and research agenda. *J Med Eng Technol.* 2015;39(8):459–470.

3. Lubbers, W. Chapter 7. Emergency Procedures. In: Stone C, Humphries RL. eds. *CURRENT Diagnosis & Treatment: Emergency Medicine.* 8th ed. New York, NY: McGraw-Hill; 2017:73–77.

4. Ramanathan R, Duane TM. Urinary tract infections in surgical patients. *Surg Clin North Am.* 2014;94(6):1351–1368.

5. Corder CJ, LaGrance CA. Suprapubic bladder catheterization. *StatPearls.* Treasure Island, FL: StatPearls Publishing; 2020.

6. Clayton JL. Indwelling urinary catheters: a pathway to health care-associated infections. *AORN J.* 2017;105(5):446–452.

7. Hooton TM, Bradley SF, Cardenas DD, et al. Diagnosis, prevention, and treatment of catheter-associated urinary tract infection in adults: 2009 international clinical practice guidelines from the Infectious Diseases Society of America. *Clin Infect Dis.* 2010;50(5):625–663.

8. Nicolle LE, Gupta K, Bradley SF, et al. Clinical practice guideline for the management of asymptomatic bacteriuria: 2019 update by the Infectious Diseases Society of America. *Clin Infect Dis.* 2019;68(10):e83–3110.

9. Hsu C, Chuang Y, Chancellor M. Intravesical drug delivery for dysfunctional bladder. *Int J Urol.* 2013;20(6):552–562.

10. Intravesical Administration of Therapeutic Medication. American Urological Association. https://www.auanet.org/guidelines/intravesical-administration-of-therapeutic-medication. Accessed April 3, 2020.

CHAPTER 60

Ventilation-Perfusion Scan

Julie A. Murphy, PharmD, FASHP, FCCP, BCPS ■ Fadi Safi, MD

Background

A pulmonary ventilation-perfusion scan (V/Q scan) is a nuclear medicine scan that uses radioactive material to examine air flow (ventilation) and blood flow (perfusion) through the lungs. In respiratory physiology, Q is the letter to describe blood flow, hence the name V/Q scan. The V/Q scan may also be referred to as lung scintigraphy since a gamma camera is used to acquire images.[1]

How to Use It

A V/Q scan is used primarily to detect pulmonary embolism (PE) in situations where a chest computed tomography angiogram (CTA) cannot be obtained. Such situations include an allergy to iodinated contrast agents, kidney disease, or the need to minimize radiation exposure as in pregnancy. The effective dose of radiation exposure from a V/Q scan is 1–5 millisieverts (mSv). A CTA with radiocontrast has an approximate effective dose of 12 mSv. One sievert carries with it a 5.5% chance of eventually developing cancer. A V/Q scan can be interpreted as normal, low probability, intermediate probability, or high probability for PE. A normal V/Q scan shows no perfusion defect and excludes PE. A low probability V/Q scan (<20% probability of a PE) will show perfusion defects that match ventilation defects. An intermediate probability V/Q scan shows perfusion defects that match abnormalities on chest X-ray with a 20%–80% probability of a PE. A high probability V/Q scan will show multiple segmental perfusion defects with normal ventilation and carry >80% chance of PE (Fig. 60.1). A V/Q scan can also be used as a quantification tool to measure lung performance before lung resection surgery, such as in the case of lung cancer. The V/Q scan also represents the initial imaging procedure of choice for patients with chronic thromboembolic pulmonary hypertension (CTEPH). These patients usually have several segmental mismatched V/Q defects.[2–4]

How It Is Done

A V/Q scan is performed by a nuclear medicine technologist, and the images are reviewed by a nuclear medicine radiologist who provides a written report to the provider who requested the scan. The test is performed in a nuclear medicine department. A chest X-ray is usually required prior to V/Q scan to look for other causes of lung disease. Using the chest X-ray findings to help determine the clinical pretest probability of a PE can help increase the sensitivity of a V/Q scan. The V/Q scan is performed in two phases with each taking place immediately following one another. In the ventilation phase, the patient inhales a small dose of radioactive material (xenon-133, krypton-81m, or technetium-99m) via a nebulizer for a few minutes. The patient then lies down on a table and images of the lungs are taken by scintigraphy (gamma camera). In the perfusion phase, a different radiopharmaceutical (technetium macro aggregated albumin [Tc-99m MAA]) is administered intravenously. A second set of images of the lungs is taken via gamma camera. The entire test takes approximately 30 to 60 minutes to complete. The patient is asked

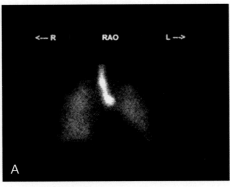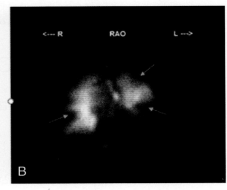

Fig. 60.1 High-probability ventilation-perfusion (V/Q) scan. (A) A normal ventilation scan. (B) A perfusion scan showing multiple segmental perfusion defects *(arrows)*.

to lie still during image capturing. The risks involved in the V/Q scan are minimal. The effective radiation dose is less than 2 mSv. Allergic reactions to the radiopharmaceuticals are rare and are treated as needed. A normal V/Q scan shows no perfusion defect and can reliably exclude PE. V/Q scans can be performed in pregnant women and a reduced dose of the intravenous radiopharmaceutical is usually used. Lactating women should avoid breastfeeding for 24 hours after the scan due to the radioactivity in the breast milk after the scan injection.[3,5–8]

Medication Implications

- Other nuclear tests that involve radioactive materials should be avoided 48 hours before and after a V/Q scan as the radioactive material from one test can interfere with the results of another test.
- No prior preparation, such as fasting, is required prior to a V/Q scan.
- If the V/Q scan is indicative of PE, anticoagulation therapy is indicated. Patient-specific factors (i.e., age, weight, creatinine clearance, concomitant medications) should be considered when deciding which agent to select (i.e., vitamin K antagonist [VKA], direct oral anticoagulant [DOAC], low-molecular-weight heparin [LMWH]). Treatment duration is determined by the most likely etiology of the PE and whether the PE was provoked or unprovoked. The most recent guidelines should be considered.[9] See Chapter 38: Lower Extremity Venous Duplex Ultrasound and Chapter 4: Anticoagulation Management in the Periprocedural Period for details about anticoagulation.
- If the V/Q scan is indicative of CTEPH, a high-quality pulmonary angiogram is necessary to confirm and define pulmonary vascular involvement in order to make a treatment decision. For all patients, lifelong anticoagulation is indicated. While bleeding rates are similar between VKAs and DOACs, recurrent venous thromboembolism rates are significantly higher with DOACs. Each patient should be evaluated for the need for pulmonary endarterectomy (treatment of choice). For inoperable cases, riociguat (soluble guanylate cyclase stimulator) is recommended and balloon pulmonary angioplasty may be considered. Riociguat may also be used after pulmonary endarterectomy for persistent/recurrent pulmonary hypertension.[10–12] Some noteworthy aspects about riociguat include the following:
    - Interactions: Due to the potential for symptomatic hypotension, concomitant administration with phosphodiesterase type-5 (PDE5) inhibitors (e.g., sildenafil, tadalafil, etc.), nitrates, or nitric oxide donor agents (e.g., amyl nitrite) is contraindicated. Patients taking concomitant strong cytochrome P450 inhibitors and P-glycoprotein/breast cancer

resistance protein (BCRP) inhibitors should be initiated on a lower than usual dose and cautiously titrated. Smoking requires higher than maximum doses of riociguat be used. Riociguat and antacids should be separated by 1 hour.[13,14]

- Adverse effects: A decrease in blood pressure is expected. If the patient develops signs or symptoms of hypotension, then a dose reduction should be considered. In trials, serious bleeding (e.g., vaginal bleeding, catheter site bleeding, subdural hematoma, hematemesis, intra-abdominal bleeding) occurred in 2.4% of riociguat patients. Serious hemoptysis occurred in 1% of patients with one fatality. Riociguat is contraindicated in patients with pulmonary veno-occlusive disease as it may worsen cardiovascular status.[14,15]
- Pregnancy: Riociguat is contraindicated in pregnancy due to the risk for fetal harm. Women of reproductive potential must have a negative pregnancy test prior to therapy initiation, receive monthly pregnancy tests, and be advised of the use of appropriate contraception while using riociguat and for 1 month after discontinuation.[14,15]
- Females: Regardless of age, riociguat is only available to female patients through a restricted access program (Adempas Risk Evaluation and Mitigation Strategy Program).[14]

References

1. Moore AJE, Wachsmann J, Chamarthy MR, et al. Imaging of acute pulmonary embolism: an update. *Cardiovasc Diagn Ther*. 2018;8(3):225–243.
2. Anderson DR, Kahn SR, Rodger MA, et al. Computed tomographic pulmonary angiography vs ventilation-perfusion lung scanning in patients with suspected pulmonary embolism: a randomized controlled trial. *JAMA*. 2007;298(23):2743–2753.
3. PIOPED investigators. Value of the ventilation/perfusion scan in acute pulmonary embolism. Results of the prospective investigation of pulmonary embolism diagnosis (PIOPED). *JAMA*. 1990;263(20):2753–2759.
4. Tunariu N, Gibbs SJ, Win Z, et al. Ventilation-perfusion scintigraphy is more sensitive than multidetector CTPA in detecting chronic thromboembolic pulmonary disease as a treatable cause of pulmonary hypertension. *J Nucl Med*. 2007;48(5):6804.
5. Bajc M, Neilly JB, Miniati M, et al. EANM guidelines for ventilation/perfusion scintigraphy: part 1. Pulmonary imaging with ventilation/perfusion single photon emission tomography. *Eur J Nucl Med Mol Imaging*. 2009;36(8):1356–1370.
6. Tirada N, Dreizin D, Khati NJ, et al. Imaging in pregnant and lactating patients. *RadioGraphics*. 2015;35:1751–1765.
7. Chernecky CC, Berger BJ. Lung scan, perfusion and ventilation (V/Q scan) – diagnostic. In: Chernecky CC, Berger BJ, eds. *Laboratory Tests and Diagnostic Procedures*. 6th ed. St. Louis, MO: Elsevier Saunders; 2013:738–740.
8. Herring W. Nuclear medicine: understanding the principles and recognizing the basics. In: Herring W, ed. *Learning Radiology*. 3rd ed. Philadelphia, AP: Elsevier; 2016:e1–e18.
9. Holbrook A, Schulman S, Witt DM, et al. Evidence-based management of anticoagulant therapy: Antithrombotic therapy and prevention of thrombosis, 9th ed: American College of Chest Physicians evidence-based clinical practice guidelines. *Chest*. 2012;141(2 Suppl):e152S–e184S.
10. Kim NH, Delcroix M, Jais X, et al. Chronic thromboembolic pulmonary hypertension. *Eur Respir J*. 2019;53:1801915.
11. Bunclark K, Newnham M, Chiu YD, et al. A multicenter study of anticoagulation in operable chronic thromboembolic pulmonary hypertension. *J Thromb Haemost*. 2020;18(1):114–122.
12. Ghofrani HA, D'Armini AM, Grimminger F, et al. CHEST-1 Study Group. Riociguat for the treatment of chronic thromboembolic pulmonary hypertension. *N Engl J Med*. 2013;369(4):319–329.
13. Ghofrani HA, Galiè N, Grimminger F, et al. Riociguat for the treatment of pulmonary arterial hypertension. *N Engl J Med*. 2013;369(4):330–340.
14. Adempas (riociguat) package insert. Whippany, NJ: Bayer HealthCare Pharmaceuticals Inc.; 2013 Oct (revised 1/2018).
15. Bishop BM. Riociguat for pulmonary arterial hypertension and chronic thromboembolic pulmonary hypertension. *Am J Health Syst Pharm*. 2014;71(21):1839–1844.

INDEX

Page numbers followed by "*f*" indicate figures, "*t*" indicate tables, and "*b*" indicate boxes.